STEP-UP

TO

OBSTETRICS AND GYNECOLOGY

STEP-UP

TO

OBSTETRICS AND GYNECOLOGY

Frank W. Ling, MD
Clinical Professor
Department of Obstetrics and Gynecology
Vanderbilt University School of Medicine and Meharry
Medical College
Nashville, Tennessee
Partner, Women's Health Specialists
Germantown, Tennessee
Director, The Foundation for Exxcellence in Women's
Health Care
Dallas, Texas

Russell R. Snyder, MD
Vice-Chair and Director, Division of Gynecology
Department of Obstetrics and Gynecology
University of Texas Medical Branch
Galveston, Texas
Director, The Foundation for Exxcellence in Women's
Health Care
Dallas, Texas

Sandra Ann Carson, MD
Adjunct Professor of Obstetrics and Gynecology
Alpert Medical School of Brown University
Providence, Rhode Island
Director, American Board of Obstetrics and Gynecology
Dallas, Texas

Wesley C. Fowler, Jr., MD
Associate Dean for Medical Alumni Affairs
Professor of Obstetrics And Gynecology
University of North Carolina School of Medicine
Chapel Hill, North Carolina
President, The Foundation for Exxcellence in Women's
Health Care
Dallas, Texas

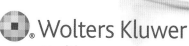
. Wolters Kluwer
Health

Philadelphia • Baltimore • New York • London
Buenos Aires • Hong Kong • Sydney • Tokyo

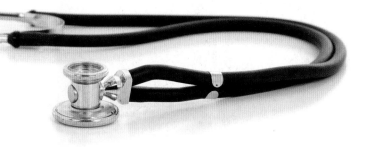

Acquisitions Editor: Tari Broderick
Product Development Editor: Jennifer Verbiar
Production Project Manager: Marian Bellus
Design Coordinator: Holly McLaughlin
Manufacturing Coordinator: Margie Orzech
Prepress Vendor: Absolute Service, Inc.

1st Edition

9 8 7 6 5 4 3 2 1

Printed in China

Library of Congress Cataloging-in-Publication Data

Step-up to obstetrics and gynecology / [edited by] Frank W. Ling, Russell R. Snyder, Sandra Ann Carson, Wesley C. Fowler. — 1st edition.
    p. ; cm. — (Step-up series)
  Includes bibliographical references and index.
    ISBN 978-1-4511-1244-3 (alk. paper)
  I. Ling, Frank W., editor. II. Snyder, Russell R. editor. III. Carson, Sandra A. (Sandra Ann), editor. IV. Fowler, Wesley C., Jr., 1940- editor. V. Series: Step up series.
  [DNLM: 1. Pregnancy Complications—Examination Questions. 2. Pregnancy Complications--Outlines. 3. Genital Diseases, Female—Examination Questions. 4. Genital Diseases, Female—Outlines. WQ 18.2]
  RG111
  618.076—dc23
                    2014008800

LWW.com

Section Editors

FRANK W. LING, MD
Section 2: *Obstetrics*
Clinical Professor
Department of Obstetrics and Gynecology
Vanderbilt University School of Medicine and
    Meharry Medical College
Nashville, Tennessee
Partner, Women's Health Specialists, PLLC
Germantown, Tennessee
Director, The Foundation for Exxcellence in Women's
    Health Care
Dallas, Texas

RUSSELL R. SNYDER, MD
Section 1: *Overview of Women's Health*
Section 3: *Gynecology*
Vice-Chair and Director, Division of Gynecology
Department of Obstetrics and Gynecology
University of Texas Medical Branch
Galveston, Texas
Director, The Foundation for Exxcellence in Women's
    Health Care
Dallas, Texas

SANDRA ANN CARSON, MD
Section 4: *Reproductive Endocrinology and Infertility*
Adjunct Professor of Obstetrics and Gynecology
Alpert Medical School of Brown University
Providence, Rhode Island
Director, American Board of Obstetrics and
    Gynecology
Dallas, Texas

WESLEY C. FOWLER, JR., MD
Section 5: *Gynecologic Oncology*
Associate Dean for Medical Alumni Affairs
Professor of Obstetrics And Gynecology
University of North Carolina School of Medicine
Chapel Hill, North Carolina
President, The Foundation for Exxcellence in
    Women's Health Care
Dallas, Texas

Contributing Authors

MICHAEL T. ADLER, MD
Chapter 25: *Postterm Pregnancy and Intrauterine Fetal Demise*
Chapter 26: *Obstetric Procedures*
Assistant Professor of Obstetrics and Gynecology
Department of Obstetrics and Gynecology
University of Texas Medical School at Houston
Houston, Texas

PAMELA D. BERENS, MD
Chapter 2: *The Obstetrician/Gynecologist's Role in Screening and Preventive Care*
Chapter 14: *Postpartum Care/Complications*
Professor, Vice Chair of Clinical Affairs
Department of Obstetrics and Gynecology
University of Texas Medical School at Houston
Houston, Texas

MOSTAFA A. BORAHAY, MD, FACOG
Chapter 34: *Dysmenorrhea and Chronic Pelvic Pain*
Assistant Professor
Women's Reproductive Health Research (WRHR) Scholar
Department of Obstetrics and Gynecology
University of Texas Medical Branch
Galveston, Texas

AMY M. BURKETT, MD
Chapter 18: *Hypertension in Pregnancy*
Department of Obstetrics and Gynecology
Summa Health Systems
Northeastern Ohio Universities College of Medicine
Akron, Ohio

CHRISTINNE CANELA, MD
Chapter 41: *Hirsutism and Virilization*
Physician Director of Medical Quality
Department of Obstetrics and Gynecology
Carilion Roanoke Memorial Hospital
Roanoke, Virginia

BETTY CHOU, MD
Chapter 16: *Common Medical and Surgical Problems in Pregnancy*
Chapter 20: *Fetal Growth Abnormalities: Fetal Growth Restriction and Macrosomia*
Director, Johns Hopkins Women's Services at Odenton
Assistant Professor
Department of Obstetrics and Gynecology
Johns Hopkins Bayview Medical Center
Baltimore, Maryland

ALICE CHUANG, MD
Chapter 45: *Cell Biology and Principles of Cancer Therapy*
Chapter 46: *Gestational Trophoblastic Neoplasia*
Chapter 50: *Ovarian and Adnexal Disease*
Associate Professor
Department of Obstetrics and Gynecology
University of North Carolina
Chapel Hill, North Carolina

LESLIE CLARK, MD
Chapter 45: *Cell Biology and Principles of Cancer Therapy*
Resident
Department of Obstetrics and Gynecology
University of North Carolina
Chapel Hill, North Carolina

BRENDAN D. CONNEALY, MD
Chapter 6: *Endocrinology of Pregnancy*
Chapter 12: *Immediate Care of Newborn*
MFM Fellow
Department of Obstetrics and Gynecology
University of Texas Medical School at Houston
Houston, Texas

DOUGLAS R. DANFORTH, PHD
Chapter 5: *Reproductive Physiology*
Associate Professor
Department of Obstetrics and Gynecology
The Ohio State University Medical Center
Columbus, Ohio

JILL EDWARDSON, MD, MPH
Chapter 16: *Common Medical and Surgical Problems in Pregnancy*
Assistant Professor
Department of Obstetrics and Gynecology
Johns Hopkins Medical Center
Baltimore, Maryland

CYNTHIA B. EVANS, MD
Chapter 42: *Menopause*
Associate Professor
Department of Obstetrics and Gynecology
The Ohio State University Medical Center
Columbus, Ohio

JASON FRANASIAK, MD
Chapter 49: *Cancer of the Uterine Corpus*
Physician at Reproductive Medicine Associates of New Jersey
Obstetrics and Gynecology
Gladstone, New Jersey

MELISSA M. GOIST, MD
Chapter 15: *Ectopic Pregnancy*
Assistant Professor
Department of Obstetrics and Gynecology
The Ohio State University Medical Center
Columbus, Ohio

SUSAN GOLDSMITH, MD
Chapter 8: *Preconception and Antepartum Care*
Assistant Professor
Department of Obstetrics and Gynecology
Northwestern University Feinberg School of Medicine
Chicago, Illinois

MATTHEW GRACE, MD
Chapter 47: *Benign Vulvar Disease*
Assistant Professor
Department of Obstetrics and Gynecology
University of North Carolina
Chapel Hill, North Carolina

CATHERINE HANSEN, MD, MPH
Chapter 37: *Sexual Function and Dysfunction*
Assistant Professor
Department of Obstetrics and Gynecology
University of Texas Medical Branch
Galveston, Texas

GERI D. HEWITT, MD
Chapter 39: *Puberty*
Assistant Professor
Department of Obstetrics and Gynecology
The Ohio State University Medical Center
Columbus, Ohio

JAOU-CHEN HUANG, MD
Chapter 43: *Infertility*
Reproductive Endocrinologist
Department of Obstetrics and Gynecology
Memorial Hermann Hospital
Houston, Texas

NANCY A. HUEPPCHEN, MD
Chapter 16: *Common Medical and Surgical Problems in Pregnancy*
Chapter 20: *Fetal Growth Abnormalities: Fetal Growth Restriction and Macrosomia*
Director of Medical Education
Associate Professor
Department of Obstetrics and Gynecology
Johns Hopkins University School of Medicine
Baltimore, Maryland

PATRICIA HUGUELET, MD, FACOG
Chapter 17: *Infectious Diseases in Pregnancy*
Assistant Professor
Department of Obstetrics and Gynecology
University of Colorado, Anschutz Medical Center
Aurora, Colorado

ANDREW F. HUNDLEY, MD
Chapter 32: *Pelvic Support Defects, Urinary Incontinence, and Urinary Tract Infection*
Division Director, Female Pelvic Medicine and Reconstructive Surgery
Department of Obstetrics and Gynecology
The Ohio State University Medical Center
Columbus, Ohio

MICHELLE M. ISLEY, MD, MPH
Chapter 28: *Sterilization*
Assistant Professor
Department of Obstetrics and Gynecology
The Ohio State University Medical Center
Columbus, Ohio

CHERYL J. JOHNSON, MD
Chapter 1: *The Woman's Health Examination*
Department of Obstetrics and Gynecology
Summa Health System
Ohio State University
Akron, Ohio

BENJAMIN A. KASE, MD
Chapter 7: *Maternal–Fetal Physiology*
Department of Obstetrics and Gynecology
Tripler Army Medical Center
Honolulu, Hawaii

AMANTIA KENNEDY, MD
Chapter 46: *Gestational Trophoblastic Neoplasia*
Assistant Professor
Department of Obstetrics and Gynecology
University of North Carolina
Chapel Hill, North Carolina

SAMI GOKHAN KILIC, MD, FACOG, FACS
Chapter 36: *Gynecologic Procedures*
Assistant Professor
Department of Obstetrics and Gynecology
University of Texas Medical Branch
Galveston, Texas

EDUARDO LARA-TORRE, MD
Chapter 41: *Hirsutism and Virilization*
Chapter 44: *Premenstrual Syndrome and Premenstrual
    Dysphoric Disorder*
Residency Program Director
Department of Obstetrics and Gynecology
Carilion Roanoke Memorial Hospital
Roanoke, Virginia

FRANK W. LING, MD
Chapter 35: *Breast Disorders*
Clinical Professor
Department of Obstetrics and Gynecology
Vanderbilt University School of Medicine and
    Meharry Medical College
Nashville, Tennessee
Partner, Women's Health Specialists
Germantown, Tennessee
Director, The Foundation for Exxcellence in Women's
    Health Care
Dallas, Texas

QUINN LIPPMANN, MD, MPH
Chapter 48: *Cervical Dysplasia and Carcinoma*
Oth Post-MD
Department of Reproductive Medicine
University of California San Diego
San Diego, California

AMANDA B. MURCHISON, MD
Chapter 22: *Preterm Labor*
Chapter 23: *Third-Trimester Bleeding*
Assistant Residency Program Director
Department of Obstetrics and Gynecology
Carilion Roanoke Memorial Hospital
Roanoke, Virginia

JESSICA L. NYHOLM, MD
Chapter 11: *Intrapartum Fetal Surveillance*
Assistant Professor
Department of Obstetrics, Gynecology and Women's
    Health
University of Minnesota
Minneapolis, Minnesota

SILKA PATEL, MD
Chapter 13: *Abnormal Labor and Malpresentation*
Assistant Professor
Department of Obstetrics and Gynecology
Johns Hopkins School of Medicine
Baltimore, Maryland

PAMELA A. PROMECENE, MD
Chapter 3: *Ethics in Obstetrics and Gynecology*
Chapter 10: *Normal Labor and Delivery*
Associate Professor of Obstetrics and Gynecology–
    Clinical
Assistant Dean for Graduate Medical Education
Department of Obstetrics and Gynecology
University of Texas Medical School at Houston
Houston, Texas

TRACY L. PROSEN, MD
Chapter 19: *Multifetal Gestation*
Assistant Professor
Department of Obstetrics, Gynecology and Women's
    Health
University of Minnesota
Minneapolis, Minnesota

KELLIE S. RATH, MD
Chapter 4: *Embryology and Anatomy*
OhioHealth Gynecologic Cancer Surgeons
Columbus, Ohio

BRITTON D. RINK, MD
Chapter 9: *Prenatal Diagnosis, Genetic Disorder
    Assessment, and Teratology*
Director, Prenatal Genetics and Ultrasound
Assistant Professor
Department of Obstetrics and Gynecology
The Ohio State University Medical Center
Columbus, Ohio

ANA M. RODRIGUEZ, MD
Chapter 27: *Contraception*
Assistant Professor
Department of Obstetrics and Gynecology
University of Texas Medical Branch
Galveston, Texas

JACQUELINE ROHL, MD, MPH
Chapter 29: *Reproductive Tract Congenital
    Anomalies*
Assistant Professor
Department of Obstetrics and Gynecology
The Ohio State University Medical Center
Columbus, Ohio

ANDREW J. SATIN, MD
Chapter 13: *Abnormal Labor and Malpresentation*
The Dorothy Edwards Professor and
Director of Gynecology and Obstetrics
Obstetrician/Gynecologist-in-Chief
Johns Hopkins Hospital
Johns Hopkins Medicine
Baltimore, Maryland

JONATHAN SCHAFFIR, MD
Chapter 33: *Endometriosis*
Assistant Professor
Department of Obstetrics and Gynecology
The Ohio State University Medical Center
Columbus, Ohio

RUSSELL R. SNYDER, MD
Chapter 40: *Amenorrhea and Abnormal Uterine Bleeding*
Vice-Chair and Director, Division of Gynecology
Department of Obstetrics and Gynecology
University of Texas Medical Branch
Galveston, Texas
Director, The Foundation for Exxcellence in Women's
    Health Care
Dallas, Texas

KATHERINE STRAFFORD, MD
Chapter 30: *Reproductive Tract Benign Conditions*
Assistant Professor
Department of Obstetrics and Gynecology
The Ohio State University Medical Center
Dublin, Ohio

OLGA F. SWANSON, MD
Chapter 31: *Vulvovaginitis and Sexually Transmitted
    Diseases*
Obstetrics and Gynecology
Houston Heights Women's Healthcare Center
Houston, Texas

JEFF R. TEMPLE, PHD
Chapter 38: *Sexual Assault and Domestic Violence*
Assistant Professor
Department of Obstetrics and Gynecology
University of Texas Medical Branch
Galveston, Texas

CHESNEY THOMPSON, MD
Chapter 17: *Infectious Diseases in Pregnancy*
Professor and Vice-Chair
Chief of General Obstetrics and Gynecology
Department of Obstetrics and Gynecology
University of Colorado
Aurora, Colorado

PATRICE M. WEISS, MD
Chapter 44: *Premenstrual Syndrome and Premenstrual
    Dysphoric Disorder*
Department Chair
Department of Obstetrics and Gynecology
Carilion Roanoke Memorial Hospital
Roanoke, Virginia

HOLLY A. WEST, MPAS, PA-C
Chapter 40: *Amenorrhea and Abnormal Uterine Bleeding*
Assistant Professor
Department of Obstetrics and Gynecology
University of Texas Medical Branch
Galveston, Texas

YASUKO YAMAMURA, MD
Chapter 21: *Isoimmunization*
Chapter 24: *Premature Rupture of Membranes*
Assistant Professor
Department of Obstetrics, Gynecology and Women's
    Health
University of Minnesota
Minneapolis, Minnesota

MATT ZERDEN, MD
Chapter 50: *Ovarian and Adnexal Disease*
Fellow
Department of Obstetrics and Gynecology
University of North Carolina
Chapel Hill, North Carolina

Preface

The Foundation for EXXcellence in Women's Health Care and these medical authors and educators proudly present this first edition of *Step-Up to Obstetrics and Gynecology*. Designed to aid the medical student to prepare for end-of-rotation and national standardized examinations, it aims to present the depth and breadth of obstetrics and gynecology in a concise outline format. It will enhance but not replace standard textbooks and other sources, which were developed for the learner during the core clerkship in the specialty.

We expect *Step-Up to Obstetrics and Gynecology* will be an effective learning tool for future physicians dedicated to serving their female patients regardless of the specialty they choose. Key concepts and facts are reinforced with "Quick Hits" in the margins, and important concepts are supplemented with clinical photographs, illustrations, tables, and algorithms. Patient-oriented clinical scenarios presented in the form of multiple-choice questions allow the student to self-assess their knowledge.

Supported in part by the American Board of Obstetrics and Gynecology, Inc., the Foundation for EXXcellence in Women's Health Care is dedicated to promoting the health of women and the professional development of their physicians. The two "Xs" in the Foundation's name is a constant reminder of our focus. We sincerely hope that those who use *Step-Up to Obstetrics and Gynecology* find it to be all that we planned.

Frank W. Ling, MD
Russell R. Snyder, MD
Sandra Ann Carson, MD
Wesley C. Fowler, MD
Nancy B. Dent, PhD, Executive Director,
The Foundation for EXXcellence
in Women's Health Care
January 2014

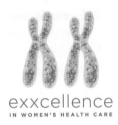

exxcellence
IN WOMEN'S HEALTH CARE

Contents

Overview of Women's Health

SECTION

1

Overview of
Women's Health

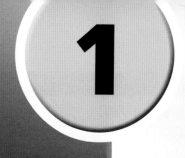

The Woman's Health Examination

I. Medical History

A. Chief complaint (CC): concise statement for reason of visit

B. History of present illness (HPI): chronologic description of present illness
  1. Quality
  2. Radiation
  3. Duration
  4. Alleviating factors
  5. Exacerbating factors

C. Review of systems (ROS): inventory of *all* body systems (Box 1.1)

D. Gynecologic history
  1. Menstrual history
     a. Age at **menarche** (age at which menses began)
     b. Last menstrual period (LMP)
     c. Previous menstrual period (PMP): establishes days between cycles
     d. Cycle length
     e. Cycle flow
        i. Clotting
        ii. Number of pads or tampons
     f. Menstrual pain (**dysmenorrhea**)
     g. Abnormal uterine bleeding (**AUB**)
        i. Irregular (**metrorrhagia**)
        ii. Heavy (**menorrhagia**)
        iii. Intermenstrual
        iv. Postcoital
        v. Postmenopausal
        vi. Midcycle spotting (mittelschmerz)
        vii. Breakthrough bleeding (BTB) if on hormonal therapy to control cycles
     h. Premenstrual symptoms
        i. **Physical**
           (a) Fluid retention
           (b) Bloating
           (c) Breast tenderness
           (d) Headaches
           (e) Pain
        ii. **Emotional**
           (a) Mood fluctuations
           (b) Food cravings
           (c) Anxiety
           (d) Nervousness
           (e) Sleep disturbances
           (f) Libido changes

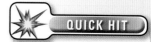

QUICK HIT

A gynecologic evaluation is an important part of primary health care and preventative medicine for women.

The Woman's Health Examination

BOX 1.1

Review of Systems (ROS)

1. CONSTITUTIONAL	☐ NEGATIVE ☐ FEVER	☐ WEIGHT LOSS ☐ FATIGUE	☐ WEIGHT GAIN ☐ OTHER	TALLEST HEIGHT_____
2. EYES	☐ NEGATIVE ☐ OTHER	☐ VISION CHANGE	☐ GLASSES/CONTACTS	
3. EAR, NOSE, AND THROAT	☐ NEGATIVE ☐ HEADACHE	☐ ULCERS ☐ HEARING LOSS	☐ SINUSITIS ☐ OTHER	
4. CARDIOVASCULAR	☐ NEGATIVE ☐ EDEMA	☐ ORTHOPNEA ☐ PALPITATION	☐ CHEST PAIN ☐ OTHER	☐ DIFFICULTY BREATHING ON EXERTION
5. RESPIRATORY	☐ NEGATIVE ☐ SHORTNESS OF BREATH	☐ WHEEZING	☐ HEMOPTYSIS ☐ COUGH	☐ OTHER
6. GASTROINTESTINAL	☐ NEGATIVE ☐ CONSTIPATION	☐ DIARRHEA ☐ FLATULENCE	☐ BLOODY STOOL ☐ PAIN	☐ NAUSEA/VOMITING/INDIGESTION ☐ FECAL INCONTINENCE ☐ OTHER
7. GENITOURINARY	☐ NEGATIVE ☐ FREQUENCY ☐ DYSPAREUNIA ☐ ABNORMAL VAGINAL BLEEDING	☐ HEMATURIA ☐ INCOMPLETE EMPTYING ☐ ABNORMAL OR PAINFUL PERIODS	☐ DYSURIA ☐ ABNORMAL VAGINAL DISCHARGE	☐ URGENCY ☐ INCONTINENCE ☐ PMS ☐ OTHER
8. MUSCULOSKELETAL	☐ NEGATIVE ☐ MUSCLE OR JOINT PAIN	☐ MUSCLE WEAKNESS	☐ OTHER	
9a. SKIN	☐ NEGATIVE ☐ DRY SKIN	☐ RASH ☐ PIGMENTED LESIONS	☐ ULCERS ☐ OTHER	
9b. BREAST	☐ NEGATIVE ☐ DISCHARGE	☐ MASTALGIA ☐ MASSES	☐ OTHER	
10. NEUROLOGIC	☐ NEGATIVE ☐ TROUBLE WALKING	☐ SYNCOPE ☐ SEVERE MEMORY PROBLEMS	☐ SEIZURES	☐ NUMBNESS ☐ OTHER
11. PSYCHIATRIC	☐ NEGATIVE ☐ SEVERE ANXIETY	☐ DEPRESSION ☐ OTHER	☐ CRYING	
12. ENDOCRINE	☐ NEGATIVE ☐ HOT FLASHES	☐ DIABETES ☐ HAIR LOSS	☐ HYPOTHYROID ☐ HEAT/COLD INTOLERANCE	☐ HYPERTHYROID ☐ OTHER
13. HEMATOLOGIC/LYMPHATIC	☐ NEGATIVE ☐ BLEEDING	☐ BRUISES ☐ ADENOPATHY	☐ OTHER	
14. ALLERGIC/IMMUNOLOGIC	(SEE FIRST PAGE)			

American College of Obstetricians and Gynecologists

Copyright © 2005 (AA322) 12345/98765

(From Beckmann CRB, Ling FW, et al. *Obstetrics and Gynecology*, 7th ed. Baltimore: Lippincott Williams & Wilkins; 2014.)

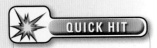

Premenstrual symptoms always occur in the second half of the menstrual cycle (luteal phase or secretory phase).

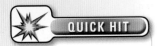

Menopause is always a retrospective diagnosis consisting of 12 consecutive months of amenorrhea.

    i. Perimenopausal/menopausal symptoms
       i. Vasomotor symptoms (hot flushes or hot flashes); typically occur during or are worse while asleep
      ii. Mood changes
     iii. Sleep disruption
     iv. Changes in libido
      v. Decreased vaginal lubrication
2. Sexual history
  a. Sexual orientation: men, women, both
  b. Lifetime partners
  c. Sexual function: desire, arousal, plateau, orgasm, resolution
  d. Satisfaction with sexual function
  e. Contraception (current and past)
    i. Problems
    ii. Complications
   iii. Satisfaction
   iv. Types
     (a) Barrier
     (b) Hormonal
     (c) Implants

BOX 1.2

Common Terms Used to Describe Parity

Gravida	A woman who is or has been pregnant
Primigravida	A woman who is in or who has experienced her first pregnancy
Multigravida	A woman who has been pregnant more than once
Nulligravida	A woman who has never been pregnant and is not now pregnant
Primipara	A woman who is pregnant for the first time or who has given birth to only one child
Multipara	A woman who has given birth two or more times
Nullipara	A woman who has never given birth or who has never had a pregnancy progress beyond the gestational age of an abortion

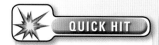

QUICK HIT

Of pregnancies in the United States, 55% are unintended.

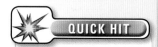

QUICK HIT

The acronyms STI (sexually transmitted infection) and STD (sexually transmitted disease) are used interchangeably.

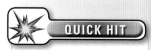

QUICK HIT

Parity is the number of pregnancies in which the fetus is over 20 weeks' gestation prior to delivery.

(d) Sterilization
(e) Emergency
- v. History of sexually transmitted infections and current high-risk behaviors
  - (a) Human papillomavirus (HPV) infection
  - (b) Gonorrhea
  - (c) Chlamydia
  - (d) Herpes simplex virus (HSV)
  - (e) Human immunodeficiency virus (HIV) infection
  - (f) Hepatitis B virus infection
  - (g) Hepatitis C virus infection
  - (h) Syphilis

E. Obstetric history
   1. **Gravidity** equals number of total pregnancies (Box 1.2)
   2. **Parity** equals births
      a. Term births
         i. Early Term – between 37 weeks 0 days and 38 weeks 6 days
         ii. Full Term – between 39 weeks 0 days and 40 weeks 6 days
         iii. Late Term – between 41 weeks 0 days and 41 weeks 6 days
         iv. Post Term – from 42 weeks 0 days and beyond
      b. Preterm births
         i. Preterm – between 32 weeks o days and 36 weeks 6 days
         ii. Early Preterm – prior to 32 weeks 0 days
      c. Abortions/miscarriages/ectopic pregnancies
      d. Live births
         i. Gestational age
         ii. Route of delivery
         iii. Birth weight
         iv. Infant: gender and neonatal complications
         v. Pregnancy complications
         vi. Breastfeeding
         vii. History of infertility or treatment for infertility
      e. Stillbirths
F. Past medical history (PMH)
   1. Diagnoses
   2. Surgeries
   3. Hospitalizations
G. Current medications/allergies
H. Allergies or intolerance
I. Family history (FH)
   1. Cancers
   2. Heart disease, hypertension, stroke
   3. Diabetes
   4. Osteoporosis
   5. Hereditary diseases

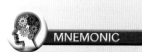

MNEMONIC

Florida **P**ower **A**nd **L**ight
In the GxPxxxx system, G is gravidity and P is parity with the following numbers describing:
Full term deliveries
Preterm deliveries
Abortions or ectopic pregnancies
Living children

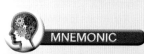

MNEMONIC

TABOO
Tobacco/drugs (nicotine, caffeine, marijuana, cocaine, etc.)
Alcohol: amount and type
"**B**eat-up": sexual abuse and domestic violence
OTC (over-the-counter) supplements (calcium, multivitamin, folic acid)
Organ donation: seat belt use, advanced directives

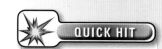

QUICK HIT

All women of reproductive age should be encouraged to take 0.4 mg (400 mcg) of folic acid (folate) daily.

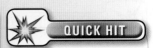

Overweight and obese individuals (BMI >25) are at increased risk for cancer and poor reproductive health outcomes.

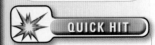

An accurate examination complements the history, provides additional information, and helps determine diagnoses and guide management. It also provides an opportunity to educate and reassure the patient.

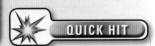

Tumors often distort the normal anatomy of the breast, causing disruption of shape, contour, or symmetry of the breast or position of the nipple.

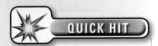

The upper outer quadrant is where 50% of malignant breast lesions occur.

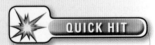

A great time to educate and remind patients about regular breast self-examination (BSE) is during the breast exam.

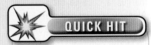

If there is swelling in the Bartholin gland area, palpate between thumb and forefinger at 8 o'clock and 4 o'clock positions. If urethritis is suspected, milk the urethra and culture any discharge.

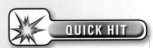

A common error during bimanual exam is failure to make effective use of the abdominal hand.

J. Social history (SH)
  1. Health hazards at work or home
  2. Seat belt use
  3. Nutrition, diet, exercise
K. Immunization history

II. Physical Examination (Box 1.3)

A. Vital signs
  1. Body mass index (BMI) = height (meters squared)/weight (kilograms)
  2. Blood pressure (sitting)
  3. Temperature
  4. Respiration
  5. Pulse
  6. Waist circumference or waist–hip ratio
  7. General appearance

B. General physical examination
  1. Extent based on patient expectation and what is being managed by other health care professionals
  2. Exam as indicated by medical history and ROS (see Box 1.1)

C. Breast examination (Figure 1.1)
  1. Inspection for shape, contour, and asymmetry in sitting position
    a. Arms at side
    b. Arms over head
    c. Arms pressed against hips (lean forward)
  2. Inspection of skin, areola, and nipple
  3. Palpation
    a. Lymph nodes, while seated: supraclavicular, infraclavicular, lateral, central, subscapular, pectoral, and axillary
    b. Breast exam, supine
      i. Entire breast in radial or spiral pattern
      ii. Palpable mass: document position, size, shape, consistency, mobility, and tenderness
    c. Nipple expression: if fluid expressed, send for culture, sensitivity, and cytopathology

D. **Pelvic examination**, lithotomy position
  1. **Inspection** of external genitalia (Figure 1.2)
    a. Mons pubis: note hair distribution, excoriation, inflammation, and lice
    b. Clitoris
    c. Labia majora: note swelling, bruises, or varicosities
    d. Labia minora
    e. Urethral meatus
    f. Introitus: note inflammation, discharge, ulceration, nodules
      i. Skene glands: periurethral (Figure 1.3)
      ii. Bartholin glands: greater vestibular
    g. Perineum
    h. Perianal region
  2. **Speculum** examination (Figure 1.4)
    a. Insert speculum at oblique angle with gentle downward pressure
    b. Inspect cervix and os: note color, position, shape, discharge, surface character, and any abnormalities (bleeding, ulceration, masses, cysts, nodules)
    c. Obtain specimens for culture or cytology
      i. Pap test: endocervical and ectocervical cells
      ii. Cultures or DNA probes (e.g., gonorrhea, chlamydia, HPV testing)
      iii. Wet mount: vaginal swab in 2 mL 0.9% NaCl for microscopy
    d. Inspect vagina as speculum is removed: note color, discharge, odor, masses, and ulcerations

BOX 1.3

Physical Examination

The Woman's Health Examination

| PATIENT NAME: | BIRTH DATE: / / | ID NO.: | DATE: / / |

CONSTITUTIONAL

● VITAL SIGNS (RECORD ≥ 3 VITAL SIGNS):

HEIGHT: _____ WEIGHT: _____ BMI: _____ BLOOD PRESSURE (SITTING): _____ TEMPERATURE: _____ PULSE: _____ RESPIRATION: _____

● GENERAL APPEARANCE (NOTE ALL THAT APPLY):

☐ WELL-DEVELOPED ☐ OTHER ☐ NO DEFORMITIES ☐ OTHER
☐ WELL-NOURISHED ☐ OTHER ☐ WELL-GROOMED ☐ OTHER
☐ NORMAL HABITUS ☐ OBESE ☐ OTHER

NECK

● NECK ☐ NORMAL ☐ ABNORMAL _____
● THYROID ☐ NORMAL ☐ ABNORMAL _____

RESPIRATORY

● RESPIRATORY EFFORT ☐ NORMAL ☐ ABNORMAL _____
● AUSCULTATED LUNGS ☐ NORMAL ☐ ABNORMAL _____

CARDIOVASCULAR

● AUSCULTATED HEART
   SOUNDS ☐ NORMAL ☐ ABNORMAL _____
   MURMURS ☐ NORMAL ☐ ABNORMAL _____
● PERIPHERAL VASCULAR ☐ NORMAL ☐ ABNORMAL _____

GASTROINTESTINAL

● ABDOMEN ☐ NORMAL ☐ ABNORMAL _____
● HERNIA ☐ NONE ☐ PRESENT _____
● LIVER/SPLEEN
   LIVER ☐ NORMAL ☐ ABNORMAL _____
   SPLEEN ☐ NORMAL ☐ ABNORMAL _____
● STOOL GUAIAC, IF INDICATED ☐ POSITIVE ☐ NEGATIVE

LYMPHATIC

● PALPATION OF NODES (CHOOSE ALL THAT ARE APPLICABLE)
   NECK ☐ NORMAL ☐ ABNORMAL _____
   AXILLA ☐ NORMAL ☐ ABNORMAL _____
   GROIN ☐ NORMAL ☐ ABNORMAL _____
   OTHER SITE ☐ NORMAL ☐ ABNORMAL _____

SKIN

● INSPECTED/PALPATED ☐ NORMAL ☐ ABNORMAL _____

NEUROLOGIC/PSYCHIATRIC

● ORIENTATION ☐ TIME ☐ PLACE ☐ PERSON ☐ COMMENTS
● MOOD AND AFFECT ☐ NORMAL ☐ DEPRESSED ☐ ANXIOUS ☐ AGITATED ☐ OTHER

GYNECOLOGIC (AT LEAST 7)

● BREASTS ☐ NORMAL ☐ ABNORMAL _____
● EXTERNAL GENITALIA ☐ NORMAL ☐ ABNORMAL _____
● URETHRAL MEATUS ☐ NORMAL ☐ ABNORMAL _____
● URETHRA ☐ NORMAL ☐ ABNORMAL _____
● BLADDER ☐ NORMAL ☐ ABNORMAL _____
● VAGINA/PELVIC SUPPORT ☐ NORMAL ☐ ABNORMAL _____
● CERVIX ☐ NORMAL ☐ ABNORMAL _____
● UTERUS ☐ NORMAL ☐ ABNORMAL _____
● ADNEXA/PARAMETRIA ☐ NORMAL ☐ ABNORMAL _____
● ANUS/PERINEUM ☐ NORMAL ☐ ABNORMAL _____
● RECTAL ☐ NORMAL ☐ ABNORMAL _____
(SEE ALSO "STOOL GUAIAC" ABOVE)

● TOTAL NUMBER OF BULLETED (●) ELEMENTS EXAMINED:

American College of Obstetricians and Gynecologists

(From Beckmann CRB, Ling FW, et al. *Obstetrics and Gynecology*, 7th ed. Baltimore: Lippincott Williams & Wilkins; 2014.)

FIGURE
1.1 Breast examination.

Inspection

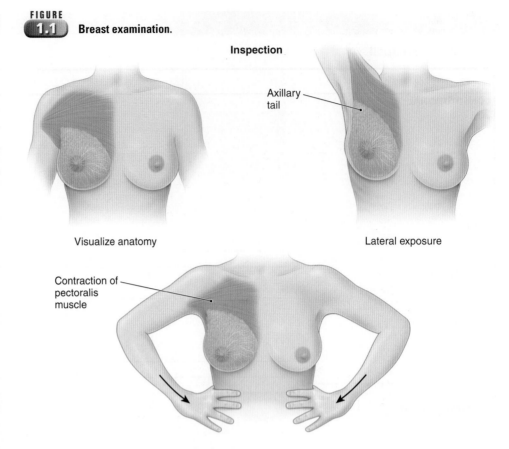

Visualize anatomy

Axillary tail

Lateral exposure

Contraction of pectoralis muscle

Breast palpation techniques

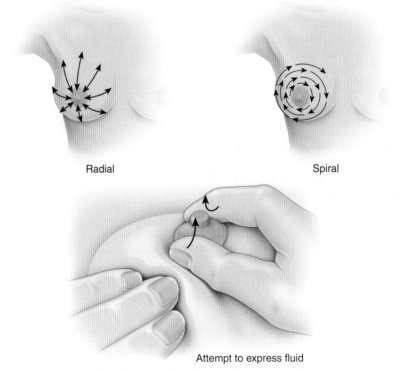

Radial

Spiral

Attempt to express fluid

(From Beckmann CRB, Ling FW, et al. *Obstetrics and Gynecology*, 7th ed. Baltimore: Lippincott Williams & Wilkins; 2014.)

FIGURE 1.2 Female external genitalia.

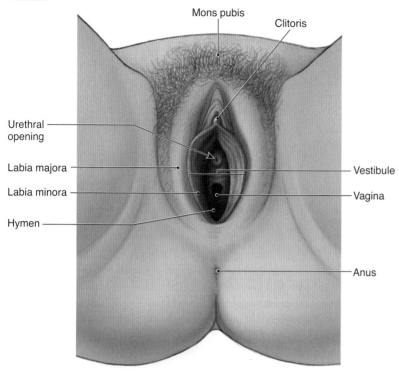

Mons pubis
Clitoris
Urethral opening
Labia majora
Labia minora
Hymen
Vestibule
Vagina
Anus

(From Beckmann CRB, Ling FW, et al. *Obstetrics and Gynecology*, 7th ed. Baltimore: Lippincott Williams & Wilkins; 2014.)

FIGURE 1.3 Palpation of the Bartholin, urethral, and Skene glands.

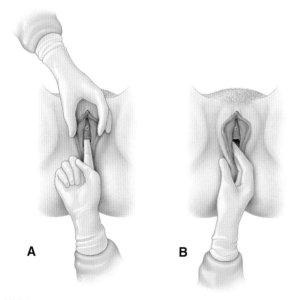

A   B

(A) Palpation of urethral and Skene glands and "milking" of urethra. **(B)** Palpation of Bartholin glands. (From Beckmann CRB, Ling FW, et al. *Obstetrics and Gynecology*, 7th ed. Baltimore: Lippincott Williams & Wilkins; 2014.)

FIGURE
1.4 Caudal view of female external genitalia during pelvic examination.

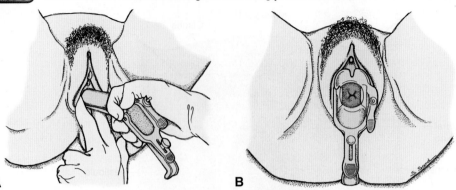

A   **B**

(A) Gloved hands of health care professional open introitus to insert speculum. **(B)** Speculum is in place within vagina and secured in its open position; ostium of uterus is visible. (From Beckmann CRB, Ling FW, et al. *Obstetrics and Gynecology*, 7th ed. Baltimore: Lippincott Williams & Wilkins; 2014.)

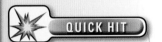

QUICK HIT

Thinking of the cervical position in the vagina as a light switch can make determining uterine position much easier (Figure 1.6). When the long axis of the cervix is in the "on" position (or high in the vagina under the pubic bone), the uterus is retroverted. When the cervix is pointing downward or in the "off" position, the uterus is anteverted.

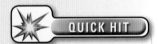

QUICK HIT

The ovaries are palpable in normal menstrual women ~half of the time, whereas palpation of ovaries in postmenopausal women is less common.

3. **Bimanual** examination (Figure 1.5)
   a. Insert lubricated fingers into vagina; place other hand on abdomen halfway between umbilicus and pubic hairline
   b. Palpate vaginal walls posteriorly, laterally, and anteriorly, noting tenderness and nodularity
   c. Palpate cervix: note position, shape, size, consistency, mobility, masses, and tenderness
   d. Palpate fornix
   e. Palpate uterus by lifting cervix upward
      i. Size
      ii. Shape
      iii. Consistency
      iv. Mobility
      v. Tenderness
      vi. Masses
      vii. Long axis: anteverted, midposition, retroverted (see Quick Hit explanation to the left)

FIGURE
1.5 Bimanual examination of the uterus and adnexa.

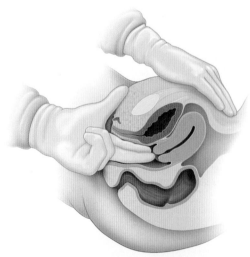

(From Beckmann CRB, Ling FW, et al. *Obstetrics and Gynecology*, 7th ed. Baltimore: Lippincott Williams & Wilkins; 2014.)

FIGURE 1.6 Thinking of the cervical position in the vagina as a light switch can make determining uterine position much easier.

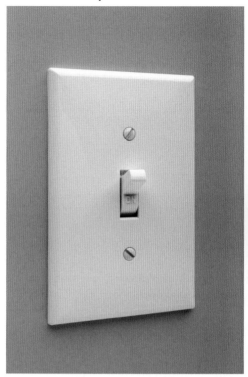 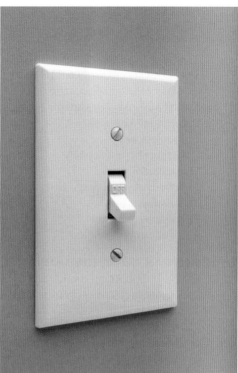

      viii. Short axis: flexion at lower uterine segment; anteflexed or retroflexed
    f. Palpate adnexal area and both ovaries
  4. **Rectovaginal** examination (Figure 1.7)
    a. Change vaginal hand glove
    b. Insert index finger into vagina and middle finger into rectum
    c. Palpate uterus, uterosacral ligaments, and adnexa
    d. Palpate rectal canal and integrity of rectal sphincter

FIGURE 1.7 Rectovaginal examination.

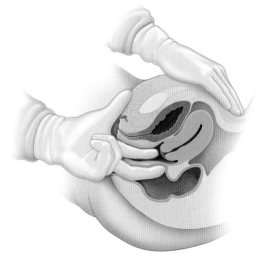

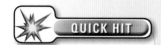 **QUICK HIT**

Rectovaginal exam allows: palpation of a mass (such as an enlarged ovary) in the pouch of Douglas; for adequate evaluation of the parametrium in patients with cervical cancer; and for assessment of the uterosacral ligaments for nodularity associated with endometriosis.

(From Beckmann CRB, Ling FW, et al. *Obstetrics and Gynecology*, 7th ed. Baltimore: Lippincott Williams & Wilkins; 2014.)

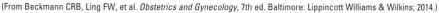

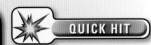

Accurately identifying problems and selecting the most likely diagnosis leads to effective management plans.

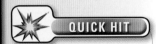

The health care provider must have the ability to interact cooperatively with a patient and *all* members of a health care team. This is a hallmark of **professionalism**.

III. Diagnosis and Management Plan

A. Assess compliance with recommended screening measures specific to women (see Chapter 2)

B. Assess risks
  1. Unintended pregnancy
  2. STDs
  3. Breast cancer (e.g., Gail model)
  4. Gynecologic malignancies
  5. Fracture risk assessment (FRAX score)

C. Differential diagnosis
  1. Problem list
  2. Diagnostic impression

D. Management plan
  1. Laboratory and diagnostic studies
  2. Treatment options
  3. Patient education
  4. Continuing care plans

V. Interpersonal and Communication Skills

A. Establish rapport and build trust by addressing culture, ethnicity, language/literacy, socioeconomic status, spirituality/religion, age, sexual orientation, and disability

B. Teamwork
  1. Patient
  2. Patient support network
  3. Health care team

C. Communicate exam findings in well-organized written and oral reports

The Woman's Health Examination

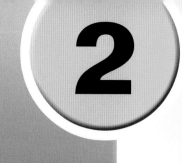

The Obstetrician/Gynecologist's Role in Screening and Preventive Care

I. Primary Prevention

A. Attempt to eliminate risk factors for disease and prevent its occurrence

B. Includes health education and behavioral interventions to promote **healthier lifestyle**

  1. Fitness and nutrition
  2. Hygiene
  3. Smoking cessation
  4. Personal safety
  5. Sexuality

C. **Immunizations**

  1. Request new patients to provide vaccination records
  2. Ages 13–18 years
      a. DTaP (diphtheria, tetanus, acellular pertussis) booster (once between ages 11 and 16 years)
      b. Hepatitis B series (if not previously immunized)
      c. Human papillomavirus (HPV) series for ages 9–26 years (given at 0, 2, and 6 months if not previously immunized)
      d. Meningococcal vaccine (prior to high school if not previously immunized)
      e. Influenza vaccine annually
      f. High-risk groups may additionally need
          i. Hepatitis A series (if not previously immunized)
          ii. Pneumococcal pneumonia vaccine (once if not previously immunized)
          iii. Measles, mumps, rubella (MMR) series (if not already immunized)
          iv. Varicella series (if not already immunized)
  3. Ages 19–39 years
      a. Td (tetanus-diphtheria) booster once every 10 years (Tdap substituted, if no prior adult immunization for pertussis)
      b. HPV series (for ages 26 years and younger if not previously immunized)
      c. Influenza vaccine annually
      d. High-risk groups may additionally need
          i. MMR (if susceptible by serologic testing)
          ii. Varicella series (if susceptible by serologic testing)
          iii. Hepatitis A series
          iv. Hepatitis B series
          v. Pneumococcal pneumonia vaccine
          vi. Meningococcal vaccine
  4. Ages 40–64 years
      a. Td booster once every 10 years (Tdap if no prior adult immunization for pertussis)
      b. Influenza vaccine annually
      c. Herpes zoster (once for women age 60 years and older if not previously immunized)

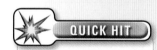

QUICK HIT

Because of the increasing prevalence of pertussis in the United States, it is currently recommended that all pregnant women receive a dose of Tdap after 27 weeks of pregnancy to protect their newborn.

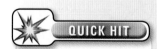

QUICK HIT

Because newborns do not get their first pertussis vaccination until age 2 months, it is important that grandparents and adults who will have close contact to newborns get immunized to pertussis.

The Obstetrician/Gynecologist's Role

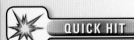

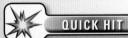

Findings from history, physical, and laboratory results guide interventions and counseling and may indicate further targeted screenings or evaluations.

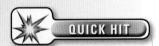

For cancer screening, the test must be shown to lower the mortality rate of the disease in the screened population compared to the unscreened population.

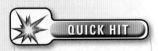

Not every disease can be detected by screening tests, and screening tests are not feasible for every disease.

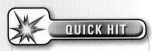

An effective screening test should be both *sensitive* (it has a high detection rate) and *specific* (it has a low false-positive rate).

d. High-risk groups
   i. MMR
   ii. Varicella series (if susceptible by serologic testing)
   iii. Hepatitis A series (if susceptible by serologic testing)
   iv. Hepatitis B series
   v. Pneumococcal pneumonia vaccine
   vi. Meningococcal vaccine
5. Age 65 years and older
   a. Td booster once every 10 years (Tdap if no prior adult immunization for pertussis)
   b. Herpes zoster (once if not previously immunized)
   c. Influenza vaccine annually
   d. Pneumococcal pneumonia vaccine once unless risk factors, then every 5 years
   e. High-risk groups may additionally need
      i. Hepatitis A series
      ii. Hepatitis B series
      iii. Meningococcal vaccine

II. Secondary Prevention
A. Periodic assessments conducted at regular intervals including screening, evaluation, and counseling
   1. Thorough medical history
   2. Physical examination
   3. Appropriate laboratory testing
B. Characteristics of screening tests
   1. Purpose is to detect presence of disease in asymptomatic individuals
      a. Asymptomatic period should be long enough to allow detection
      b. Disease should be prevalent enough to justify screening
      c. Early treatment (in asymptomatic stage) should be available
      d. Treatment provides sufficient effect on quality/quantity of life
   2. Criteria for testing
      a. Sensitivity: proportion of *affected* individuals that test *positive* on test (true +)
      b. Specificity: proportion of *unaffected* individuals that test *negative* on test (true −)
      c. Safe
      d. Affordable
      e. Acceptable to patients
   3. Criteria for population to be tested
      a. High disease prevalence in population
      b. Accessible
      c. Compliant with testing and treatment
C. Cancer screening (Boxes 2.1 and 2.2)
   1. **Breast cancer**
      a. Characteristics and assessment
         i. Most common cancer in U.S. women (excludes skin cancer)
         ii. 2nd leading cancer-related death in women (1st is lung cancer)

BOX 2.1

Most Common Malignancies in U.S. Women (2009)

1. Breast
2. Lung
3. Colorectal
4. Endometrial
5. Thyroid

(Adapted from Centers for Disease Control and Prevention. United States cancer statistics (USCS) 2009 top ten cancers. Accessed at http://apps.nccd.cdc.gov/uscs/toptencancers.aspx.)

BOX 2.2

Leading Cancer Mortalities in U.S. Women (2009)

1. Lung
2. Breast
3. Colorectal
4. Pancreas
5. Ovary

(Adapted from Centers for Disease Control and Prevention. United States cancer statistics (USCS) 2009 top ten cancers. Accessed at http://apps.nccd.cdc.gov/uscs/toptencancers.aspx.)

---

      iii. Lifetime risk 12.5%

      iv. Assess risk with thorough history; screening recommendations differ based on risks

      v. Breast Cancer Risk Assessment Tool: computer program to estimate an individual patient's risk

  b. Screening for average-risk women

    i. American Congress of Obstetricians and Gynecologists (the Congress)

      (a) Annual clinical breast examination for all women

      (b) Screening mammography

        (i) Ages 40+ every 1–2 years

        (ii) Ages 50+ annually

    ii. American Cancer Society (ACS)

      (a) Clinical breast examination

        (i) Ages 20–39 every 3 years

        (ii) Ages 40+ annually

      (b) Screening mammography: ages 40+ annually

    iii. Magnetic resonance imaging (MRI) and ultrasound currently have no role in routine screening

  c. Screening for very high–risk women (>20% lifetime risk): MRI is also recommended in addition to yearly mammography

  d. Palpable breast mass

    i. Diagnostic mammogram recommended in women 30+ years (even if recent screening mammogram normal); may be appropriate in some younger women

    ii. Normal mammogram should *not* preclude further workup (sensitivity of mammogram 90% or less in some studies)

    iii. Ultrasound to delineate cystic versus solid mass

      (a) Cystic mass may be aspirated if symptomatic

      (b) Solid mass: consider biopsy

  e. Biopsy

    i. Fine-needle aspiration (FNA) biopsy

    ii. Core needle biopsy

    iii. Excisional biopsy

2. **Cervical cancer**

  a. Characteristics and assessment

    i. Cervical intraepithelial neoplasia (CIN) (cervical dysplasia) is precursor lesion to cervical cancer

      (a) CIN 1 regresses spontaneously ~2/3 of the time

      (b) CIN 2 and 3 are more likely to progress to cancer over time (average time from dysplasia to cancer is >10 years)

    ii. Pap testing (exfoliative cytology) allows early diagnosis in most cases

      (a) Slide or liquid-based testing methods

      (b) With or without high-risk HPV testing

  b. Screening recommendations

    i. Initiate cytology screening at age 21 years, unless immunocompromised patient (e.g., AIDS)

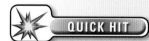

QUICK HIT

Although still recommended, neither clinical breast exam nor breast self-examination have been shown to lower the mortality of breast cancer.

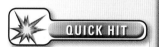

QUICK HIT

Mammogram is normal in 10%–20% of palpable breast cancers.

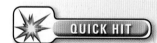

QUICK HIT

Because an FNA specimen is a cytology specimen, it is both less sensitive and specific than a core needle biopsy, which provides a **histopathologic** diagnosis.

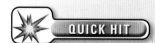

QUICK HIT

A core biopsy can be done directly on a palpable lesion but will need to be image guided if the lesion is only detected by imaging (e.g., ultrasound guided, stereotactic mammographic guided).

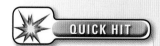

QUICK HIT

HPV testing is only done for the known serotypes with a high risk for developing CIN. Currently, the high-risk group comprises 14 serotypes to include types 16 and 18.

ii. Ages 21–30 years
   (a) Cervical cytology testing every 3 years
   (b) High-risk HPV testing does not influence management in this age group and is not recommended
iii. Age 30 years and older
   (a) If testing with cytology alone, the screening interval should remain every 3 years
   (b) If co-testing with cervical cytology and high-risk HPV testing, then a negative result on both tests reduces the screening interval to every 5 years
   (c) Women with immunosuppression, human immunodeficiency virus (HIV) infection, or Diethylstilbestrol (DES) exposure should continue annual screening even with negative results
   (d) Women with a history of CIN 2 or worse should continue screening for 20 years after the original diagnosis
iv. Women age 65 years and older with no prior history of CIN can discontinue screening
v. Women who have undergone hysterectomy
   (a) Supracervical hysterectomy: continue screening as noted above
   (b) Total hysterectomy (removal of cervix and uterus)
      (i) Women with no history of CIN do not require continued screening
      (ii) Women with a history of prior CIN 2 or 3 should continue recommended screening

3. **Ovarian cancer**
   a. Characteristics and assessment
      i. Leading cause of death from gynecologic malignancy in United States
      ii. 5th leading cause of cancer death in women
      iii. Disease is spread beyond ovary at diagnosis 75% of the time
      iv. Overall 5-year survival ~45%
      v. 90% are epithelial tumors
      vi. Risk factors
         (a) Genetic disposition
         (b) Family cancer syndrome (5%–10% of ovarian cancers)
            (i) *BRCA1*: lifetime risk ovarian cancer 40%–60%
            (ii) *BRCA2*: lifetime risk ovarian cancer 15%–25%
            (iii) Lynch II syndrome: lifetime risk ovarian cancer 3%–14%
         (c) Increasing age
            (i) Reproductive factors such as late menopause
            (ii) Risk reduction with use of oral contraceptives, pregnancy, breastfeeding, tubal ligation, or hysterectomy
            (iii) Risk increased by history of endometriosis, infertility, and menopausal hormone therapy
   b. Testing
      i. Tumor markers
         (a) CA-125 glycoprotein antigen (only useful for epithelial types of ovarian tumors). See Chapter 50 for other types of ovarian tumors.
            (i) Lacks adequate specificity for screening average-risk women
            (ii) Sensitivity up to 80% in advanced disease (lower with early-stage disease)
            (iii) Specificity limited
               (1) Elevated in 1% of healthy women
               (2) Elevated by endometriosis, pelvic infection, fibroids, other malignancies, ascites, other diseases
      ii. Pelvic ultrasound
         (a) Transvaginal ultrasound (TVUS) provides improved visualization of ovaries compared to abdominal imaging
         (b) Sensitivity 75%+
         (c) Specificity 94%–99% (performs more poorly, however, at detecting early-stage disease)

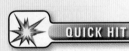

QUICK HIT

In general, the risk of ovarian cancer is linked to the number of ovulations during women's reproductive years, such that early menarche and late menopause increase risk, and breastfeeding and combination oral contraceptives decrease risk.

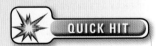

QUICK HIT

There is currently no recommended screening test for ovarian cancer in average-risk women.

c. Screening recommendations
   i. Average-risk population: screening with CA-125 testing or TVUS *not* recommended
   ii. Increased-risk populations
      (a) + Family history but no specific high-risk pattern known: counsel regarding poor positive predictive value of testing and risk of false-positive results and costs
      (b) + Family history of suspected hereditary ovarian cancer syndrome: refer for genetic counseling; consider testing for *BRCA1* and *BRCA2*
         (i) Consider offering to women of Ashkenazi Jewish heritage with single family member with breast or ovarian cancer
         (ii) For women with known *BRCA1* and *BRCA2* mutation, consider referral to specialist familiar with surveillance protocols (may include every 6 months CA-125 and TVUS); preventative measures should also be offered (e.g., combination oral contraceptives and risk-reducing salpingo-oophorectomy once childbearing is completed)

4. **Colorectal cancer**
   a. Characteristics: 3rd leading cause of cancer deaths in women (after lung and breast)
   b. Screening recommendations
      i. All women at average risk beginning at age 50 years
      ii. Colonoscopy: preferred method every 10 years
      iii. Alternative testing
         (a) Annual fecal occult blood testing (FOBT) or fecal immunochemical testing (FIT); patient collects and returns 3 home stool samples for analysis
         (b) Flexible sigmoidoscopy every 5 years (misses right-sided lesions—65% of advanced colon cancer in women)
         (c) Both FOBT and flexible sigmoidoscopy
         (d) Double-contrast barium enema every 5 years

D. Screening for sexually transmitted diseases (STDs); see also Chapter 31
   1. Risk factors
      a. History of multiple sex partners
      b. Sex partner with multiple sexual contacts
      c. Sexual contact of someone with culture-proven STD
      d. History of prior STDs
      e. Attendance at STD clinic
      f. Developmental disability
      g. Illicit drug use
      h. CIN or history of HPV
   2. **HIV**
      a. Testing recommended for all women at least once; no consensus regarding frequency of repeat testing
      b. Targeted testing recommended for women with risk factors
      c. Encourage routine testing prior to initiating new sexual relationship (both woman and her prospective partner)
      d. Annual testing recommended for woman who
         i. Injects drugs
         ii. Has sex partner who injects drugs
         iii. Has sex partner who is HIV positive
         iv. Exchanges sex for drugs
         v. Has been diagnosed with another STD in past year
         vi. Has had more than 1 partner since last HIV test
      e. Screening test
         i. Enzyme-linked immunosorbent assay (ELISA) on blood (most common test)
         ii. ELISA can also be performed on urine or saliva
         iii. Reactive (+) test requires supplementary confirmatory test (Western blot)

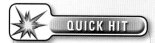

Cancer screening tests are not currently available for endometrial, vaginal, or vulvar cancers.

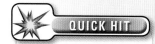

Although there is no screening test for endometrial adenocarcinoma, it is the most commonly diagnosed gynecologic malignancy but the least frequent gynecologic cancer mortality. This is because it has an **early warning sign**, abnormal uterine bleeding, which triggers evaluation and diagnosis with an endometrial biopsy.

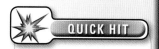

FOBT of a single stool sample from a physician examination is not adequate and not recommended for screening.

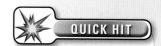

Due to the risks related to STDs in pregnancy, screening for HIV, chlamydia, gonorrhea, hepatitis B, and syphilis is recommended for all pregnant women.

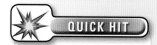

Even without known risk factors, all women who desire STD screening should be tested.

The Obstetrician/Gynecologist's Role

3. **Chlamydia** (*Chlamydia trachomatis*)
    a. Characteristics
        i. Most commonly reported bacterial STD in United States
        ii. >1.2 million cases reported to CDC for 2009
        iii. Many cases unreported; people may be unaware of infection
        iv. 10%–15% of untreated cases develop pelvic inflammatory disease (PID)
        v. Potential long-term complications include
            (a) Infertility
            (b) Ectopic pregnancy
            (c) Chronic pelvic pain
    b. Screening recommendations
        i. Sexually active women age ≤25 years: annually
        ii. Women 26 years and older who are high risk for infection: annually
        iii. All pregnant women
    c. Screening test
        i. Nucleic acid amplification tests (NAATs): high sensitivity and specificity
        ii. Endocervical swab, vaginal swab, or urine testing
4. **Gonorrhea** (*Neisseria gonorrhoeae*)
    a. Characteristics
        i. >300,000 cases reported to CDC in 2009
        ii. Less than half of cases reported
        iii. Symptoms may include
            (a) Vaginal discharge
            (b) Burning with urination
            (c) Spotting between periods
        iv. Most women asymptomatic
        v. Most common cause of PID
        vi. Can also spread to blood or joints
        vii. Long-term complications
            (a) Infertility
            (b) Ectopic pregnancy
            (c) Chronic pelvic pain
    b. Screening recommendations
        i. Sexually active women age ≤25 years: annually
        ii. Women age 26 years and older who are high risk for infection: annually
        iii. All pregnant women
    c. Screening test: same as for chlamydia
5. **Syphilis** (*Treponema pallidum*)
    a. Characteristics
        i. Approximately 10,000 cases diagnosed in United States in 2006
        ii. Primary stage
            (a) Usually single painless sore (chancre) but can be multiple
            (b) Last 3–6 weeks
            (c) Heals without treatment (but disease progresses)
        iii. Secondary stage
            (a) Characteristic red or brown rash (usually nonpruritic) on palms of hands or soles of feet
            (b) Condylomata lata – wart-like, broad based papules on vulva, perineum, or anus; highly contagious
            (c) Other symptoms may include fever, swollen lymph nodes, sore throat, hair loss, headache, weight loss, muscle pain, fatigue
            (d) Rash and symptoms resolve without treatment (but disease progresses)
        iv. Latent stage: asymptomatic (may last years)
        v. Tertiary stage
            (a) ~15% of untreated individuals
            (b) May be 10–20 years after contracting disease

QUICK HIT

Because of their prevalence and the fact that they can be asymptomatic and cause significant long-term complications, all sexually active women 25 years old and younger should be screened for *C. trachomatis* and *N. gonorrhoeae* annually.

(c) Damage to internal organs including heart, nerves, brain, eyes, blood vessels, bones, joints

(d) May result in death

b. Screening recommendations

  i. Annual screening for women who are high risk for infection

  ii. Pregnant women

   (a) All pregnant women as early as possible in pregnancy

   (b) All pregnant women again at delivery

   (c) High-risk women additionally retest early 3rd trimester

c. Screening tests

  i. Initial nontreponemal test

   (a) Venereal Disease Research Laboratory (VDRL) test

   (b) Rapid plasma reagin (RPR)

   (c) Specificity for nontreponemal tests is decreased by other conditions: pregnancy, collagen vascular disease, advanced cancer, malaria, and rickettsial disease

  ii. Confirmatory treponemal test for all initial +

   (a) *T. pallidum* particle agglutination (TP-PA)

   (b) microhemagglutination assay (MHA-TP)

  iii. Many institutions are now screening with immunoglobulin G (IgG) antibody for syphilis; if positive, titers are performed with nontreponemal tests

E. Screening for metabolic and cardiovascular diseases

  1. **Osteoporosis**

   a. Characteristics

    i. 13%–18% U.S. women age 50 years and older

    ii. Bone mineral density (BMD) is indirect measure of bone fragility and is a surrogate measure of woman's fracture risk

    iii. 37%–50% U.S. women age 50 years and older have osteopenia (low BMD)

   b. Screening recommendations (the College)

    i. All women beginning at age 65 years

    ii. Younger postmenopausal women with 1+ risk factor

    iii. Risk factors for osteoporotic fracture

     (a) Prior fracture

     (b) Family history

     (c) Caucasian

     (d) Dementia

     (e) Poor nutrition

     (f) Smoking

     (g) Low body mass

     (h) Estrogen deficiency

      (i) Early menopause (age <45 years)

      (ii) Prolonged premenopausal amenorrhea (>1 year)

     (i) Prolonged low calcium

     (j) Poor eyesight despite correction

     (k) History of falls

     (l) Inadequate physical activity

    iv. Postmenopausal women with personal history of fracture should have BMD testing and treatment if osteoporotic

    v. Consider more frequent testing with

     (a) Cushing disease

     (b) Hyperparathyroidism

     (c) Hypophosphatasia

     (d) Inflammatory bowel disease

     (e) Lymphoma

     (f) Leukemia

     (g) Long-term corticosteroid usage

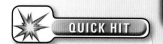

QUICK HIT

Women without risk factors need BMD testing beginning at age 65 years.

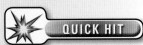

QUICK HIT

An online calculation tool called the **FRAX score** is very useful to assess a woman's 10-year risk of both hip fracture and major osteoporotic fracture. It takes into account T score as well as risk factors, ethnicity, age, and BMI.

      (h) Phenobarbital
      (i) Phenytoin
      (j) Lithium
      (k) Long-term heparin

  c. Screening test
    i. Dual-energy X-ray absorptiometry (DXA)
      (a) Hip
      (b) Spine
    ii. **T score**
      (a) Standard deviation from peak BMD of normal, young adult
      (b) World Health Organization (WHO) definition
        (i) Normal T score > -1.0
        (ii) **Osteopenia** (low bone mass) T score ≤ -1.0 to > -2.5
        (iii) **Osteoporosis** T score ≤ -2.5
    iii. **Z score**: standard deviation from mean BMD of sex-, race-, and age-matched population (**not clinically useful**)
    iv. Measurements vary between sites and machines
  d. Preventive strategies
    i. Calcium: 1,000–1,500 mg/d (in two divided doses)
    ii. Vitamin D: 400–800 IU/d
    iii. Weight-bearing, muscle-strengthening exercise
    iv. Smoking cessation
    v. Moderate alcohol intake
    vi. Fall prevention strategies

2. **Diabetes mellitus**
  a. Screening recommendations
    i. Routine testing at age 45 years, every 3 years
    ii. Begin screening at younger age and more frequently with risk factors
      (a) Body mass index (BMI) ≥ 25
      (b) + Family history
      (c) Habitual physical inactivity
      (d) Gave birth to newborn >9 lb
      (e) History of gestational diabetes
      (f) Hypertension
  b. Screening tests
    i. Random blood sugars (>200 mg/dL is diabetes)
    ii. Fasting blood sugar (>100 mg/dL, needs additional testing; >126, diabetes)
    iii. 2-hour post 75-gram glucose challenge (140–199, impaired glucose tolerance; ≥ 200 mg/dL, diabetes)
    iv. HbA1c >6.0% (needs additional testing)

3. **Thyroid disease**: routine screening at age 50 years, every 5 years
  a. TSH or
  b. TSH with reflex to fT4 (if TSH is high or low a fT4 is automatically performed by the lab)

4. **Hypertension**
  a. Characteristics
    i. 30% adults age 20 years and older
    ii. Systolic blood pressure (BP) ≥ 140 mm Hg
    iii. Diastolic BP ≥ 90 mm Hg
    iv. Long-term complications
      (a) Heart disease
      (b) Cerebrovascular accident (CVA)
      (c) Mortality
  b. Screening recommendations: begin screening at age 13 years
    i. Every 2 years with normal values
    ii. Annual screening with borderline pressures

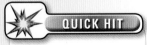

QUICK HIT

A 1% reduction in cholesterol levels results in a 2% reduction in coronary heart disease.

5. **Lipid disorders**
   a. Characteristics
      i. 1 in 5 adults have elevated total cholesterol ≥240
      ii. Abnormal levels linked to
         (a) Atherosclerosis
         (b) Cardiovascular disease
         (c) Cerebrovascular disease
   b. Screening recommendations
      i. Routine screening beginning at age 45 years, every 5 years
      ii. Begin earlier screening with risk factors
         (a) Family history of familial hyperlipidemia
         (b) Family history of premature cardiovascular disease
            (i) age <50 years for men
            (ii) age <60 years for women
         (c) Diabetes mellitus
         (d) Multiple coronary heart disease risk factors (such as smoking, hypertension, etc.)
   c. Screening tests
      i. Total cholesterol
      ii. Low-density lipoprotein (LDL)
      iii. High-density lipoprotein (HDL)
      iv. Triglycerides
6. **Obesity**
   a. Characteristics
      i. Increased risk
         (a) Heart disease
         (b) Type 2 diabetes
         (c) Hypertension
         (d) Cancers of endometrium, colon, and breast
         (e) Sleep apnea
         (f) Osteoarthritis
         (g) Gallbladder disease
         (h) Depression
         (i) Death (BMI >30 = 2-fold increased risk)
   b. Screening recommendations
      i. Measurement of height, weight, and calculation of BMI recommended as part of periodic assessments
      ii. Waist circumference >35 inches in women
      iii. Waist–hip ratio of >0.8
   c. Definitions
      i. Underweight: BMI <18.5
      ii. Normal weight: BMI 18.5–24.9
      iii. Overweight: BMI 25–29.9
      iv. Obesity (class I): BMI 30–34.9
      v. Obesity (class II): BMI 35–39.9
      vi. Extreme obesity: BMI ≥40

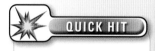

QUICK HIT

Women without risk factors should have a lipid profile performed every 5 years beginning at age 45 years.

The Obstetrician/Gynecologist's Role

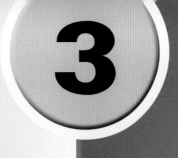

3 Ethics in Obstetrics and Gynecology

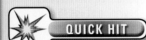

QUICK HIT

Autonomy is the moral foundation for informed consent in the practice of medicine.

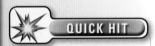

QUICK HIT

Paternalism is attempting to override patient autonomy to promote what the clinician perceives as a patient's best interest.

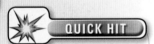

QUICK HIT

Justice is the obligation to treat equally those who are alike or similar.

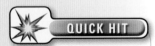

QUICK HIT

Feminist ethics challenges decisions biased by attitudes and traditions about gender roles that are embedded in our culture.

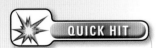

QUICK HIT

Case-based reasoning asserts precedence over primacy of ethical principles.

I. Ethical Framework(s)

A. Purpose: ensure that decision making and situation evaluation can be done systematically rather than based on physician's emotions, personal biases, or social pressures

B. **Principle-based ethics**
1. **Autonomy:** individual's right to make choices, hold views, and take action
2. **Beneficence:** promote well-being of others
3. **Nonmaleficence:** do no harm
4. **Justice:** fairly rendering what is due to others; important criteria include need, effort, contribution, and merit

C. Other ethical frameworks
1. **Virtue-based ethics:** character qualities that guide decisions that achieve others' well-being
   a. Trustworthiness
   b. Prudence
   c. Fairness
   d. Fortitude
   e. Temperance
   f. Integrity
   g. Self-effacement
   h. Compassion
2. **Ethics of care:** responsibilities that arise from personal attachments
   a. Commitment
   b. Empathy
   c. Compassion
   d. Caring
   e. Love
3. **Feminist ethics:** considers how gender distorts traditional analysis
4. **Communitarian ethics:** considers shared values and community goals
5. **Case-based reasoning:** considers precedents set in specific cases

II. Ethical Foundations

A. Patient–physician relationship: patient welfare is priority
B. Physician conduct and practice
1. Physician must be honest with patients, colleagues, and self
2. Avoid misrepresentation
3. Maintain medical competence
4. Avoid any behavior diminishing capability to practice
5. Respond to evidence of questionable conduct by others
C. Avoid conflict of interest (COI)
1. Recognize real or perceived COI
2. Publicly disclose COI

D. Professional responsibilities: maintain professional relationships with other health care providers
   1. Honesty
   2. Integrity
   3. Fairness
   4. Share mutual respect
E. Societal responsibilities to greater community
   1. Respect for laws
   2. Membership in medical societies
   3. Uphold dignity of profession
F. **Informed consent**
   1. Education of patient with consideration of capacity to understand
   2. Discussion of all options/alternatives
   3. Discussion of risks and benefits
   4. Uncover physician biases to maintain objectivity
   5. Answer all questions

III. Ethical Considerations in Obstetrics and Gynecology
A. Maternal rights *versus* fetal rights
   1. Laws protecting fetus may challenge maternal rights (e.g., incarceration for maternal drug use)
   2. Maternal rights take precedence over fetal rights
   3. Ensure maternal comprehension of harmful behaviors and refer mother to treatment programs
   4. Balance maternal autonomy and fetal beneficence
B. Justice (e.g., equalizing access to prenatal care)
   1. Universal screening for risky behaviors
      a. Drug and alcohol use
      b. Smoking
      c. Domestic violence
      d. Sexually transmitted infections
   2. Fair distribution of resources
C. Maternal–fetal conflict
   1. Women's autonomous decisions should be respected
   2. Obstetrician should present balanced information regarding expected outcomes of mother and fetus
      a. Fetal reasons for recommendation
      b. Explore barriers to accept recommendations
      c. Foster development/acceptance of health-promoting behavior

IV. Guidelines for Ethical Decision Making
A. Identify decision makers
   1. Generally, patient is presumed to have authority
   2. Surrogate decision maker if patient is incapable or legally incompetent
      a. Individual with durable power of attorney
      b. Family members may have to make proxy decision
      c. Court-appointed guardian
B. Collect data; establish facts
   1. Goal is objectivity
   2. Consultants may be necessary
C. Identify all medically appropriate options
D. Evaluate options according to values and principles involved
E. Identify conflicts and set priorities
   1. Define problem in terms of ethical principles
   2. Weigh principles underlying each argument
   3. Study similar cases and ascertain differences and similarities
F. Select option that can be best justified
G. Reevaluate decision after it is acted on

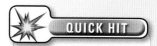

QUICK HIT

Veracity, or *honesty*, at all times is a fundamental precept.

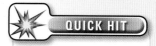

QUICK HIT

Obtaining informed consent encourages ongoing and open communication of relevant information.

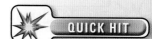

QUICK HIT

A patient's right to make health care decisions includes the right to refuse recommended treatment.

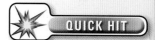

QUICK HIT

In medical care, maternal rights take precedence over fetal rights.

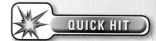

QUICK HIT

Pregnant women screened for psychosocial issues each trimester are less likely to have low-birth-weight or preterm babies.

Ethics in Obstetrics and Gynecology

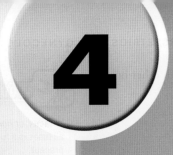

4 Embryology and Anatomy

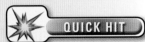

Through the first trimester of pregnancy, the fetal gonads, genital ducts, and genitalia are in an undifferentiated stage, in which it is not possible to determine sex based on appearance.

I. Embryology

A. Early stages (Figure 4.1)
1. Intermediate mesoderm
   a. 4th week: urogenital ridges develop along posterior body wall
   b. Gives rise to ovaries, fallopian tubes, uterus, upper portion of body wall, and urinary system
2. Ectoderm
   a. Genital swellings arise in pelvic region
   b. Gives rise to external genitalia
3. Genetic sex: determined by sperm (X or Y) fertilizing oocyte (X)
   a. Y chromosome: *SRY* (sex-determining gene on Y) encodes testis-determining factor (TDF)
   b. X chromosome: *WNT4* (ovarian development gene)
4. Phenotypic sex
   a. **Undifferentiated stage**
      i. **Gonads** become ♂ or ♀ by 7th week
      ii. **External genitalia** become ♂ or ♀ by 12th week
   b. **Androgens influence external genitalia development**
      i. Crucial for development of male genitalia
      ii. Excess causes ambiguity of female genitalia

FIGURE 4.1 Early development of the urogenital system.

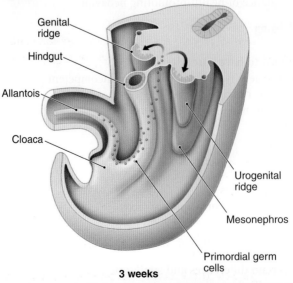

3 weeks

Beginning at approximately 3 weeks of gestation, urogenital ridges arise along the posterior wall of the coelomic cavity. Primordial germ cells migrate across the allantois into the genital ridges. (Modified from Sadler TW. *Langman's Medical Embryology*, 10th ed. Baltimore: Lippincott Williams & Wilkins; 2006:240–241.)

B. Differentiated organ development
1. Gonads (Figure 4.2)
   a. Initially undifferentiated primordial germ cells
      i. 3rd week: start in yolk sac
      ii. 5th week: migrate along allantois to reach gonadal ridges (see Figure 4.1)
      iii. 6th week: associate with primary sex cords
   b. Ovary
      i. Primordial germ cells → become oogonia → undergo 1st meiotic division to primary oocyte → arrest until puberty
      ii. Primary sex cords degenerate → secondary sex cords/cortical cords form → surround each primary oocyte → become primordial follicles
      iii. **Gubernaculum** (mesenchymal condensation attached to caudal end of gonad) → supports descent into pelvis → then becomes adult ovarian and round ligaments
   c. Testis
      i. Primary sex cords → become seminiferous cords → develop into rete testis and seminiferous tubules
      ii. Tunica albuginea → surface covering of testis
      iii. Gubernaculum supports descent to developing scrotum → becomes adult scrotal ligament holding testis in place
2. Genital duct development within urogenital ridge
   a. 2 pairs of ducts: **mesonephric** (Wolffian) and **paramesonephric** (Müllerian) → both present in undifferentiated stage
   b. Female
      i. Mesonephric ducts disappear; can leave behind remnants
      ii. **Paramesonephric ducts**: bilateral tubes
         (a) Fuse caudally to form uterus, cervix, upper vagina → meet **vaginal plate** and fuse with lower vagina (posterior wall of urogenital sinus)
         (b) As these ducts fuse, they carry folds of peritoneum with them to form broad ligaments
         (c) Cranially, they remain separate to form fallopian tubes
   c. Male
      i. Testes (Sertoli cells) secrete **anti-Müllerian hormone (AMH)** to inhibit development of paramesonephric ducts
      ii. **Mesonephric ducts** form epididymis, ductus deferens, and ejaculatory ducts
3. External genitalia (Figure 4.3)
   a. Dependent on presence or absence of androgen and estrogen
   b. Genital tubercle → clitoris or penis
   c. Labioscrotal swellings → labia majora or scrotum
   d. Urogenital folds → labia minora or spongy urethra
   e. **Cloaca** (dilation of caudal end of hindgut) → divided into **urogenital sinus** and **anorectal canal** separated by **urorectal septum** → become vaginal and rectal openings

II. Anatomy
A. Abdominal wall
1. Layers
   a. Skin
   b. Subcutaneous layer (fat, Camper's and Scarpa's fascia)
   c. Musculoaponeurotic layer (Figure 4.4)
      i. Above arcuate line (**rectus muscle between layers**): see Figure 4.4A
         (a) Anterior rectus sheath: aponeurosis of external and internal (splits) oblique muscles
         (b) Posterior rectus sheath: aponeurosis of internal oblique (splits) and transverse abdominal muscles
      ii. Below arcuate line (**rectus muscle below fascia**): rectus sheath composed of aponeurosis of all 3 muscles (see Figure 4.4B)
   d. Peritoneum

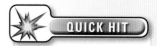

Primary oocyte development is arrested in the diplotene stage of prophase I until puberty.

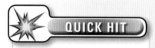

Gonads become structurally male or female by week 7.

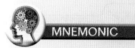

Think **"wolfman"** to remember that the *mesonephric*, or **Wolffian**, ducts are responsible for the male genital ducts. Therefore, the *paramesonephric*, or Müllerian, ducts must be female.

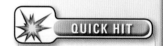

Gartner duct cysts can form in the sidewall of the vagina. They are remnants of the mesonephric ducts that did not completely regress during development.

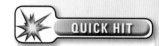

Without AMH in a genetic male, the Müllerian system develops, leading to undescended testes and the presence of a small, underdeveloped uterus in a male infant or adult.

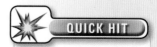

In congenital adrenal hyperplasia (CAH), decreased cortisol production results in increased androgen production. In females, this leads to ambiguous genitalia (neither normal male nor normal female).

Embryology and Anatomy

Embryology and Anatomy

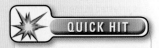

QUICK HIT

Failure of the urogenital folds to fuse in the male leads to hypospadias. Hypospadias should always be excluded before circumcision because the foreskin can be used in reconstruction.

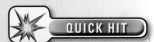

QUICK HIT

A persistent cloaca is a complex anorectal and genitourinary malformation in which the rectum, vagina, and urinary tract meet and fuse, creating a cloaca, a single common channel.

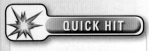

QUICK HIT

At 15 weeks, male and female fetuses can be differentiated on ultrasound.

FIGURE 4.2 Development of the gonads and their migration to their adult locations.

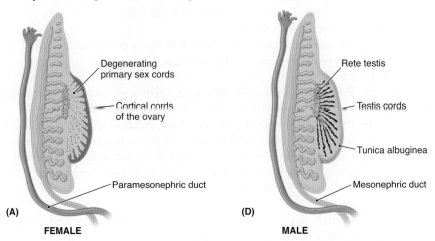

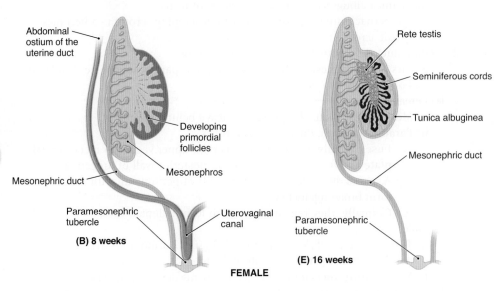

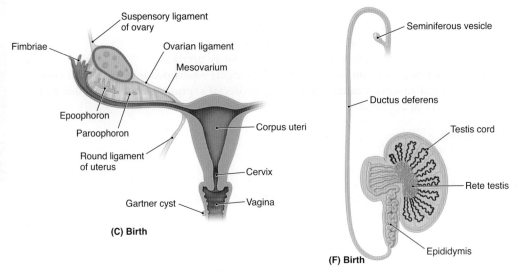

At approximately 6 weeks of gestation, the gonads have differentiated into either male or female (**A** and **B**). In female embryos, the paramesonephric ducts develop into the uterus, uterine tubes, and part of the vagina (**C** and **D**). In male embryos, the mesonephric ducts develop into the main genital tracts (ductus deferens) (**E** and **F**). (Modified from Sadler TW. *Langman's Medical Embryology,* 10th ed. Baltimore: Lippincott Williams & Wilkins; 2006:243, 245.)

FIGURE 4.3 Comparison of the development of male and female external genitalia.

FEMALE   MALE

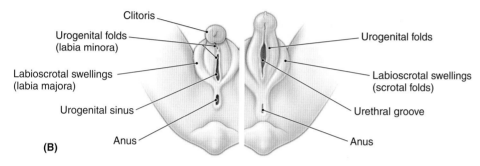

Genital tubercle
Urogenital folds
Labioscrotal swellings
Anus

(A)

Genital tubercle
Urogenital folds
Labioscrotal swellings
(scrotal folds)
Anus

7 weeks

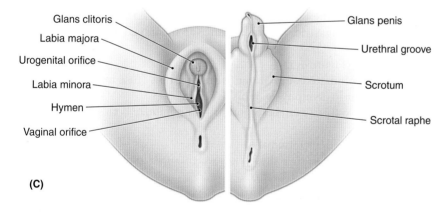

Clitoris
Urogenital folds
(labia minora)
Labioscrotal swellings
(labia majora)
Urogenital sinus
Anus

(B)

Urogenital folds
Labioscrotal swellings
(scrotal folds)
Urethral groove
Anus

10 weeks

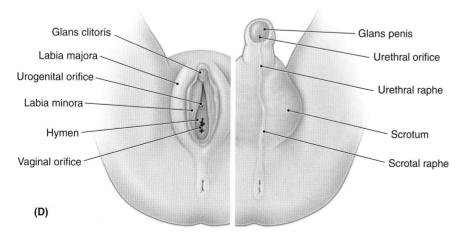

Glans clitoris
Labia majora
Urogenital orifice
Labia minora
Hymen
Vaginal orifice

(C)

Glans penis
Urethral groove
Scrotum
Scrotal raphe

12 weeks

Glans clitoris
Labia majora
Urogenital orifice
Labia minora
Hymen
Vaginal orifice

(D)

Glans penis
Urethral orifice
Urethral raphe
Scrotum
Scrotal raphe

Near term

(A) Early in gestation, the genital tubercle develops along with labioscrotal swellings and urogenital folds. **(B)** Shortly thereafter, the genital tubercle enlarges in both the male and female embryo. **(C)** The posterior commissure forms, effectively dividing genitals from anus. **(D)** Without the influence of a Y chromosome, the phallus regresses in relative size to form the clitoris.

Embryology and Anatomy

FIGURE 4.4 Cross-section of lower abdominal wall.

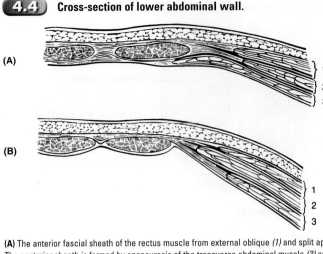

(A)

(B)

(A) The anterior fascial sheath of the rectus muscle from external oblique *(1)* and split aponeurosis of internal oblique *(2)* muscles. The posterior sheath is formed by aponeurosis of the transverse abdominal muscle *(3)* and split aponeurosis of the internal oblique muscle. **(B)** Lower portion of the abdominal wall below arcuate line (linea semicircularis) with absence of a posterior fascial sheath of the rectus muscle and all of the fascial aponeuroses *(1, 2, 3)* forming the anterior rectus muscle sheath. (From Rock JA, Jones HW. *TeLinde's Operative Gynecology*, 9th ed. Baltimore: Lippincott Williams & Wilkins; 2003.)

> **QUICK HIT**
>
> Care must be taken when placing lateral trocars at the time of laparoscopic surgery to avoid injury of the **inferior epigastric** vessels.

2. Blood supply
   a. Skin and subcutaneous tissues (from femoral vessels)
      i. **Superficial epigastric:** runs from femoral artery to umbilicus
      ii. **External pudendal:** runs medially to mons pubis
      iii. Superficial circumflex iliac: runs laterally to flank
   b. Muscles (from external iliac vessels and runs parallel to above)
      i. Deep circumflex iliac: runs laterally to flank
      ii. **Inferior epigastric:** runs along anterior abdominal wall in rectus muscle
B. Bony pelvis
   1. Composed of (Figure 4.5)
      a. Paired **innominate** bones: **ilium, ischium, pubis** (fuse in adolescence) → join anteriorly (**symphysis pubis**)
      b. **Sacrum:** 5–6 fused vertebrae (join with innominate bones via sacroiliac joints)
   2. Divided into (by linea terminalis)
      a. Greater pelvis (false) → distributes weight of abdominal organs and gravid uterus (see Figure 4.5, orange)
      b. Lesser pelvis (true) → contains pelvic viscera (see Figure 4.5, purple)

FIGURE 4.5 The bony pelvis.

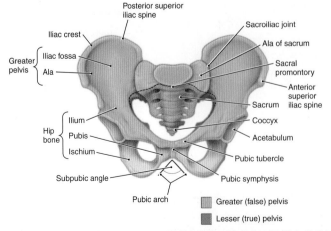

The greater and lesser pelves are color coded. (From Moore KL, Dalley AF. *Clinically Oriented Anatomy*, 5th ed. Baltimore: Lippincott Williams & Wilkins; 2006: Fig. 3.3B)

FIGURE
4.6 **Clinical pelvimetry.**

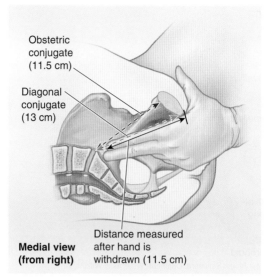

Obstetric
conjugate
(11.5 cm)

Diagonal
conjugate
(13 cm)

Distance measured
after hand is
withdrawn (11.5 cm)

**Medial view
(from right)**

(From Moore KL, Dalley AF. *Clinically Oriented Anatomy*, 5th ed. Baltimore: Lippincott Williams & Wilkins; 2006: Fig. B3.2.)

3. Pelvimetry → important measurements in obstetrics (Figure 4.6)
  a. Pelvic inlet
    i. **Obstetric conjugate:** should be >10 cm
      (a) Narrowest fixed distance that fetal head passes through during birth
      (b) Cannot measure directly on pelvic exam
    ii. **Diagonal conjugate**
      (a) Used as surrogate measure for above (obstetric conjugate)
      (b) Distance between lower border of pubis and sacral promontory (at level of ischial spines)
      (c) **Must be >11.5 cm** to accommodate fetal head
  b. Midpelvis
    i. **Interspinous diameter:** distance between ischial spines
    ii. Should be >10 cm
  c. Pelvic outlet
    i. **Transverse diameter** (distance between 2 ischial tuberosities): >11cm
    ii. Anteroposterior (pubic arch to tip of sacrum) 9.5–11 cm
    iii. Posterior sagittal: line between transverse diameter to tip of sacrum
4. Classifications (Figure 4.7)
  a. **Gynecoid** (most common, **40%–50%**): round in shape; ideal for vaginal delivery
  b. **Anthropoid (25%):** long oval
  c. **Android (20%):** wedge or heart shaped; least favorable for vaginal delivery
  d. **Platypelloid (2%–5%):** wide oval
C. Vulva and perineum (Figure 4.8)
  1. Vulva
    a. **Labia majora** (outer folds): adipose tissue, hair follicles, sebaceous and sweat glands
    b. **Labia minora** (inner folds): sebaceous and sweat glands, no hair/adipose tissue
      i. Merge with prepuce above clitoris
      ii. Fuse below clitoris to form frenulum
    c. **Clitoris:** composition: crura (2) and glans
    d. **Vestibule**
      i. Urethral opening: between clitoris and vagina
      ii. Vaginal opening
      iii. Skene ducts (anterior): paraurethral glands
      iv. Bartholin glands (posterior)

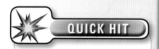

QUICK HIT

During a new obstetric physical exam, the diagonal conjugate should be assessed and noted if <11.5 cm.

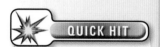

QUICK HIT

The most common shape of pelvis is the gynecoid pelvis.

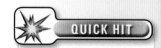

QUICK HIT

The two areas that typically have sebaceous glands without hair follicles are the labia minora and the areola of the breast.

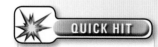

QUICK HIT

Bartholin glands can become blocked and lead to cyst or abscess formation. In women age >40 years, excision, rather than the more conservative treatment of incision with Word catheter drainage or marsupialization, should be undertaken to rule out carcinoma.

Embryology and Anatomy

FIGURE
4.7 Caldwell-Moloy pelvic types.

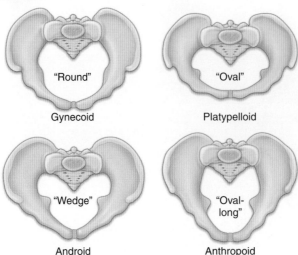

Gynecoid — "Round"

Platypelloid — "Oval"

Android — "Wedge"

Anthropoid — "Oval-long"

(From Beckmann CRB, Ling FW, et al. *Obstetrics and Gynecology*, 7th ed. Baltimore: Lippincott Williams & Wilkins; 2014.)

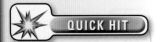

  e. Muscles (Figure 4.9)
   i. **Ischiocavernosus:** laterally and diagonally
   ii. **Bulbocavernosus:** medially
   iii. **Superficial transverse** perineal: horizontally
2. Perineum
 a. Surface area of trunk between thighs and buttocks from coccyx to symphysis pubis
 b. Also refers to superficial compartment deep to this area
3. **Urogenital diaphragm:** vulva lies on diaphragm; vulvar muscles are superficial to diaphragm (see Figure 4.9)
 a. Muscles (levator ani)
  i. **Pubococcygeus**
  ii. **Puborectalis**
  iii. **Iliococcygeus**
 b. Fascia
  i. Urogenital diaphragm
  ii. Endopelvic fascia
 c. Ligaments
  i. Uterosacral ligaments
  ii. Cardinal ligaments (broad ligament)

FIGURE
4.8 External female genitalia.

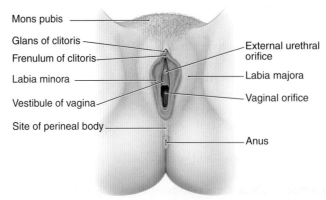

Mons pubis

Glans of clitoris

Frenulum of clitoris

Labia minora

Vestibule of vagina

Site of perineal body

External urethral orifice

Labia majora

Vaginal orifice

Anus

(From Beckmann CRB, Ling FW, et al. *Obstetrics and Gynecology*, 7th ed. Baltimore: Lippincott Williams & Wilkins; 2014.)

FIGURE 4.9 The urogenital diaphragm with the skin and subcutaneous fat cut away.

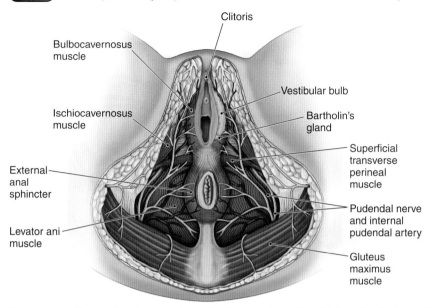

Clitoris

Bulbocavernosus muscle

Vestibular bulb

Ischiocavernosus muscle

Bartholin's gland

Superficial transverse perineal muscle

External anal sphincter

Levator ani muscle

Pudendal nerve and internal pudendal artery

Gluteus maximus muscle

The musculature, blood supply, and nerve supply constitute the external part of the pelvic floor. (From Beckmann CRB, Ling FW, et al. *Obstetrics and Gynecology*, 7th ed. Baltimore: Lippincott Williams & Wilkins; 2014.)

4. Blood vessels and nerves: leave pelvis through greater sciatic foramen
   a. Internal pudendal artery
      i. Clitoral branch
      ii. Perineal branch
      iii. Inferior hemorrhoidal
   b. Pudendal nerve (S2–S4): motor and sensory
D. Vagina
   1. Extends from vestibule to uterus
      a. Stratified, **nonkeratinized** squamous epithelium
      b. Smooth muscle inner layer
      c. Support: tendinous arch connects rugae to pelvic fascia (weakens with age and childbirth)
   2. Hymen: fold of mucosal-covered connective tissue (fragments with sexual activity and childbirth)
   3. Blood supply
      a. Vaginal artery (from internal iliac, anterior division)
      b. Branches from internal pudendal, uterine, middle rectal arteries
      c. Likely some contribution from inferior hemorrhoidal artery
E. Uterus: lies between bladder and rectum, 6–8 cm (Figure 4.10)
   1. **Cervix and isthmus**
      a. **Cervical os (external os):** opening to uterus
      b. **Squamocolumnar junction (SCJ):** squamous epithelium → simple columnar mucinous epithelium (migrates up with age)
      c. **Endocervix:** lined by **mucinous epithelium,** it traverses lower uterine segment
      d. **Internal cervical os:** transition from mucinous to endometrioid epithelium and underlying fibrous tissue of cervix to smooth muscle of uterine body
      e. Blood supply: cervical branch of uterine artery
   2. Body of uterus
      a. Uterine **fundus:** most cephalic portion of uterus
      b. Uterine **cornu:** entry of fallopian tubes
   3. Layers
      a. **Endometrium:** columnar, **endometrioid epithelium** forming glands and underlying endometrial stroma; changes with menstrual cycle

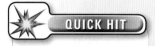

QUICK HIT

The vaginal epithelium is very responsive to estrogenic stimulation and becomes atrophic in postmenopausal women.

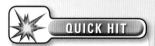

QUICK HIT

The SCJ (junction between the squamous epithelium of the cervix and the mucinous epithelium of the endocervix) is where squamous metaplasia is constantly taking place and the area most susceptible to human papillomavirus (HPV) infection and development of dysplasia.

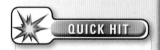

QUICK HIT

The **transformation zone (TZ)** starts at the SCJ and extends outward onto the ectocervix to the point wherever the original squamous epithelium was. As such, it represents a "concept" and is not really a geographically identifiable landmark.

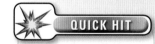

QUICK HIT

The presence of endometrial glands and stroma in the myometrium (uterine wall) is referred to as *adenomyosis.*

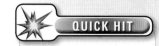

QUICK HIT

The presence of endometrial glands and stroma anywhere outside of the uterus is *endometriosis.*

Embryology and Anatomy

FIGURE
4.10   **Internal female reproductive organs.**

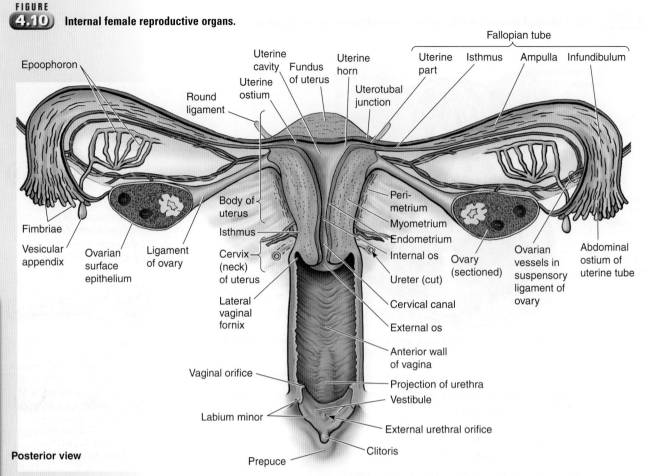

Posterior view

(From Moore KL, Dalley AF. *Clinically Oriented Anatomy*, 5th ed. Baltimore: Lippincott Williams & Wilkins; 2006: Fig. 3.39A&B.)

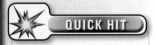

QUICK HIT

A frequent "pimp" question during a hysterectomy concerns Sampson's artery, which runs along the round ligament.

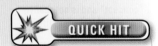

QUICK HIT

Uterine position is clinically important for the clinician to know in order to avoid perforation when performing procedures like endometrial biopsy or intrauterine device insertion.

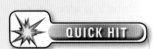

QUICK HIT

Applying traction to the cervix with an instrument called a *tenaculum*, when performing a procedure, can often straighten the axis and, to some extent, the angle.

b. **Myometrium:** smooth muscle layer; contracts with menses and childbirth
c. **Serosa** (also referred to as *perimetrium*): thin coelomic epithelial layer contiguous with peritoneum
4. Ligamentous support (see Figure 4.10)
   a. **Uterosacral ligament:** posterior lower uterine segment to sacrum
   b. **Broad ligament (cardinal ligament):** lateral uterus to pelvic sidewall and contains
      i. Uterine artery and veins
      ii. Distal ureter
   c. **Round ligament** (homolog of gubernaculum testis): arise on lateral and anterior uterine fundus and enter retroperitoneum via internal inguinal ring and attach to labia majora
   d. **Ovarian ligament:** uterine cornu to ovary
5. Uterine position (Figure 4.11)
   a. Position of uterus relative to **straight axis**
      i. **Anteverted:** most common
      ii. **Midplane**
      iii. **Retroverted:** *normal variant in 20% of women*
   b. **Angle** of cervix to uterine fundus
      i. **Anteflexed**
      ii. **Retroflexed**
6. Blood supply (Figure 4.12)
   a. **Uterine artery:** anterior division of internal iliac (hypogastric artery)—primary
      i. Runs at level of internal cervical os
      ii. Ureter is 1.5–3 cm from this location (common area of injury)
   b. **Ovarian artery**—secondary

FIGURE 4.11 Uterine position.

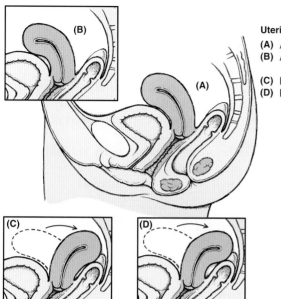

Uterine position
(A) Anteverted
(B) Anteverted and anteflexed
(C) Retroverted
(D) Retroverted and retroflexed

(A) Anteverted. **(B)** Anteverted and anteflexed. **(C)** Retroverted. **(D)** Retroverted and retroflexed. (From Neil O. Hardy, Westpoint, CT.)

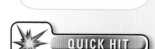

QUICK HIT

Pelvic adhesive disease (e.g., surgery, infection, endometriosis) can cause an anteverted uterus to become permanently fixed and retroverted, which can lead to chronic pain, dyspareunia, and dysmenorrhea being referred to the lower back.

QUICK HIT

Because the right gonadal vein drains obliquely into the vena cava but the left gonadal vein drains into the left renal artery at a **right angle**, a varicocele is more common on the left side in men.

QUICK HIT

Most ectopic pregnancies occur in the ampullary portion of the fallopian tube.

F. Ovary: 3–5 cm
   1. Ovarian ligament (caudal portion of ovary): attaches to uterus
   2. **Infundibulopelvic ligament** (cephalad portion of ovary; suspensory ligament)
      a. Attaches to pelvic side wall
      b. Carries ovarian artery and vein
   3. Blood supply
      a. Ovarian artery (directly from aorta)
      b. Ovarian vein
         i. Right: drains directly into inferior vena cava
         ii. Left: drains into left renal vein
      c. Branches of uterine artery and vein running in broad ligament below fallopian tube
G. Fallopian tube: 7–14 cm (see Figure 4.10)
   1. **Interstitial (cornual)**: traverses uterine cornu into endometrial cavity
   2. **Isthmus**: narrow and straight proximal portion
   3. **Ampulla**: larger diameter with numerous and complex internal plical folds

FIGURE 4.12 Relative locations of the ureter and uterine artery.

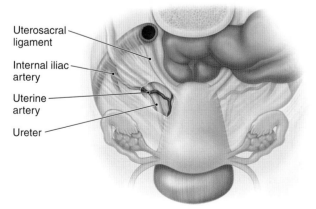

Uterosacral ligament

Internal iliac artery

Uterine artery

Ureter

During pelvic surgery, it is important to correctly identify the ureter in order to avoid injury to the uterine artery. (From Beckmann CRB, Ling FW, et al. *Obstetrics and Gynecology*, 7th ed. Baltimore: Lippincott Williams & Wilkins; 2014.)

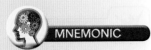

Because the ureter travels under the uterine artery, it is frequently referred to as "water under the bridge" during gynecologic surgery.

4. **Infundibulum:** distal end, fringed by fimbriae that sweep oocytes into tubal lumen
5. Ciliated, columnar epithelium of **serous type**
6. Blood supply: uterine and ovarian artery branches

H. Ureter
   1. Carries urine from kidney to bladder (see Figure 4.12)
   2. Easily injured during gynecologic surgery
   3. **Course of ureter**
      a. Crosses over bifurcation of external and internal iliac arteries
      b. Courses medially below ovarian vessels and along pelvic sidewall
      c. Enters broad ligament and courses under uterine artery (at level of internal cervical os)
      d. ~1 cm from external cervical os before coursing anteriorly to bladder
   4. Blood supply from nearby vessels

I. Blood supply of pelvis and abdominal wall (venous system follows) (Figure 4.13)
   1. **Common iliac artery**
      a. **External iliac artery** – becomes femoral artery
         i. Inferior epigastric artery
         ii. Femoral artery
         iii. Superficial epigastric artery
         iv. Superficial circumflex iliac artery
         v. External pudendal artery

FIGURE 4.13 Blood supply of the pelvis.

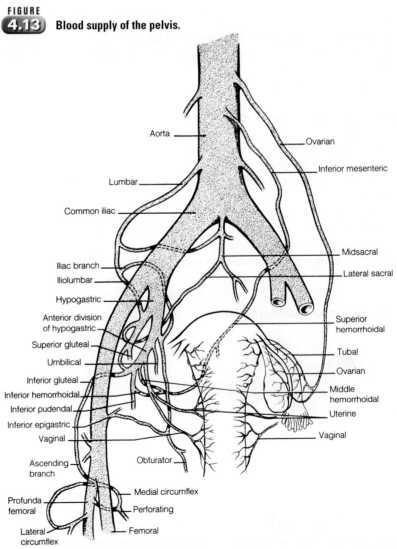

(From Rock JA, Jones HW. *TeLinde's Operative Gynecology*, 9th ed. Baltimore: Lippincott Williams & Wilkins; 2003.)

    b. **Internal iliac artery**
        i. **Anterior division**
           (a) Uterine
           (b) Superior vesicle
           (c) Vaginal
           (d) Middle rectal
           (e) Internal pudendal
           (f) Inferior gluteal
           (g) Obturator
           (h) Inferior vesicle
       ii. **Posterior division**
           (a) Iliolumbar
           (b) Lateral sacral
           (c) Superior gluteal
  2. Collaterals from inferior mesenteric artery circulation

III. Development Anomalies (see Chapter 29, which discusses congenital anomalies of the reproductive tract in detail)

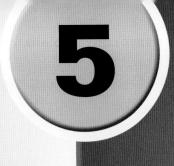

5 Reproductive Physiology

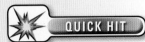

QUICK HIT

GnRH is what causes release of the "gonadotropins" luteinizing hormone (LH) and follicle-stimulating hormone (FSH) from the pituitary. Some endocrine conditions are called *hypergonadotropic* or *hypogonadotropic*; for example, menopause is called hypergonadotropic because the FSH is persistently elevated.

I. Endocrine Regulation of Female Reproduction

A. Normal reproductive function requires coordinated interaction of hypothalamus, pituitary, and ovary (Figure 5.1)

B. Hypothalamic endocrinology

1. **Gonadotropin-releasing hormone (GnRH)** is secreted in pulses (Figure 5.2) from arcuate nucleus of hypothalamus

2. Frequency of GnRH pulses regulated by steroid milieu

   a. Estrogen (E) increases pulse frequency from 1 pulse/hr in early follicular phase to 2 pulses/hr in late follicular phase

   b. Progesterone (P) decreases pulse frequency to 1 pulse/3 hr in luteal phase

FIGURE 5.1 Normal reproductive function requires coordinated interaction of the hypothalamus, pituitary, and ovaries.

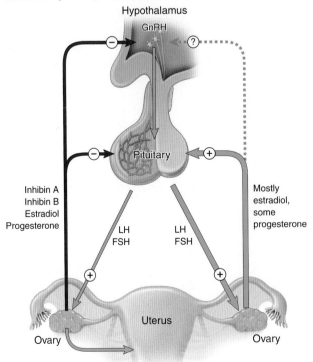

Hypothalamic gonadotropin-releasing hormone (GnRH) stimulates pituitary luteinizing hormone (LH) and follicle-stimulating hormone (FSH) secretion, which stimulates follicular growth (FSH), follicular estrogen production (LH/FSH), oocyte maturation (LH), ovulation (LH), and corpus luteum formation to produce progesterone (LH). Ovarian steroids prepare the uterine endometrium for implantation and, along with inhibins, feedback to regulate pituitary gonadotropin secretion. (From Beckmann CRB. *Obstetrics and Gynecology*, 7th ed. Baltimore: Lippincott Williams & Wilkins; 2014.)

FIGURE
5.2 GnRH secretion from the hypothalamus is pulsatile.

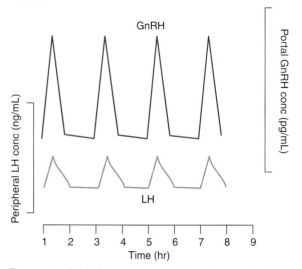

The arcuate nucleus in the hypothalamus contains a pulse generator that stimulates gonadotropin-releasing hormone (GnRH) secretion in a regular pulsatile fashion. The frequency of GnRH pulses (and, as a result, luteinizing hormone [LH] pulses) is modulated by the steroid environment. Estrogen increases and progesterone decreases the frequency of the pulse generator. Follicle-stimulating hormone (FSH) is also secreted in pulses but, because of a longer half-life and tonic (non–GnRH dependent) secretion, it is less tightly controlled by GnRH. (Modified from Rhoades & Bell, Medical Physiology: Principles for Clinical Medicine, 4th edition. Baltimore: Lippincott Williams & Wilkins, 2013.)

    c. GnRH neurons do not contain steroid receptors; therefore, estrogen and progesterone modulation of pulse frequency is via interneurons

  3. GnRH reaches pituitary via hypophyseal–portal system

  4. Short half-life of GnRH (2–4 minutes) ensures that pituitary stimulation is also pulsatile; GnRH is not measurable in peripheral circulation

  5. GnRH stimulates both **luteinizing hormone (LH)** and **follicle-stimulating hormone (FSH)** secretion from pituitary

C. Pituitary endocrinology

  1. Single-cell type (gonadotrope) secretes both LH and FSH

  2. Both gonadotropins share **common α subunit** and have **unique β subunit**

  3. LH has relatively short half-life (20 minutes) compared to FSH (3–4 hours); thus, LH in circulation is more pulsatile than FSH

  4. LH is similar to human chorionic gonadotropin (hCG) in structure and function, but hCG has much longer half-life (10–30 hours) compared to LH

  5. LH secretion almost completely regulated by GnRH; FSH secretion also has basal (autonomous) component

  6. GnRH stimulation of pituitary *must* be pulsatile in order to produce physiologic gonadotropin secretion

    a. Constant GnRH stimulation results in desensitization and down-regulation of pituitary GnRH receptors

    b. Result is decreased gonadotropin secretion

  7. GnRH analogs can stimulate or inhibit pituitary gonadotropin secretion

    a. **GnRH antagonists** (e.g., nafarelin) compete with endogenous GnRH for pituitary GnRH receptors, resulting in decreased GnRH stimulation of pituitary and therefore decreased pituitary gonadotropin secretion

    b. **GnRH agonists** (e.g., leuprolide)

      i. Initially (10–14 days) stimulate pituitary gonadotropin secretion (classic hormone agonist action)

      ii. After 10–14 days, gonadotropin secretion eventually declines as a result of down-regulation and desensitization of pituitary GnRH receptors due to constant stimulation (occupancy) of GnRH receptors by agonist (Figure 5.3)

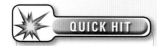

QUICK HIT

hCG is clinically used instead of LH to achieve LH-like effects (induce ovulation or follicular maturation) because it is cheaper and has a longer half-life.

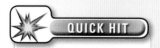

QUICK HIT

Molar pregnancies are associated with extremely high hCG levels. Again, because of the similarity to LH, the ovarian follicles in the ovaries can be overstimulated in molar pregnancies to produce enlarged bilateral theca lutein ovarian cysts up to 20 cm in size.

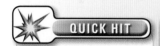

QUICK HIT

GnRH agonists and antagonists are designed with specific amino acids that resist degradation; therefore, GnRH analogs have much longer half-lives than native GnRH and will not have the physiologic pulsatile effect.

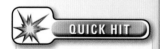

QUICK HIT

GnRH antagonists are generally used for shorter duration clinical situations because they cannot be administered orally and require at least twice-daily dosing.

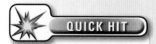

QUICK HIT

GnRH agonists are often used for long-term inhibition of LH/FSH secretion rather than GnRH antagonists because the different mechanism of action allows for less frequent administration of agonists (e.g., intramuscular [IM] every 3 months).

Reproductive Physiology

FIGURE
5.3 Gonadotropin-releasing hormone (GnRH) analogs have different mechanisms of action.

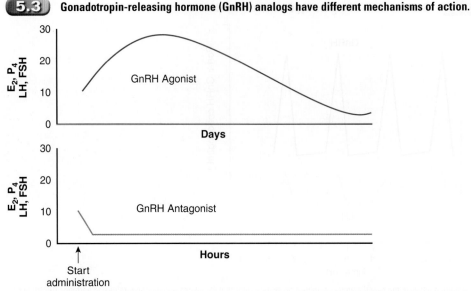

GnRH **agonists** cause a transient (few days) stimulation of pituitary gonadotropin (and therefore ovarian steroid) secretion. Due to their long action, GnRH analogs result in continued stimulation of GnRH receptors, which eventually result in desensitization and down-regulation of the receptor. As a result, gonadotropin secretion declines. In contrast, GnRH **antagonists** result in immediate inhibition (within minutes, hours) of gonadotropin secretion because they simply compete with native GnRH for its receptor.

C. Ovarian endocrinology
  1. 2 cell (granulosa and theca)/2 gonadotropin (LH and FSH) regulation of estrogen production (Figure 5.4)
  2. **Granulosa cells** also make inhibin, activin, and follistatin
    a. Inhibin regulates pituitary FSH
    b. Activin and follistatin may be more important locally in ovary
  3. Follicular estrogen and inhibin feedback to regulate pituitary FSH secretion during follicular phase
  4. After ovulation, granulosa cells become **corpus luteum**, which makes progesterone
  5. Luteal progesterone (along with estrogen and inhibin) feedback to regulate pituitary LH (and FSH) during luteal phase

II. Ovarian Structure and Function
  A. Ovary contains follicles in various stages of development (Figure 5.5 and Table 5.1)
  B. Follicle numbers decline throughout life
    1. Follicles do not get replenished or replaced
    2. At all stages of development, follicles undergo **atresia** (apoptotic process to remove growing and nongrowing follicles)
    3. Follicle numbers decline to 100,000–500,000 by puberty
    4. Very few (<0.1%) will ovulate during reproductive life span
    5. Few, if any, follicles remain at menopause
  C. **Preantral** follicular growth is slow (Figure 5.6)
    1. Primordial follicles can remain "dormant" for decades
    2. Signals for initiation of follicle growth remain poorly understood
    3. Growth from primordial to early antral follicle takes many months
    4. This stage does *not* require gonadotropin stimulation
  D. **Antral** follicle growth is very rapid
    1. Final maturation from early antral to preovulatory occurs during follicular phase of menstrual cycle; <2 weeks
    2. Requires FSH
    3. Preovulatory follicle is complex structure designed to support final oocyte maturation (Figure 5.7)

Reproductive Physiology

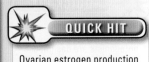

Ovarian estrogen production requires two gonadotropins (LH and FSH) and two cell types (granulosa and theca cells) working together.

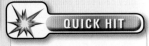

Females are born with their entire complement of primordial follicles, which is normally ~1–2 million at birth.

FIGURE
5.4 **Two-cell two-gonadotropin regulation of gonadal steroid secretion.**

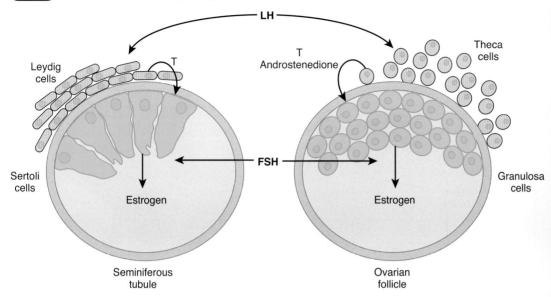

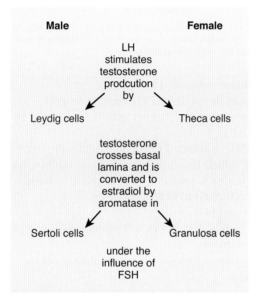

Analogous structures in male are shown for comparison.

E. Follicle growth and oocyte maturation are **dyssynchronous** (Figure 5.8)
 1. **Oocyte** begins meiosis in utero and remains arrested in 1st meiotic division until midcycle LH surge; therefore, all follicles in ovary contain *primary* oocytes
 2. Although all oocytes in ovary are exposed to midcycle elevation of LH, only oocyte in preovulatory follicle will respond by completing **meiosis I** to become secondary oocyte
 3. **Secondary oocyte** becomes arrested in **meiosis II** until fertilization

III. Menstrual Cycle Regulation *(Figure 5.9)*
 A. Initiation of menstrual flow is defined as day 1
 B. **Menstrual phase**: ~days 1–5
 1. Corpus luteum from previous cycle undergoes **luteolysis**
 a. Progesterone falls, causing endometrial destabilization and shedding
 b. 20–60 mL of blood and endometrial tissue; does not clot

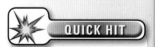

Primary oocytes are arrested in prophase of the 1st meiotic division until the midcycle elevation of LH.

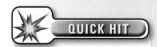

Fertility declines with aging due primarily to the fact that oocyte quality declines with age. Oocytes that are ovulated near menopause have been arrested in meiosis I for decades.

Reproductive Physiology

FIGURE 5.5 Illustration of follicular growth, ovulation, and corpus luteum formation and demise.

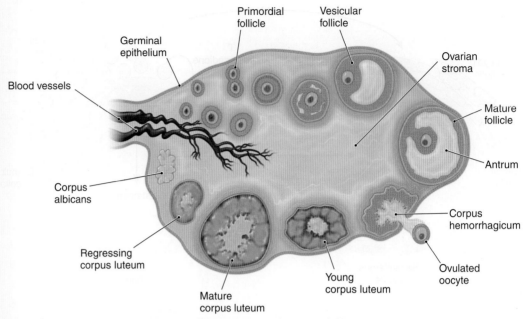

The ovary contains follicles at various stages of development and, during the luteal phase, a corpus luteum. This is a composite illustration; not all structures (e.g., preovulatory follicle, corpus luteum) are present in the ovary at the same time. (From Beckmann CRB. *Obstetrics and Gynecology*, 7th ed. Baltimore: Lippincott Williams & Wilkins; 2014.)

C. **Follicular phase**: ~days 6–14
   1. Duration can be variable (7–18 days in length)
   2. Recruitment: previously growing follicles rescued by intercycle rise in FSH (Figure 5.10)
   3. Single follicle is selected to become dominant (see Figure 5.10)
   4. Dominant follicle produces estradiol and inhibin, which suppress FSH
   5. Estrogen feedback switches from negative to positive during late follicular phase to induce **GnRH/LH/FSH surge**

D. **Ovulation**: ~day 14
   1. LH surge begins ~35 hours and peaks ~11 hours prior to ovulation
   2. LH surge induces
      a. Completion of meiosis I by preovulatory oocyte
      b. Ovulation
      c. Luteinization of remaining granulosa and thecal cells to form corpus luteum

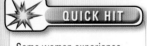

QUICK HIT

Some women experience a twinge of pain called **mittelschmerz** at the time of ovulation when the oocyte is extruded from the ovarian capsule.

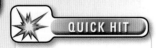

QUICK HIT

Secondary oocytes are arrested in metaphase of the 2nd meiotic division until fertilization occurs.

TABLE 5.1	Follicle Classification			
Follicle Type	**Granulosa Cells**	**Theca Cells**	**Oocyte**	**Antrum**
Primordial	Single layer Squamoid	Not present	Small No zona pellucida	Not present
Primary	Single layer Cuboidal	Not present	Larger Early zona pellucida	Not present
Secondary	Multiple layers Cuboidal	Developing	Fully grown Zona pellucida	Not present
Tertiary	Cumulus GC Mural GC	Theca interna Theca externa	Fully grown Zona pellucida	Developing
Preovulatory/ Graafian	Cumulus GC Mural GC	Theca interna Theca externa	Fully grown Zona pellucida May be secondary	Present Fully developed

GC, granulosa cell.

FIGURE 5.6 **Follicle growth is a protracted process.**

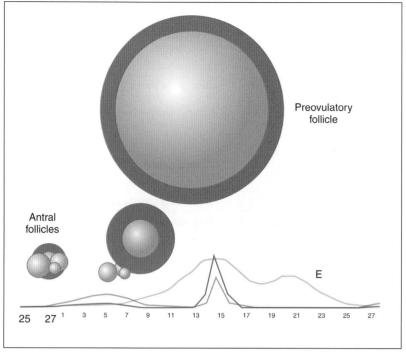

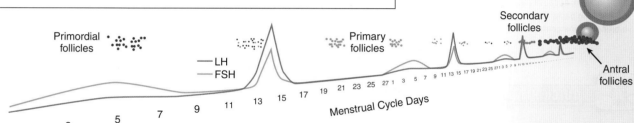

Early follicle growth (primordial → primary → secondary) takes many months and does not require gonadotropin stimulation. Once a follicle acquires an antral cavity, it becomes dependent on follicle-stimulating hormone (FSH) for continued growth and survival. The last stage of follicle growth (early antral → preovulatory) requires FSH and occurs during the follicular phase of the cycle in which the dominant follicle will ovulate.

E. **Luteal phase**: ~days 14–28
1. Duration is fairly constant: 14 days
2. **Luteinization**: formation of corpus luteum
   a. Remnant granulosa and thecal cells become granulosa-lutein and theca lutein cells
   b. Blood fills tissue: corpus luteum is also called *corpus hemorrhagicum* during 1st few days after formation
   c. Steroidogenic enzymes change to result in progesterone being primary steroid secreted; some estrogen and inhibin also produced
3. **Progesterone** prepares endometrium for implantation
4. Corpus luteum regresses at end of menstrual cycle (due to unknown mechanism) unless rescued by hCG produced by developing blastocyst
5. During pregnancy, luteal progesterone production is maintained by hCG for 7–10 weeks until placenta takes over (**luteal–placental shift**)
6. Degenerated corpus luteum called **corpus albicans**

IV. Uterine Changes Throughout Menstrual Cycle *(Figure 5.11)*
A. Uterus consists of several tissue layers
1. **Perimetrium**: outer serosal layer
2. **Myometrium**: middle thick smooth muscle layer (tunica muscularis)
   a. Estrogen stimulates and progesterone inhibits uterine myometrial contractions
   b. Prostaglandins (E_2 and $F_{2\alpha}$) also stimulate contractions

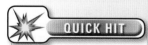

QUICK HIT

Variations in menstrual cycle length are due primarily to variation in length of *follicular phase* insofar as the *luteal phase* is constant at 14 days.

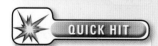

QUICK HIT

Progesterone raises basal body temperature (BBT) by 0.5°–1.0°F compared to preovulatory levels; therefore, charting BBT each morning can provide indirect evidence of ovulation.

Reproductive Physiology

FIGURE **5.7** **Mature follicle.**

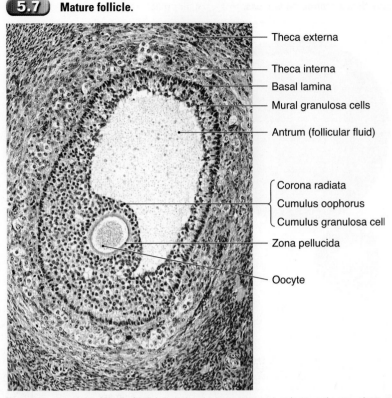

The mature, preovulatory (Graafian) follicle is designed to protect, support, and nurture the preovulatory oocyte. The oocyte sits on a stalk in a fluid-filled environment, bathed in extremely high concentration of estrogens, inhibin, and oocyte maturation inhibitor (OMI). The luteinizing hormone (LH) surge transforms the follicular (granulosa and theca) cells into progesterone-producing luteal cells, causes resumption of meiosis I by neutralizing OMI, and causes ovulation of the oocyte. (From Mills SE. *Histology for Pathologists*, 3rd ed. Philadelphia: Lippincott Williams & Wilkins; 2007.)

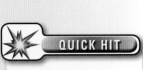

QUICK HIT

Nonsteroidal anti-inflammatory drugs can ameliorate menstrual cramps by inhibiting prostaglandin production; however, they are contraindicated for analgesia during labor for the same reason, because they can prolong parturition by inhibiting uterine contractions.

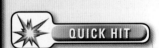

QUICK HIT

Endometrial thickness measured by ultrasound is a summation of the anterior endometrium and the posterior endometrium. Single-layer thickness can be measured by instilling saline into the endometrial cavity, with the saline creating a fluid-filled space separating the endometrial surfaces. This is called a **saline infusion sonohysterogram**.

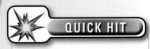

QUICK HIT

The postovulatory day of the cycle can be accurately (within 24–48 hours) determined by obtaining an endometrial biopsy during the luteal phase and examining histologic features, which is how luteal phase defects are diagnosed—mismatch with histologic cycle day compared to actual postovulatory day (see Chapter 40).

3. **Endometrium:** inner mucosal layer
   a. Layers
      i. Zona basalis: basal layer that remains intact
      ii. Zona functionalis: functional layer that changes throughout menstrual cycle in response to ovarian steroids
   b. Composition
      i. Endometrioid epithelium (glandular)
      ii. Endometrial stroma
B. Endometrium changes throughout menstrual cycle
   1. **Menstrual phase (days 1–5):** progesterone falls
      a. Endometrium very thin: 0.5–1.0 mm
      b. Arteries alternate constricting and dilating
      c. Blood escapes, pools, leads to tissue necrosis; most menstrual flow originates from venous system
   2. **Proliferative phase = follicular** phase (days 6–14): estrogen rises
      a. Endometrium rapidly growing due to estrogen
         i. Numerous mitotic figures seen on histologic section
         ii. Thickness 2–3 mm
      b. Proliferation of glands and stroma (zona functionalis)
      c. Glands are straight and lumens are narrow
   3. **Secretory phase = luteal phase** (days 14–28): progesterone dominant
      a. Endometrium has stopped proliferation; thickness is 5–6 mm
      b. Progesterone transforms proliferating endometrium into secreting endometrium in preparation for implantation
      c. Glands are sacculated and tortuous, secreting a thick mucus rich in glycoproteins to support implanting blastocyst
      d. Endometrial stroma becomes decidualized

FIGURE
5.8 Follicle growth and oocyte maturation are dyssynchronous.

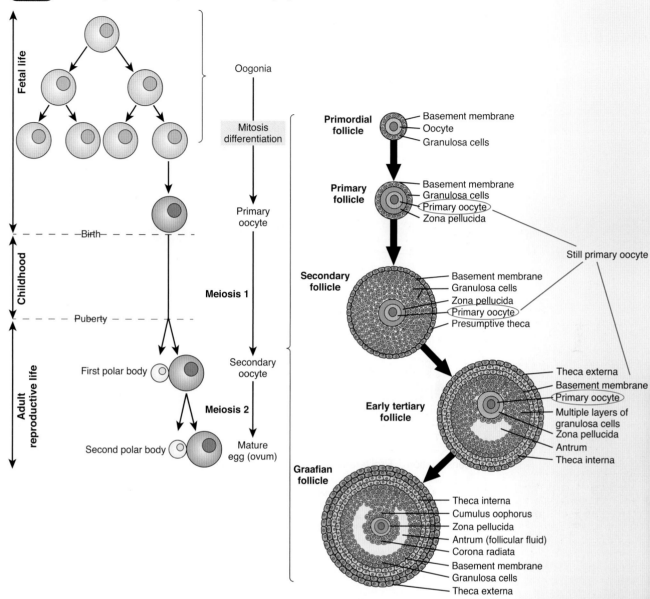

Oogonia undergo mitotic divisions during fetal life to become primary oocytes encased in primordial follicles, which populate the ovary by birth. The primary oocytes begin meiosis I and arrest in prophase. They will remain in this state until their follicle matures and becomes a preovulatory follicle. Only the oocyte in the preovulatory follicle will complete meiosis I in response to the midcycle luteinizing hormone (LH) surge. Thus, follicle growth is occurring (from primordial through preovulatory) while oocyte maturation has halted. (Modified from Rhoades & Bell, Medical Physiology: Principles for Clinical Medicine, 4th edition. Baltimore: Lippincott Williams & Wilkins, 2013.)

V. Endocrine Effects on Other Reproductive Tissues

A. Oviduct
1. Estrogen stimulates oviductal secretions and ciliogenesis
2. Progesterone counteracts estrogen action in oviduct (and many other reproductive tissues)

B. Vagina
1. Estrogen stimulates vaginal epithelium and glycogen production
2. Estrogen increases vaginal lubrication, which facilitates intercourse

C. Cervix/endocervix
1. Endocervical glands secrete mucus in response to estrogen and progesterone
   a. Estrogen causes cervical secretions to be thin, watery, and abundant
      i. Production is maximal at ovulation
      ii. Facilitates sperm penetration through cervix and uterus to aid sperm transport to oviduct for fertilization of ovum

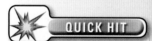

QUICK HIT

One mechanism of action of continuous progesterone contraceptives and combination oral contraceptives is progesterone's effects on tubal motility and cervical mucus.

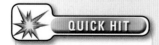

QUICK HIT

A common complaint of postmenopausal women is vaginal dryness, which results from decreased estrogen production by the ovaries.

FIGURE
5.9   **Menstrual cycle.**

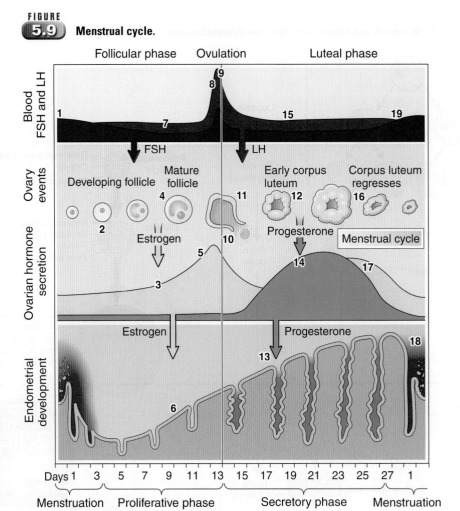

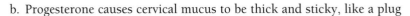

1. Follicle-stimulating hormone (FSH) + luteinizing hormone (LH) ↑. *2.* Multiple early antral follicles grow and make estrogen (E). *3.* Serum E ↑. *4.* One follicle becomes dominant. *5.* Serum E ↑↑↑. *6.* E stimulates endometrial proliferation. *7.* FSH ↓ due to (−) feedback of E + inhibin. *8.* E feedback switches from (−) to (+). *9.* LH surge is triggered. *10.* Oocyte completes 1st meiotic division. *11.* Ovulation occurs. *12.* Corpus luteum (CL) forms and makes progesterone (P) and some E. *13.* P transforms proliferative to secretory endometrium. *14.* Serum P ↑↑↑ and inhibin ↑. *15.* FSH and LH are inhibited. *16.* CL begins to regress (cause unknown). *17.* Serum P and E fall. *18.* Endometrium destabilizes and sloughs. *19.* FSH + LH ↑. (Modified with permission from McConnell TH. *The Nature of Disease Pathology for the Health Professions*. Philadelphia: Lippincott Williams & Wilkins; 2007.)

    b. Progesterone causes cervical mucus to be thick and sticky, like a plug
       i. Production decreases during luteal phase
       ii. Inhibits bacteria from entering uterus, thereby protecting developing embryo
       iii. Inhibits sperm penetration
    c. Ovulatory mucus: at transition from copious, watery mucus of proliferative phase to thick mucus of luteal phase, mucus becomes more viscous and "stringy"

D. Breast
    1. Estrogen stimulates breast growth at puberty and during pregnancy
    2. Changes during menstrual cycle are due to cyclical progesterone; breast tenderness increases during luteal phase and nearing menstruation
    3. Elevated progesterone during pregnancy inhibits lactation; fall in placental steroids at parturition allows lactation to commence

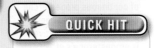

QUICK HIT

The stretchability of cervical mucus is called **spinnbarkeit**. Just before ovulation, it is maximal at 8–10 cm, and this is the basis for the natural, or rhythm, method of contraception.

FIGURE
5.10 Follicle recruitment and selection.

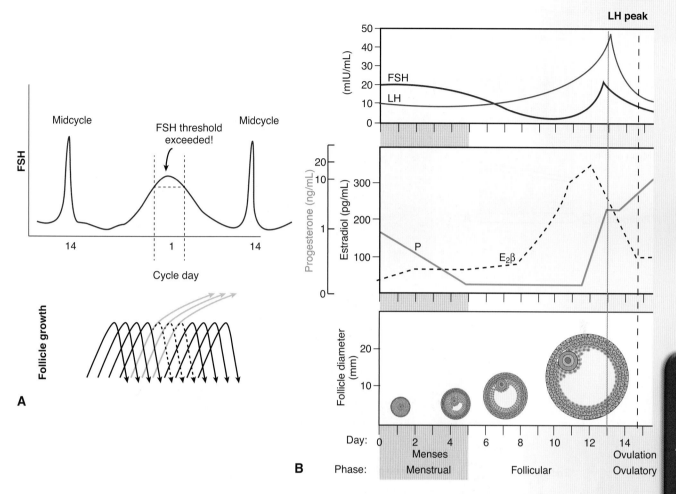

Follicle Recruitment

(A) Follicles start growing every day beginning at birth. Once a follicle acquires an antrum, it becomes dependent on follicle-stimulating hormone (FSH) for survival. Those follicles (the cohort) that acquire an antrum when FSH is high enough (during the intercycle rise in FSH) can continue to grow (they become recruited). From this cohort, one follicle will be selected and become the dominant follicle. The remaining follicles in the cohort will undergo atresia.

How Is the Dominant Follicle Selected?

(B) Follicles are selected based on these criteria: enhanced vascularity, increased number of FSH receptors, and enhanced cyclic adenosine monophosphate (cAMP) responsiveness to utilize FSH, all which increase ability to utilize FSH. Estradiol and inhibin feedback to reduce FSH. Selected follicle can survive declining FSH levels; others in the cohort cannot. (Modified from Rhoades & Bell, Medical Physiology: Principles for Clinical Medicine, 4th edition. Baltimore: Lippincott Williams & Wilkins, 2013.)

FIGURE 5.11 Uterine changes throughout the menstrual cycle.

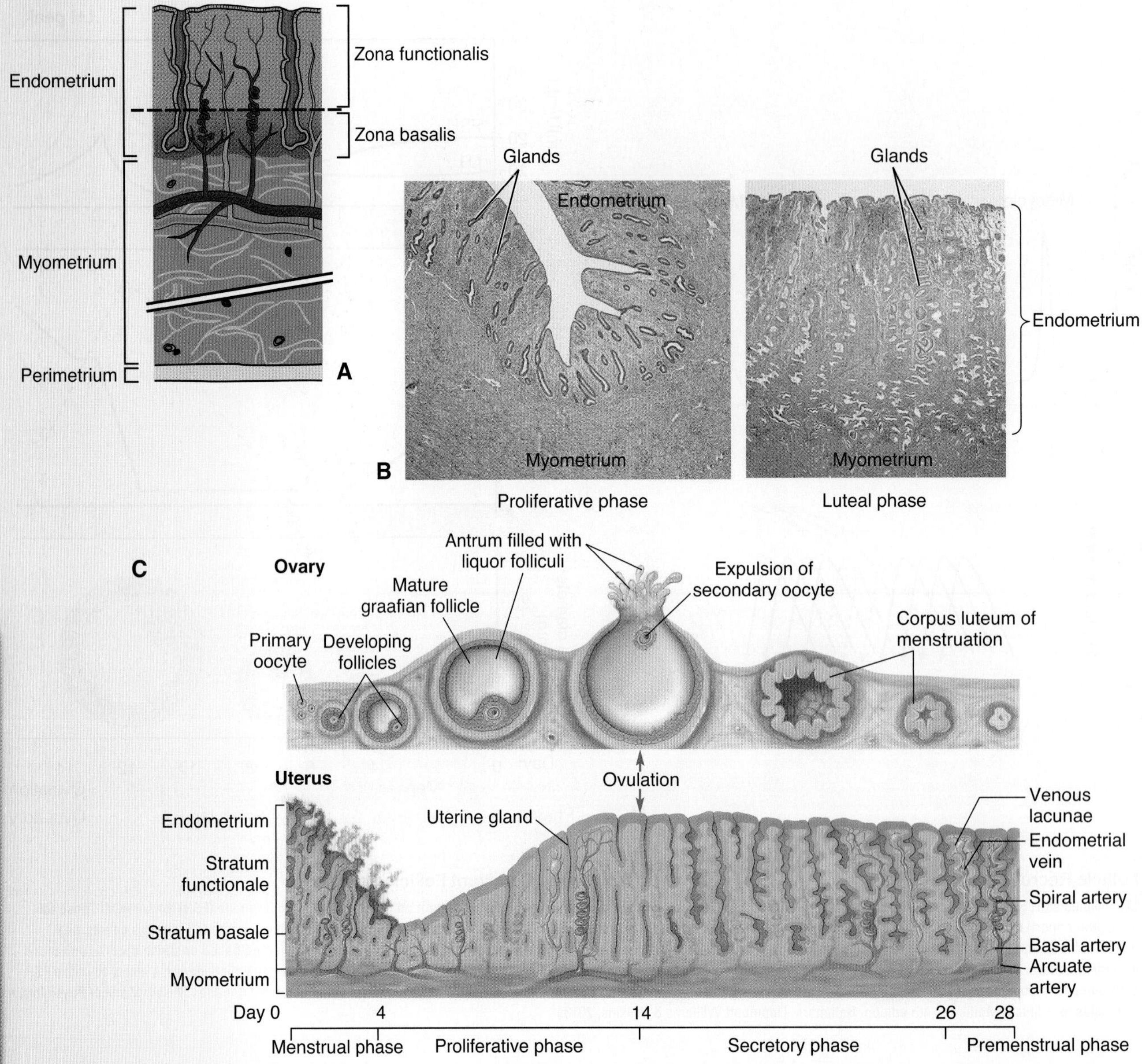

(A) Of the three layers in the uterus, only the endometrial layer (B) changes morphology throughout the menstrual cycle in response to ovarian steroids. (C) In the endometrium, the basal layer remains intact and the functional layer proliferates in response to estrogen, secretes glycoproteins in response to progesterone, and sloughs at the end of the menstrual cycle when progesterone falls. (Used with permission from A and C, Anatomical Chart Co. B, Mills SE. *Histology for Pathologists*, 3rd ed. Philadelphia: Lippincott Williams & Wilkins; 2007.)

Obstetrics

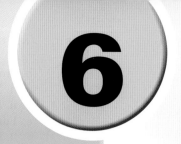

Endocrinology of Pregnancy

I. Fetal–Maternal–Placental Unit

A. Fetal component: **adrenal gland** = major endocrine gland of fetus
   1. Cortex
      a. Outer definitive (adult) zone
         i. Becomes zona fasciculata, glomerulosa, and reticularis in adult
         ii. Secretes glucocorticoids and mineralocorticoids in fetus
      b. Inner (fetal) zone
         i. Secretes androgens during fetal life
         ii. Involutes at delivery; disappears by 1 year of life
   2. Medulla: synthesizes and stores catecholamines

B. Placental component: produces steroid and peptide hormones
   1. Maternal circulation precursors → converted to progesterone
   2. Fetal androgens: precursors for estrogen production
      a. Lack 17α-hydroxylase
      b. Unable to convert progesterone to estrogen

C. Maternal component
   1. Ovary: major producer of **progesterone** in early pregnancy (up to 8 weeks)
   2. Hypothalamus and posterior pituitary: produce and release **oxytocin**
      a. Responsible for uterine contractions
      b. Source of milk letdown
   3. Anterior pituitary: produces prolactin (responsible for milk production)

II. Pregnancy Hormones

A. Peptide hormones
   1. **Human chorionic gonadotropin (hCG)**
      a. Structure
         i. α Subunit: shared with luteinizing hormone (LH) and thyroid-stimulating hormone (TSH)
         ii. β Subunit: specific and unique
      b. Detection
         i. Increases 8 days after ovulation if pregnancy occurs
         ii. Detectable in urine and serum (basis of pregnancy tests)
         iii. hCG values peak at 60–90 days of pregnancy; declines to steady state at 15 weeks' gestation
         iv. Presence of hCG in nonpregnant state: hydatidiform mole, choriocarcinoma, embryonal carcinoma
         v. Function of hCG in pregnancy
            (a) Maintains corpus luteum in first 8 weeks of pregnancy, which ensures progesterone until production shifted to placenta
            (b) Weak stimulating effect on thyroid (similar α subunit)
   2. Human placental lactogen
      a. Structure: single-chain polypeptide; resembles prolactin and pituitary growth hormone in structure

    b. Produced by placenta
      i. Serum levels increased during pregnancy with increasing placental weight
      ii. Low values noted in threatened abortion and growth restriction
    c. Functions as insulin antagonist
      i. Decreases maternal glucose utilization, thereby ensuring available glucose for the fetus
      ii. May be a cause of increased insulin resistance and diabetes in later gestation
  3. Corticotropin-releasing hormone (CRH)
    a. Produced by placenta
    b. Stimulates fetal adrenocorticotropic hormone (ACTH) production → fetal adrenal production of dehydroepiandrosterone sulfate (DHEA-S) → precursor for placental estrogen production
    c. As gestation age increases, fetal cortisol production stimulates placental CRH production (positive feedback loop); important role in activation and amplification of labor
  4. Prolactin
    a. Produced by anterior pituitary; increases during pregnancy due to estrogen stimulation of pituitary lactotrophs
    b. Stimulates postpartum milk production
B. Steroid hormones
  1. Progesterone: most important progestational hormone
    a. Production
      i. Corpus luteum: up to 6–8 weeks of gestation
      ii. Placenta: beyond 8 weeks' gestation; uses cholesterol precursors from maternal circulation (Figure 6.1)
    b. Function
      i. Promotes uterine quiescence
        (a) Suppresses placental CRH
        (b) Inhibits cytokines and prostaglandins
        (c) Prevents uterine contractions
      ii. May be important in establishing immune tolerance to products of conception
  2. Estrogen
    a. Production (Figure 6.2)
      i. Requires interaction of fetal DHEA-S, maternal (cholesterol) and placental (conversion to estrogen) units; placenta lacks all the necessary enzymes to synthesize estrogens directly
      ii. Estriol (E_3)
        (a) 90% of placental E_3 production is dependent on fetal precursors
        (b) Maternal serum E_3 concentrations thought by some to be index of fetal well-being
    b. Function
      i. Implicated in increasing myometrial contractions and excitability
      ii. May cause cervical ripening prior to onset of labor
  3. Androgens
    a. Production
      i. Fetal zone of adrenal cortex
        (a) Predominantly DHEA
        (b) Stimulated by ACTH and hCG (early pregnancy)
      ii. Fetal testis; predominantly testosterone converted in target cells to dihydrotestosterone (DHT)
    b. Function
      i. DHEA: precursor for estradiol (E_2) and E_3 production
      ii. Testosterone: development and differentiation of male external genitalia
  4. Glucocorticoids (cortisol)
    a. Production
      i. Outer definitive (adult) zone of the adrenal cortex
      ii. Placental CRH → fetal pituitary ACTH → fetal adrenal cortisol → placental CRH

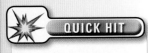

QUICK HIT

If surgical removal of the corpus luteum is needed prior to 7 weeks, progesterone supplementation is required.

QUICK HIT

E_3 is the most abundant estrogen in human pregnancy.

FIGURE 6.1 **Adrenal steroid biosynthetic pathway.**

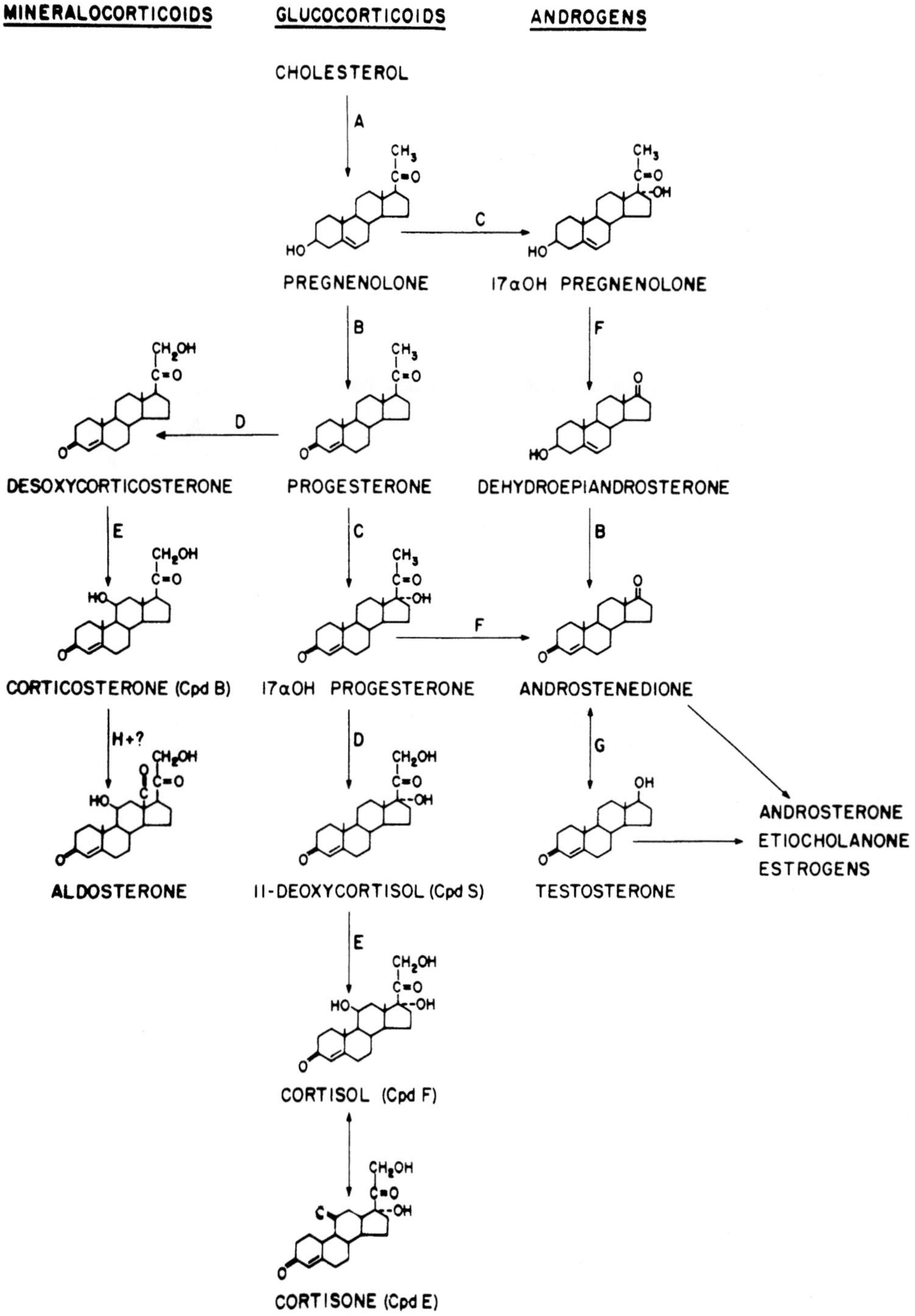

The classic enzyme terminology is represented by the alphabetical letters with the appropriate cytochrome P450 oxidases in parentheses. *A*, 20, 22-desmolase (P450scc); *B*, 3β-hydroxysteroid dehydrogenase: *C*, 17α-hydroxylase (P450c17); *D*, 21-hydroxylase (P450c21); *E*, 11-hydroxylase (P450c11); *F*, 17, 20-lyase (P450c17); *G*, 17-keto reductase; *H+*, 18-hydroxylase +18-oxidase (P450c11). (From MacDonald MG, Seshia MMK, et al. *Avery's Neonatology Pathophysiology & Management of the Newborn*, 6th ed. Philadelphia: Lippincott Williams & Wilkins; 2005.)

  b. Function
     i. Promotes differentiation of type II alveolar cells → synthesis and release of surfactant into the alveoli
     ii. Activation of labor (see below); increases release of placental CRH and prostaglandins

FIGURE
6.2 Placental estrogen synthesis from fetal and maternal precursors.

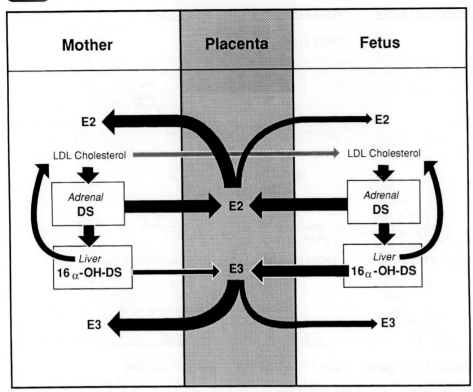

After 20 weeks of gestation, the fetal compartment supplies most steroid precursors for placental estrogen production. The fetal adrenal uses low-density lipoprotein cholesterol, produced by the fetal liver or transferred from the maternal compartment, to synthesize dehydroepiandrosterone sulfate (DS). DS is converted to 16α-OH-DS in the fetal liver. DS and 16α-OH-DS undergo placental metabolism to estradiol (E_2) and estriol (E_3), respectively, which are released predominantly on the maternal side. (From MacDonald MG, Seshia MMK, et al. *Avery's Neonatology Pathophysiology & Management of the Newborn*, 6th ed. Philadelphia: Lippincott Williams & Wilkins; 2005.)

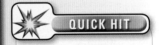
QUICK HIT

Interestingly, impairment of oxytocin production (diabetes insipidus) does not interfere with labor.

5. Additional hormones and transmitters
   a. Oxytocin
      i. Produced in the supraoptic and paraventricular nuclei of hypothalamus → migrates to posterior pituitary where it is released in response to birth canal distention and mammary stimulation
      ii. Function
         (a) Causes uterine contractions
         (b) Causes milk letdown in response to mammary stimulation
   b. Relaxin
      i. Produced in ovary; peak concentration in maternal circulation at 10 weeks' gestation
      ii. Functions as an angiogenic peptide
         (a) Facilitates implantation of embryo
         (b) Associated with cervical softening in pregnancy
   c. Prostaglandins and leukotrienes (PGE_2, $PGF_{2\alpha}$, thromboxane A2)
      i. Biologically active *lipids*, not hormones
      ii. Synthesized in endometrium, myometrium, fetal membranes, decidua, and placenta
         (a) Phospholipase A2 hydrolyzes glycerophospholipids in trophoblastic membrane → arachidonic acid
         (b) Cyclooxygenase 2 (COX2) expressed in the amnion (increases with gestational age) metabolize arachidonic acid to prostaglandins
         (c) Lipoxygenase metabolize arachidonic acid to leukotrienes

iii. Function
   (a) PGE_2 and $PGF_{2\alpha}$ cause uterine and smooth muscle contractions
      (i) PGE_2 (cervical ripening); $PGF_{2\alpha}$ (uterine contractions)
      (ii) When used pharmacologically may cause nausea, vomiting, diarrhea
      (iii) Can be used pharmacologically as induction agents, abortifacients, or in treatment of postpartum hemorrhage
   (b) Phospholipase A2 activity
      (i) May lead to premature labor
      (ii) Increased in setting of infections (uterine, cervical, urinary tract)

III. Maternal Metabolism

A. Angiotensin–aldosterone system
   1. Aldosterone production
      a. Mineralocorticoid synthesized in the zona glomerulosa of adrenal cortex
         i. Renin (kidney) converts angiotensinogen to angiotensin I, which is further metabolized to angiotensin II (angiotensin-converting enzyme)
         ii. Angiotensin II stimulates aldosterone production
      b. Main source in pregnancy is maternal adrenal gland
      c. Aldosterone secretion decreased in patients with preeclampsia
   2. Function
      a. Stimulates absorption of sodium and secretion of potassium in the distal tubule of kidney; maintains electrolyte balance
      b. Increase in pregnancy likely due to estrogen and progesterone stimulation of renin
B. Calcium metabolism
   1. Absorption increased in pregnancy
   2. Total serum calcium declines due to decline of serum albumin (of which 50% of total calcium is bound)
   3. Free (ionized) calcium remains stable throughout pregnancy due to increased maternal production of parathyroid hormone (PTH)
   4. Fetal calcium metabolism
      i. Late pregnancy maternal PTH enhances maternal intestinal absorption of calcium and bone resorption and decreases urinary calcium excretion
         (a) Coincides with maximal fetal skeletal calcification
         (b) Calcium ions actively transported across placenta to facilitate this process and results in increased fetal serum calcium
            (i) Results in fetal parathyroid suppression
            (ii) Results in increased calcitonin production → improved calcium for calcification of skeleton
      ii. Postpartum fetal serum calcium declines while serum phosphorous concentration rises → both normalize to adult levels within 1 week

IV. Parturition (Childbirth)

A. Hormonal regulation
   1. ACTH → adrenal gland → cortisol → placenta → increased estrogen and decreased progesterone
   2. Increased estrogen-to-progesterone ratio leads to
      a. Increased prostaglandins
      b. Myometrial gap junction formation
      c. Cervical ripening
      d. Onset of labor
B. Myometrial contractions
   1. Smooth muscle contraction triggered by hormonal stimuli
   2. Oxytocin and prostaglandins bind receptors → activation of phospholipase C → hydrolyzes phospholipids → release of calcium from sarcoplasmic reticulum
   3. Contractions spread as current flows from cell to cell via gap junctions; estradiol and prostaglandins increase gap junctions at parturition

Endocrinology of Pregnancy

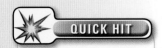

C. Phases of parturition
1. Phase 0: quiescence; maintained by progesterone
2. Phase 1: activation; signaled by
   a. Myometrial stretch from growing fetus
   b. Fetal hypothalamic–pituitary–adrenal axis (HPA) signals fetal maturation
3. Phase 2: stimulation
   a. Increase in estrogen at end of pregnancy
      i. Placental CRH promotes fetal cortisol and DHEA-S production
      ii. Adrenal androgens (DHEA-S) precursor for placental estrogen production
      iii. Increased presence of estrogen-dependent receptors: oxytocin receptors, prostaglandin receptors, and COX
   b. Alterations in progesterone receptors may result in functional progesterone withdrawal
   c. Leads to cascade of biological processes of parturition
      i. Cervical ripening
      ii. Uterine contractions
      iii. Decidual/fetal membrane activation
4. Phase 3: involution; expulsion of fetus → increase in oxytocin's effect
   a. Facilitates placental separation and delivery
   b. Continued uterine contractions prevent bleeding from large venous sinuses in exposed placental bed
   c. Uterine involution: process by which uterus returns to prepregnant size (completed by 6 weeks' postpartum)

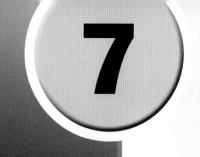

Maternal–Fetal Physiology

I. Maternal Physiology

A. Cardiovascular system
1. Earliest and most dramatic changes
2. Goal to ↑ fetal oxygenation/nutrition
3. Anatomy
    a. Enlarging uterus elevates diaphragm, displaces heart upward and laterally (Figure 7.1)
    b. Increase in myocardial mass (left ventricle and left atrium)
4. Function
    a. Blood volume begins increasing by 6–8 weeks' gestational age; peaks at 32 weeks' gestation, 45% above nonpregnant volume
    b. Cardiac output (CO) ↑ 30%–50% above nonpregnant state
    c. By 8 weeks' gestation, CO already increased by 15%–25%
    d. CO can decrease in late pregnancy due to compression of inferior vena cava (IVC) by gravid uterus
    e. Decrease in systemic vascular resistance (SVR)
    f. Pulse increases as pregnancy advances by 10–18 beats/min above baseline
    g. Labor can ↑ CO by 40% above pregnant state, likely due to pain

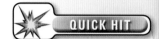

QUICK HIT

Among pregnant women, 10% will become dizzy or light-headed when suddenly standing after lying supine. This is called *IVC syndrome* and is due to decreased venous return.

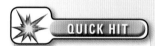

QUICK HIT

The uterus receives 20% of CO at term versus 2% in the 1st trimester.

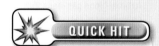

QUICK HIT

Blood pressure begins decreasing by 7 weeks, reaches the nadir (10 mm Hg) at 24–32 weeks, and increases to nonpregnant values at term.

FIGURE 7.1 Changes in the outline of the heart, lungs, and thoracic cage.

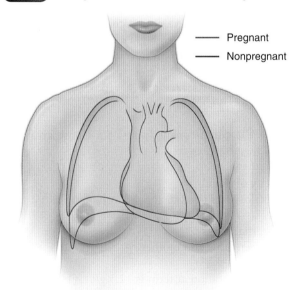

Pregnant

Nonpregnant

(Adapted from Bonica JJ, McDonald JS, eds. *Principles and Practice of Obstetric Analgesia and Anesthesia*, 2nd ed. Baltimore: Williams & Wilkins; 1995:47, Fig. 2.)

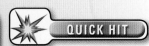

Maternal–Fetal Physiology

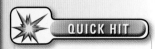
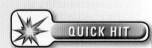
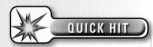
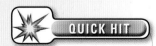
    h. CO ↑ 60%–80% within 10–15 minutes following delivery
      i. Release of vena cava compression
      ii. Autotransfusion of uteroplacental blood
      iii. Rapid mobilization of extravascular fluid
  5. Physical exam changes
    a. Low-grade systolic ejection murmur due to increased turbulence of expanded blood volume
    b. Distended neck veins
    c. Increased 2nd heart sound split with inspiration
    d. S_3 gallop commonly heard after mid-pregnancy
    e. Changes in diagnostic tests
      i. Chest X-ray: cardiac silhouette appears enlarged; may be mislabeled as "cardiomegaly"
      ii. electrocardiogram (EKG): slight left-axis deviation is common

B. Respiratory system
  1. Anatomy
    a. Diaphragm elevates 4 cm in late pregnancy
    b. Chest diameter and circumference widen
  2. Function
    a. 20% greater O_2 consumption above nonpregnant state
    b. 20% reduction in residual volume and functional residual capacity of lungs
    c. Increase in minute ventilation and tidal volume
      i. Reduction in PCO_2 → respiratory alkalosis
      ii. Renal compensation (loss of bicarbonate) maintains maternal pH
  3. Symptoms: dyspnea
    a. Physiologic response to low arterial PCO_2
    b. Mucosal hyperemia, nasal stuffiness, and nose bleeds common
  4. Physical exam changes: none
  5. Diagnostic test changes
    a. PCO_2 27–32 mm Hg and bicarbonate of 18–31 mEq/L are normal
    b. Chest X-ray: may demonstrate prominent pulmonary vasculature

C. Hematologic system
  1. Anatomic changes
    a. Marked ↑ in plasma volume, red cell mass, and coagulation factors
    b. Plasma volume ↑ 50% in singletons, more in multiple gestations
    c. ↑ Red cell mass, relatively less than plasma volume (**physiologic anemia**)
    d. At term, maternal blood volume is 35% above nonpregnant state
    e. White blood cell (WBC) count ↑ slightly (even higher during labor)
    f. Platelets decrease slightly but should remain in normal nonpregnant range
    g. 50% ↑ in fibrinogen; fibrin split products; factors VII, VIII, IX, and X
    h. No change in prothrombin, factors V and XII
    i. Proteins C and S decrease
    j. Risk for thromboembolism is ↑ 2× in pregnancy and ↑ 5.5× postpartum with *increased risk lasting at least 6 weeks*
  2. Functional changes
    a. Increased O_2-carrying capacity of blood
    b. Compensated respiratory alkalosis shifts oxyhemoglobin-binding curve to left
      i. Greater O_2 affinity in maternal lungs
      ii. Greater CO_2 gradient between fetus and mother
  3. Diagnostic test changes
    a. Average hemoglobin (Hgb) concentration at term is 12.5 g/dL (14 g/dL in nonpregnant state)
    b. Iron-deficiency anemia is common, with highest frequency among pregnant teens

   c. WBC count from 5,000 to 12,000 can be normal (up to 30,000 in labor)

   d. Fibrinogen ↑ to 300–600 mg/dL (200–400 mg/dL in nonpregnant state)

   e. *No change* in clotting times

D. Renal system

  1. Anatomy

    a. Kidneys lengthen by 1 cm

    b. Renal calices, pelvis, and ureters dilate due to mechanical compression and hormones; imaging of collective system resembles hydronephrosis

    c. Right ureter usually more dilated than left; due to compression by gravid uterus and ovarian venous plexus

  2. Functional changes

    a. Drastic ↑ in renal plasma flow and glomerular filtration rate (GFR)

     i. Glomerular filtration rate (GFR) ↑ by 50% at term

     ii. Renal plasma flow can be 75% greater than nonpregnant state

     iii. Common to see trace or 1+ glucose on urine dip due to increased GFR

    b. ↑ All components of renin (↑ 10×)–angiotensin (↑ 5×)–aldosterone system; women with hypertensive disease more vulnerable

  3. Symptoms

    a. Urinary frequency: due to mass effect of gravid uterus

    b. Stress incontinence: 20% of women

    c. Infection: urinary stasis in collecting system leads to increased frequency of pyelonephritis (especially among women with asymptomatic bacteriuria)

  4. Laboratory changes

    a. Decrease in blood urea nitrogen (BUN) by 25% (8–10 mg/dL)

    b. Creatinine ↓ 0.5–0.6 mg/dL at term (0.8 mg/dL in nonpregnant women)

    c. Creatinine clearance ↑ by 30%

E. Gastrointestinal (GI) system

  1. Anatomy

    a. Mass effect from enlarging uterus displaces stomach and intestines

    b. No change in liver or biliary tract size

    c. Portal vein enlarges due to ↑ blood flow

  2. Functional changes

    a. ↓ Intestinal motility → constipation

    b. ↓ Lower esophageal sphincter tone → reflux

    c. ↓ Gallbladder contractility → gallstones and cholestasis

  3. Symptoms

    a. Nausea and vomiting

     i. Typically begins around 4–8 weeks' gestational age

     ii. May be due to ↑ human chorionic gonadotropin (hCG), ↑ progesterone, and smooth muscle relaxation in stomach

     iii. Severe nausea/vomiting (hyperemesis gravidarum) → weight loss, electrolyte imbalance, ketonemia

    b. Ptyalism

     i. Perception of excessive salivation

     ii. Likely represents inability to swallow saliva when nauseated

    c. Food craving/aversion

     i. Pica: intense craving for foods or nonfoods (e.g., clay)

     ii. Development of aversion to particular food odor or texture

    d. Gastroesophageal reflux: worsens as pregnancy advances

    e. Constipation

     i. Mechanical obstruction of colon by enlarging uterus

     ii. ↓ Intestinal motility

     iii. Increased water absorption from GI tract

    f. Itching/generalized pruritus

     i. Intrahepatic cholestasis of pregnancy, elevated bile acid concentrations

     ii. Associated with increased risk of stillbirth at term

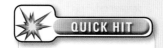

QUICK HIT

Progesterone causes smooth muscle relaxation in the GI system.

4. Physical exam changes
   a. Hemorrhoids: due to constipation, mass effect of enlarging uterus, and increased venous blood flow
   b. Gingival disease: edematous gums bleed more easily with brushing
5. Laboratory changes
   a. ↑ Alkaline phosphatase (ALP): due to placental production of ALP
   b. ↑ Serum cholesterol levels
   c. ↓ Serum albumin: hemodilution effect
   d. *No* changes to alanine aminotransferase, aspartate aminotransferase, amylase, lipase, γ-glutamyl transpeptidase
F. Endocrine system
   1. Anatomy
      a. Enlargement of thyroid gland
      b. No change in size of adrenal glands
   2. Functional changes
      a. hCG stimulates thyroid, causes transient rise in free thyroxine (T_4) in early pregnancy
      b. ↑ Serum cortisol, free cortisol, and serum aldosterone
      c. ↓ Dehydroepiandrosterone (DHEA) due to increased hepatic metabolism, conversion to estrogen
      d. ↑ Insulin resistance, possibly due to human placental lactogen's (hPL's) insulin antagonism
         i. Glycogen synthesis and storage increased, gluconeogenesis inhibited
         ii. **Postprandial hyperglycemia** (diabetogenic effect of pregnancy)
         iii. Glucose transfer to fetus/placenta via facilitated diffusion
         iv. Prolonged fasting → hypoglycemia
      e. ↑ Lipids, lipoproteins, apolipoproteins: fat stored centrally in early pregnancy
      f. No change in ionized calcium, decrease in total calcium
         i. ↑ in parathyroid hormone (PTH) leads to ↑ absorption of calcium from GI tract and ↓ renal loss of calcium
         ii. Allows for mobilization of calcium for fetal skeleton development
G. Musculoskeletal system
   1. Lumbar lordosis (anterior convexity of lower spine)
      a. Maintains center of gravity as uterus grows
      b. High frequency of low back pain
   2. Exacerbation of hernia defects (e.g., umbilical hernias)
   3. Separation of pubic symphysis
      a. Typically occurs at 28–30 weeks, mediated by relaxin
      b. Can have unsteady gait, ↑ frequency of falls
H. Skin/integument
   1. Anatomy
      a. ↑ Estrogen and progesterone cause skin changes
         i. Vascular spiders (spider angiomata) on upper torso, face, arms
         ii. Palmar erythema, present in 50% of patients
      b. Striae gravidarum >50% of patients
         i. Occur on lower abdomen, breasts, thighs
         ii. Appear pink/purple, eventually turn pale
         iii. No effective preventive therapy; cannot be eliminated
      c. Hyperpigmentation
         i. Occurs on any skin surface; commonly involves umbilicus, perineum, face (melasma), and lower abdomen (linea nigra)
         ii. Nevi can increase in size, resolve postpartum
      d. Hair changes
         i. Number of hairs in anagen (growth) phase increases
         ii. Postpartum number of hairs in telogen (resting) phase increases
            (a) Can lead to significant hair loss at 2–4 months' postpartum
            (b) Normalizes by 6–12 months' postpartum

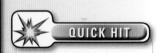

QUICK HIT

Increased thyroxine-binding globulin (TBG) causes increases in total T_4 and total T_3.

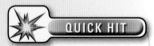

QUICK HIT

Increased lipolysis in later pregnancy provides energy during fasting periods (called *accelerated starvation of pregnancy*).

I. Reproductive tract
  1. Anatomic/functional changes
    a. Uterus
      i. Increases in size from 70 g (nonpregnant) to 1,100 g at term due to hypertrophy of myometrium
      ii. Uterine cavity accommodates up to 5 L (nonpregnant = <10 mL)
    b. Vagina: ↑ blood flow
    c. Vulva: may develop venous varicosities (typically resolve postpartum)
J. Breasts
  1. Anatomy
    a. ↑ Size over course of pregnancy
      i. Rapidly over the first 8 weeks, steadily thereafter
      ii. Total enlargement is usually 25%–50%
      iii. Nipples increase in size and pigmentation
    b. ↑ Blood flow to support lactation
  2. Functional changes
    a. Estrogen → ductal growth
    b. Progesterone → alveolar hypertrophy
    c. Colostrum: thick yellow fluid expressed from nipples in late pregnancy
    d. Lactation dependent on interplay of estrogen, progesterone, prolactin, hPL, cortisol, and insulin
K. Ophthalmic: corneal changes related to increased thickness result in blurry vision, which regresses by 8 weeks' postpartum

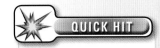

QUICK HIT

Increased blood flow leads to an increase in transudative fluid to the vagina, which, in turn, leads to physiologic discharge **(leukorrhea)** of pregnancy.

II. Fetus and Placenta

A. Placenta
  1. Unique organ of pregnancy
    a. Key role in respiratory and metabolite exchange for fetus
    b. Produces estrogen, progesterone, hCG, hPL; necessary for pregnancy, labor and delivery, and lactation
    c. Maternal fetal transfer of solutes dependent on size, ionization, and lipid solubility
  2. Gas exchange
    a. Fetal O_2 uptake and CO_2 excretion depend on uterine/placental blood flow
    b. Require adequate maternal and fetal blood-carrying capacity
  3. Metabolism
    a. Glucose
      i. Primary metabolic substrate for placenta
      ii. ~70% of glucose transferred from mother is used by placenta
      iii. Crosses via facilitated diffusion
    b. Amino acids
      i. Actively transported to fetus
      ii. Higher levels in fetus than mother
    c. Free fatty acids
      i. Limited transport to fetus
      ii. Lower levels than mother
B. Fetal circulation: oxygenated blood passes from placenta → umbilical vein → fetus (Figure 7.2)
  1. 50% of umbilical venous blood bypasses liver → ductus venosus → IVC → right atrium → across foramen ovale → left atrium → left ventricle → ascending aorta
  2. Other 50% of umbilical venous blood → portal veins → hepatic circulation → hepatic veins → IVC
  3. Blood from superior vena cava (SVC) → right atrium → right ventricle → pulmonary artery → ductus arteriosus → descending aorta → lower body → umbilical arteries → placenta
  4. Small amount of blood travels to pulmonary circulation

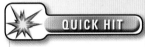

QUICK HIT

Corrective lens prescriptions should not be changed during pregnancy.

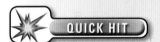

QUICK HIT

All gases cross the placenta via simple diffusion.

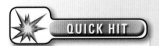

QUICK HIT

Oxygenation occurs in the placenta, not in the fetal lungs.

FIGURE 7.2 Fetal circulation at term (A) and after delivery (B).

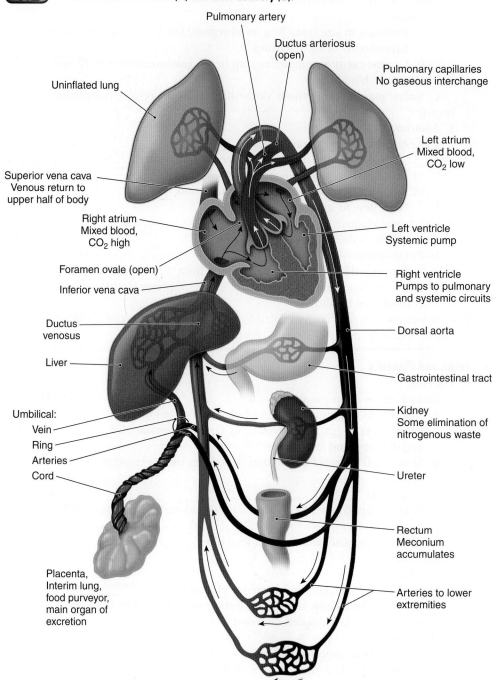

Pulmonary artery

Ductus arteriosus (open)

Pulmonary capillaries
No gaseous interchange

Uninflated lung

Left atrium
Mixed blood,
CO_2 low

Superior vena cava
Venous return to
upper half of body

Right atrium
Mixed blood,
CO_2 high

Left ventricle
Systemic pump

Foramen ovale (open)

Right ventricle
Pumps to pulmonary
and systemic circuits

Inferior vena cava

Ductus
venosus

Dorsal aorta

Liver

Gastrointestinal tract

Umbilical:
Vein
Ring
Arteries
Cord

Kidney
Some elimination of
nitrogenous waste

Ureter

Rectum
Meconium
accumulates

Placenta,
Interim lung,
food purveyor,
main organ of
excretion

Arteries to lower
extremities

A

Note the changes in function of the ductus venosus, foramen ovale, and ductus arteriosus in the transition from intrauterine to extra-uterine existence. *Red,* oxygenated blood; *pink/purple,* partially oxygenated blood; *blue,* deoxygenated blood. (From Beckmann CRB. *Obstetrics and Gynecology,* 7th ed. Baltimore: Lippincott Williams & Wilkins; 2014.)

FIGURE
7.2 *(Continued)*

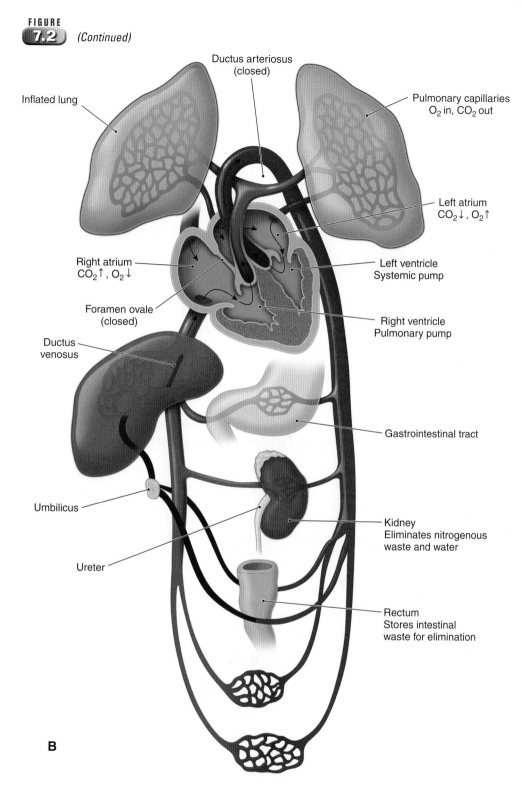

Ductus arteriosus
(closed)

Inflated lung

Pulmonary capillaries
O_2 in, CO_2 out

Left atrium
$CO_2\downarrow$, $O_2\uparrow$

Right atrium
$CO_2\uparrow$, $O_2\downarrow$

Left ventricle
Systemic pump

Foramen ovale
(closed)

Right ventricle
Pulmonary pump

Ductus
venosus

Gastrointestinal tract

Umbilicus

Kidney
Eliminates nitrogenous
waste and water

Ureter

Rectum
Stores intestinal
waste for elimination

B

C. Hgb and oxygenation
1. **Fetal Hgb** (HgF): 2α and 2β chains
   a. At all O_2 concentrations, HgF has higher O_2 affinity than HgA (adult)
   b. HgA binds 2,3 DPG more avidly than HgF (releasing more oxygen to tissues)
2. Maternal respiratory alkalosis facilitates CO_2 transfer from fetus
   a. Loss of fetal CO_2 shifts oxyhemoglobin-binding curve to right, increases Hgb O_2 affinity
   b. Maternal gain of CO_2 shifts oxyhemoglobin-binding curve to left, increases O_2 delivery to tissue
D. Kidneys
1. Become functional in 2nd trimester
2. Produce dilute hypotonic urine
3. Volume produced depends on fetal size (400–1,200 mL/day)
E. Liver
1. Anatomy: slow to develop/mature
2. Function
   a. Glycogen synthesis/storage
      i. Increase with gestational age
      ii. Premature fetuses frequently hypoglycemic
   b. Bilirubin conjugation/metabolism primarily by placenta
   c. Coagulation factor production may be deficient
   d. Vitamin K deficiency in newborn life may lead to hemorrhage
F. Thyroid
1. Becomes functional at end of 1st trimester
2. Fetal TBG, triiodothyronine (T_3), T_4 increase over gestation
3. Placenta does not transport TSH from maternal circulation
G. Gonads
1. Anatomy
   a. Differentiation of gonads → testes occurs ~6 weeks
      i. Requires presence of Y chromosome
      ii. If Y chromosome absent, develops into ovary
   b. Differentiation of gonads → ovaries occurs ~7 weeks
   c. Other genital organs depend on +/− of hormonal influence

III. Immunology of Pregnancy

A. Placenta
1. Appears to protect fetus from maternal immune system
2. Production of progesterone, estrogen, hPL, and hCG helps suppress maternal immune system response
3. Only allows immunoglobulin (Ig) G to pass to fetus, blocks/masks all others
B. Maternal
1. Normal WBC count, normal B and T cell counts, normal Ig levels
2. IgG can pass to fetus, provides passive immunity for fetus/newborn
C. Fetal
1. Gradually develops
2. Lymphocytes begin developing by 6 weeks' gestational age
3. Fetal IgG, IgM, IgD, and IgE present by 12 weeks' gestational age (production increases as pregnancy progresses)

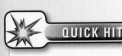

The fetal kidneys are the primary source of amniotic fluid by the middle of the second trimester.

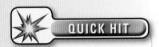

Newborns are routinely administered vitamin K at birth to prevent hemorrhage.

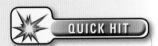

The mother is the primary source of T_3 and T_4 until 24–28 weeks' gestational age.

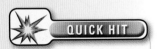

IgG is the only immunoglobulin able to cross the placenta.

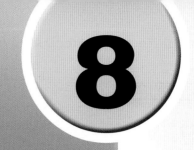

Preconception and Antepartum Care

I. Preconception Counseling

A. History (both potential parents)
  1. Medical history: hypertension, diabetes, thyroid disease, metabolic disorders
  2. Family history: congenital abnormalities, mental retardation, fragile X syndrome
B. Physical exam
C. Supplementation
  1. Prenatal vitamins: minimum 1 month prior to attempting conception
  2. Folic acid supplementation: 0.4 mg folic acid daily (4 mg folic acid daily if prior open neural tube defect)
D. Genetic screening/testing
  1. Carrier testing
     a. Sickle hemoglobinopathies (African Americans)
     b. Thalassemias
        i. α (Southeast Asian, Mediterranean, African American)
        ii β (Mediterranean, Southeast Asian, African American)
     c. Cystic fibrosis (CF): highest among Caucasians of European descent (1:29) and Ashkenazi Jews (1:25); all patients should be offered testing
  2. Ashkenazi Jewish panel: includes Tay-Sachs, Niemann-Pick, Gaucher, and Canavan diseases; familial dysautonomia; Fanconi anemia, CF, Bloom syndrome
E. Immunity/immunization status
  1. Rubella: if nonimmune or susceptible, plan vaccination at least 1 month prior to attempting conception
  2. Varicella
  3. Hepatitis B
F. Behavioral modification
  1. Food/nutrition
     a. Weight optimization: obese patients should lose weight; underweight patients should gain weight
     b. Food faddism: avoid fad diets
  2. Substance use/abuse: abstain from alcohol, tobacco, and illicit drugs
  3. Exercise should be encouraged

II. Antepartum Care

A. Diagnosing pregnancy
  1. Physical exam
     a. Uterus softens and enlarges; palpable at symphysis pubis at ~12 weeks
     b. Cervix softens (**Hegar sign**)
     c. Vagina bluish discoloration (**Chadwick sign**)
  2. Pregnancy test
     a. Urine pregnancy test
        i. Best performed on early-morning specimen, which contains highest concentration of human chorionic gonadotropin (hCG)
        ii. Turns positive around time of 1st missed period

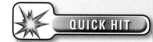

The fetal neural tube closes by 28 days after conception, so folic acid should be taken daily at least 1 month prior to attempting pregnancy.

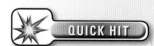

Live-virus vaccinations should be avoided during pregnancy. Influenza vaccination should be strongly recommended.

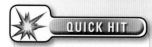

Maternal alcohol consumption is the most common preventable cause of mental retardation.

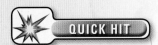

   b. Serum pregnancy test: β subunit of hCG
      i. Earlier detection than with urine pregnancy test
      ii. Serial levels can help differentiate between normal and abnormal pregnancy
   3. Ultrasound examination
      a. Abdominal ultrasound: gestational sac seen at 5–6 weeks' estimated gestational age (β-hCG of 5,000–6,000 mIU/mL)
      b. Transvaginal ultrasound: gestational sac at β-hCG of 1,500–2,000 mIU/mL
   4. Fetal heart activity detected by electronic Doppler device at <12 weeks' gestation
B. Common symptoms
   1. Nausea/vomiting usually improves by end of 1st trimester
      a. Morning sickness
         i. Dietary modification: bland food, small meals
         ii. Medications: H_1-receptor blockers, phenothiazines, vitamin B6 + doxylamine
      b. Hyperemesis gravidarum
         i. <2% of pregnancies
         ii. May require hospitalization, intravenous fluids, medications, and electrolyte replacement
   2. Headaches: further evaluation if not improved with acetaminophen
   3. Constipation: due to increased transit time, increased water absorption
      a. Dietary modifications: increase fluid intake, increase bulk (fruits, vegetables)
      b. Medications: bowel softeners (docusate), fiber supplements (psyllium), lubricants
   4. Fatigue improves in 2nd trimester
   5. Heartburn: due to relaxation of lower esophageal sphincter, delayed gastric emptying, and increased transit time of gastrointestinal tract; smaller, more frequent meals and bland foods recommended
   6. Round ligament pain/stretching groin pain improves with modified activity
   7. Hemorrhoids and varicose veins: gravid uterus causes venous congestion
      a. Treatment
         i. Support hose improves discomfort but not appearance
         ii. Sitz baths
         iii. Local preparations: topical anesthetics, steroid creams
      b. Course: regress postpartum; allow 6 months for involution
   8. Edema: common finding; may be sign of preeclampsia after 20 weeks' gestation; monitor blood pressure and urine protein
   9. Vaginal discharge: hormones cause increase in normal secretions; must distinguish from infections and ruptured membranes
C. Prenatal visits
   1. 1st visit
      a. History: chronic medical issues, past pregnancy complications, gynecologic history, genetic screening concerns, current pregnancy issues, and reproductive choice
      b. Physical exam including breast and pelvic exams
         i. Bony pelvis (clinical pelvimetry)
         ii. Cervical assessment and uterine size
      c. 1st trimester labs (Table 8.1)
      d. Risk assessment: nutrition, environmental/work hazards, domestic violence, seat belts, tobacco/drugs/alcohol
      e. Assess gestational age
         i. Determine if LMP is reliable: Does patient have regular menses and normal cycle length?
         ii. Assisted reproductive techniques (e.g., in vitro fertilization, intrauterine insemination) have known conception date
         iii. Ultrasound should be performed as soon as possible if dating is uncertain
   2. Subsequent visits
      a. For uncomplicated patients, visits occur at 4-week intervals until 28 weeks, at 2–3 week intervals until 36 weeks, and then weekly until delivery
      b. Blood pressure, weight, urine dipstick (albumin, glucose, ketones)
      c. Fundal height/fetal heart tones

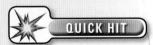

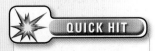

TABLE **8.1** First Trimester Prenatal Labs	
Blood type	Surface antigen of the hepatitis B virus (HBsAg)
D (Rh) type	Human immunodeficiency virus 1 and 2 antibodies
Antibody screen	Urine culture
Hemoglobin/hematocrit	Pap smear
Varicella	Hemoglobin electrophoresis[a]
Rubella	Purified protein derivative[a]
Venereal Disease Research Laboratory test/ rapid plasma reagin	Carrier screening[a]

[a]As indicated based on patient characteristics and risk factors.

3. Ultrasound
   a. 1st trimester: confirm location; most accurate assessment of gestational age (less accurate for estimated date of confinement [EDC] as gestation advances); perform nuchal translucency measurement; evaluate multiple gestations, uterine abnormalities, and pelvic masses
   b. 2nd trimester (18–20 weeks): fetal biometry, placental position, amniotic fluid volume, fetal presentation, anatomic survey
   c. 3rd trimester: only as clinically indicated for growth assessment, fetal position, or amniotic fluid volume
   d. Cervical length
4. Screening tests
   a. Genetics
      i. Screening tests
         (a) 1st-trimester screen (10–13 weeks): nuchal translucency, pregnancy-associated plasma protein-A, β-hCG
         (b) 2nd-trimester screen (15–21 weeks): triple or quadruple screen
         (c) Integrated 1st- and 2nd-trimester screen
      ii. Diagnostic tests
         (a) Chorionic villus sampling (10–13 weeks)
         (b) Amniocentesis (15 weeks' gestation and above)
   b. Gestational diabetes (24–28 weeks)
      i. Glucose challenge test: 50-g glucose load, if abnormal then
      ii. Glucose tolerance test (GTT) + fasting glucose
         (a) 3-hour GTT with 100-g glucose load
         (b) 2-hour GTT with 75-g glucose load
   c. Group B *Streptococcus* (35–37 weeks) from vagina/anal region
5. Fetal assessment techniques
   a. Fetal growth
      i. Fundal height measurement
         (a) Size > dates: suspect large-for-gestational-age fetus
         (b) Size < dates: suspect small-for-gestational-age fetus
      ii. Ultrasonography: crown–rump length, biparietal diameter, abdominal circumference, femur length
   b. Fetal well-being
      i. Fetal activity/kick counts
      ii. Nonstress test (NST): measures fetal heart rate with external transducer for minimum 20 minutes
         (a) Reactive: 2 or more fetal heart rate accelerations in 20 minutes
         (b) Nonreactive: 0 sufficient accelerations in 40 minutes
      iii. Contraction stress test: nipple stimulation or oxytocin
      iv. BPP: given 0 or 2 points for each of 5 categories (NST: amniotic fluid index, fetal heart rate, fetal movement, fetal tone, and fetal breathing movements)
      v. Umbilical artery Doppler

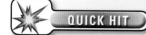

QUICK HIT

Ultrasound is most accurate in predicting gestational age when done early.

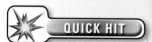

QUICK HIT

A shortened cervix as identified by transvaginal ultrasound has been correlated with increased risk of preterm delivery.

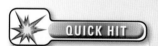

QUICK HIT

The triple screen utilizes maternal serum α-fetoprotein, estriol, and hCG, whereas the quadruple screen also includes inhibin.

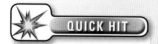

QUICK HIT

The most common cause of "abnormal" gestational size is incorrect dates.

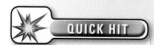

QUICK HIT

Fundal height (cm) should be roughly equivalent to the gestational age (weeks) at 16–36 weeks of gestation.

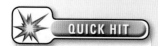

QUICK HIT

A nonreactive NST should be followed by further fetal assessment, most often a biophysical profile (BPP).

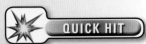

QUICK HIT

Surfactant production occurs in the **type II pneumocytes** of the fetal lungs and maintains the patency of the alveolar sacs.

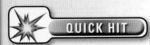

QUICK HIT

The large, polar molecules of heparin and low-molecular-weight heparin do not cross the placenta and are *not* teratogenic; therefore, they are used preferentially for anticoagulation in pregnancy over warfarin, which does cross the placenta and is a potent teratogen (see Table 8.2).

c. Fetal maturity
  i. Lecithin–sphingomyelin ratio
  ii. Phosphatidylglycerol
  iii. Lamellar body counts
6. Patient education
  a. Exercise
    i. Encourage 30 minutes of moderate exercise per day
    ii. Avoid supine exercises after 1st trimester
    iii. Contraindications include placenta previa, preeclampsia, cardio-pulmonary disease, cerclage, ruptured membranes
  b. Nutrition and weight gain
    i. Body mass index determines recommendations for total weight gain and rate of weight gain per month
    ii. Iron supplementation is recommended
  c. Sexual activity not typically restricted except in setting of placenta previa, premature rupture of membranes
  d. Travel
    i. May travel via airplane until 34–36 weeks' gestation if uncomplicated pregnancy
    ii. Patients should carry copy of their obstetric record and walk every 1–2 hours to promote circulation
  e. Teratogens (Table 8.2)
    i. Medications
      (a) Timing of medication use often determines degree of effect
      (b) U.S. Food and Drug Administration classifications: A is lowest risk; X is contraindicated in pregnancy

TABLE 8.2	**Teratogenic Effects of Medications in Pregnancy**
Drug	**Effect**
Warfarin	Easily crosses placenta; exposure between weeks 6 and 9: nasal and midface hypoplasia, stippled femoral and vertebral epiphyses; later exposure: hydrocephalus
Heparin and low-molecular-weight heparin	Not teratogenic
Phenytoin	Abnormal facies, cleft lip/palate, microcephaly, growth deficiency
Valproic acid	Spina bifida and other neural tube defects
Lithium	Cardiovascular malformations; limit exposure until after 8 weeks
Quinolones	Cartilage erosion and arthropathies in animal studies
Tetracyclines	Discoloration of deciduous teeth
Serotonin reuptake inhibitors	Paroxetine: VSD and ASD All: neonatal behavioral syndrome associated with exposure in late pregnancy
Angiotensin-converting enzyme inhibitors	Limb contractures, growth restriction, abnormalities in calvarium development
Thiazide diuretics	Fetal thrombocytopenia, bleeding, electrolyte abnormalities; can decrease breast milk production
Androgens	Exposure between 7 and 12 weeks: full masculinization; later exposure: partial masculinization
Vitamin A and retinoids	Fetal loss, congenital malformations
Nonsteroidal anti-inflammatory drugs	All: short-term use with reversible fetal effects Indomethacin: constriction of fetal ductus arteriosus and neonatal pulmonary hypertension when used near delivery
Acetaminophen	Not teratogenic

ASD, atrial septal defect; VSD, ventricular septal defect.

ii. Radiation

   (a) Normal yearly exposure is 125 mrads

   (b) 1st 2 weeks: 10 rads can produce problems

   (c) 1st trimester: 25 rads cause detectable damage

   (d) Remainder of pregnancy: 100 rads

iii. Alcohol

   (a) Most common preventable cause of mental retardation, fetal birth defects

   (b) Greatest risk is in 1st trimester

   (c) *No* established safe level of use in pregnancy; all patients should be advised not to drink alcohol

iv. Tobacco

   (a) Risks include intrauterine growth restriction, low birth weight, fetal mortality

   (b) Counsel patients to quit at every visit

v. Substance abuse

   (a) Illicit agents may reach fetus via placenta or newborn via breast milk

   (b) Monitor fetus for withdrawal symptoms

vi. Methyl mercury: limit intake of large fish such as mackerel, shark, swordfish, tilefish, and tuna (especially albacore)

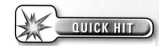

QUICK HIT

Fetal alcohol syndrome is characterized by growth restriction, central nervous system (CNS) dysfunction (microcephaly, mental retardation) and behavioral disorders, and facial abnormalities (low-set ears, midfacial hypoplasia, shortened palpebral fissures, smooth philtrum, and a thin upper lip).

Preconception and Antepartum Care

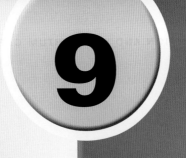

9 Prenatal Diagnosis, Genetic Disorder Assessment, and Teratology

I. Prenatal Diagnosis

A. Basic genetic principles
  1. Chromosomes
     a. Haploid (n = 23)
     b. Diploid (2n = 46)
  2. Chromosome replication and cell division
     a. Meiosis (Figure 9.1)
        i. Definition: process of cell division to produce germ cells
        ii. Results in formation of 4 gametes

FIGURE 9.1 First and second meiotic divisions.

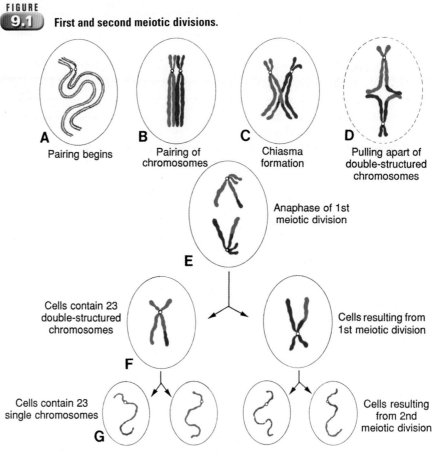

(A) Homologous chromosomes approach each other. (B) Homologous chromosomes pair, and each member of the pair consists of two chromatids. (C) Intimately paired homologous chromosomes interchange chromatid fragments (crossover). Note the chiasma. (D) Double-structured chromosomes pull apart. (E) Anaphase of the first meiotic division. (F, G) During the second meiotic division, the double-structured chromosomes split at the centromere. At completion of division, chromosomes in each of the four daughter cells are different from each other. (From Sadler T. *Langman's Medical Embryology*, 9th ed. Baltimore: Lippincott Williams & Wilkins; 2003.)

FIGURE 9.2 **Various stages of mitosis.**

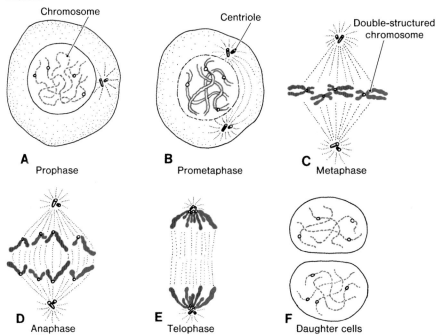

A Prophase

B Prometaphase

C Metaphase

D Anaphase

E Telophase

F Daughter cells

In prophase, chromosomes are visible as slender threads. Doubled chromatids become clearly visible as individual units during prometaphase. At no time during division do members of a chromosome pair unite. *Blue*, paternal chromosomes; *red*, maternal chromosomes. (From Sadler T. *Langman's Medical Embryology*, 9th ed. Baltimore: Lippincott Williams & Wilkins; 2003.)

iii. Meiosis 1 = reductional division from diploid to haploid

iv. Meiosis 2 = division of haploid chromosomes to form germ cells

b. Mitosis: process of cell division to replicate genetic material and produce 2 identical daughter cells (Figure 9.2)

3. Abnormalities of cell replication and cell division

a. **Polyploidy**: numerical change in whole sets of chromosomes (e.g., triploidy 69, XXY or 69, XXX)

b. **Aneuploidy**

i. Definition: extra or missing chromosome or piece of chromosome

ii. Result of **nondisjunction** during meiosis (e.g., trisomy 21)

4. Abnormalities of chromosome structure (Figure 9.3)

a. **Deletion**

i. Definition: loss of chromosome material

ii. Variable size

iii. Variable clinical outcome depending on deletion size and location

b. **Inversion**

i. Definition: reversal of DNA order between 2 breaks along 1 chromosome

ii. Inversion carriers usually normal but have risk for miscarriage and/or child born with birth defects, mental retardation

c. **Insertion**

i. Definition: portion of 1 chromosome moved into nonhomologous chromosome

ii. Result of unequal crossing-over during meiosis

iii. Variable clinical outcomes, depends on size and location

d. **Translocation**

i. Definition: exchange of material between nonhomologous chromosomes

ii. Carriers usually normal when balanced but have risk for miscarriage and/or child with birth defects; mental retardation when unbalanced

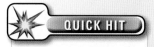

QUICK HIT

Trisomy 16 is the most common chromosomal abnormality in miscarriage.

FIGURE 9.3 Examples of common chromosome abnormalities.

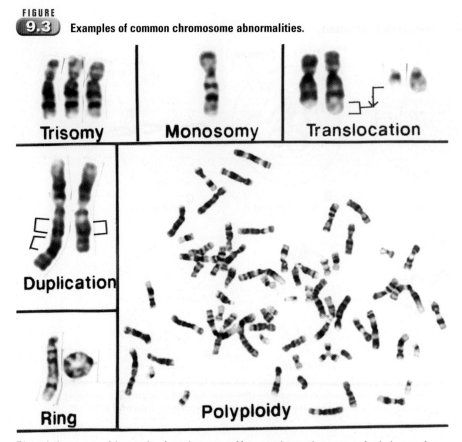

Trisomy is the presence of three copies of any chromosome. Monosomy denotes the presence of a single copy of any chromosome. Translocations involve the exchange of chromatin between any two or more nonhomologous chromosomes. Duplications produce structural abnormalities with multiple copies of genes. Deletions result in the loss of a portion of a chromosome; a ring chromosome is an example of a deletion. Polyploid cells involve 69 or 92 chromosomes or some exact multiple of the haploid chromosome number. (From McClatchey KD. *Clinical Laboratory Medicine*, 2nd ed. Philadelphia: Lippincott Williams & Wilkins; 2002.)

    iii. **Robertsonian translocation** involves exchange between specific chromosomes: 13, 14, 15, 21, and 22

    iv. Incidence of Robertsonian translocation = 1 in 1,000

    v. Genetic counseling for parent with translocation 13 or 21 given increased risk for offspring with trisomy 21 or 13

5. **Mendelian disorders** or single gene disorders

  a. Result of mutation in specific gene

  b. Demonstrate clear pattern of inheritance (Figure 9.4)

  c. Autosomal dominant

    i. Affected males and females appear in each generation

    ii. Affected mothers and fathers transmit phenotype to both sons and daughters

    iii. Affected individuals have 50% chance with each pregnancy of having affected offspring

    iv. Example: neurofibromatosis

  d. Autosomal recessive

    i. Disease appears in male and female children of unaffected parents

    ii. Carrier parents have 25% chance with each pregnancy of having affected offspring

    iii. 1 parent carrier = 50% chance with each offspring to also be carrier

    iv. Example: cystic fibrosis (CF)

  e. X-linked inheritance

    i. X chromosome present as 2 copies in females and 1 copy in males

    ii. Males will manifest disease if X chromosome carries mutation

FIGURE 9.4 Inheritance patterns of genetic disease.

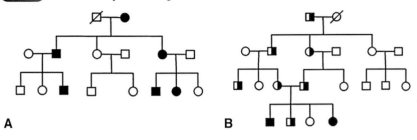

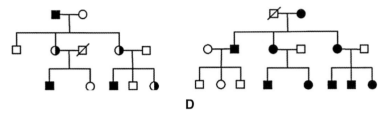

(A) Autosomal-dominant inheritance. **(B)** Autosomal-recessive inheritance. **(C)** X-linked recessive inheritance. **(D)** Mitochondrial inheritance. Affected individuals are shown as *filled circles* (female subjects) or *squares* (male subjects), and unaffected individuals are shown as *empty symbols*. Heterozygous carriers in **B** and **C** are shown as *half-filled symbols*. (From Topol EJ, Califf RM, et al. *Textbook of Cardiovascular Medicine*, 3rd ed. Philadelphia: Lippincott Williams & Wilkins; 2006.)

  iii. Example: fragile X syndrome and *FMR-1* related disorders
   (a) Heterozygous females can demonstrate cognitive impairment
   (b) Risk for **premature ovarian failure** and tremor ataxia syndrome in carriers of permutation
 f. X-linked recessive
  i. All daughters of affected male are carriers
  ii. No sons of affected male show disease or are carriers
  iii. Females can show evidence of disease with skewed X inactivation
  iv. Example: hemophilia A
 g. X-linked dominant
  i. Affected males pass disorder to all daughters but to no sons
  ii. Affected heterozygous females pass condition to half of their sons and daughters
  iii. Example: X-linked hypophosphatemic rickets
6. Multifactorial inheritance
 a. Definition: conditions caused by combination of genes and environmental influences
 b. No consistent or recognizable pattern of inheritance
 c. In general, have 3%–5% recurrence rate for couple with previously affected child
 d. Example: neural tube defects (NTDs)

II. Genetic Disorder Assessment

A. Preconception counseling: review risks associated with family history and exposures prior to and during pregnancy
B. Counseling must be nondirective and respect patient's right to accept or decline testing
 1. Advanced maternal age (Table 9.1)
  a. Aneuploidy
  b. At age 35 years, risk for Down syndrome equals risk of miscarriage from amniocentesis (~1 in 300)
 2. Advanced paternal age: age ≥45 years associated with increased risk for new-onset autosomal-dominant disorders

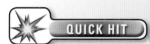

QUICK HIT

Fragile X syndrome is the most common form of inherited mental retardation and single cause of autism.

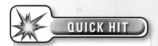

QUICK HIT

As many as 3% of all live births have a birth defect.

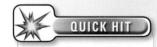

QUICK HIT

The American College of Obstetricians and Gynecologists recommends all women be offered screening and diagnostic tests for aneuploidy in pregnancy irrespective of maternal age.

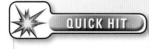

QUICK HIT

The risk for aneuploidy increases with maternal age.

Prenatal Diagnosis and Teratology

TABLE **9.1** **Risk for Chromosomal Abnormalities by Maternal Age at Term**

Age at Term	Risk for Trisomy 21[a]	Risk for Any Chromosomal Aneuploidy[b]
15	1 in 1,578	1 in 454
20	1 in 1,528	1 in 525
25	1 in 1,351	1 in 475
30	1 in 909	1 in 384
35	1 in 384	1 in 178
40	1 in 112	1 in 62
45	1 in 28	1 in 18

[a]Cuckle HA, Wald NJ, Thompson SC. Estimating a woman's risk of having a pregnancy associated with Down syndrome using her age and serum alpha-fetoprotein level. *Br J Obstet Gynecol.* 1987:387–402.
[b]Hook EB. Rates of chromosomal abnormalities at different maternal ages. *Obstet Gynecol.* 1981;58:282–285.

III. Chromosomal Aneuploidy Screening *(Table 9.2)*

A. Positive screen does not mean fetus is affected

B. Negative screen does not exclude possibility that fetus is affected

C. 1st trimester (10–13 weeks' gestation)
  1. Calculates risk for trisomy 13, 18, and 21
  2. Does not assess risk for NTDs
  3. Includes maternal serum, ultrasound, or both for composite risk
  4. Maternal serum analytes: pregnancy-associated plasma protein-A and free β-human chorionic gonadotropin (β-hCG)
  5. Ultrasound (Figure 9.5)
    a. Nuchal translucency: increased nuchal translucency associated with aneuploidy, congenital heart defects, other birth defects, and genetic conditions
    b. Nasal bone
      i. Absence of bone reflects midface hypoplasia in fetus with Down syndrome
      ii. Absent in 1% of unaffected fetuses
  6. 1st-trimester screening in twin pregnancies: 75%–80% detection rate for trisomy 21 with 5% false-positive rate

D. 2nd trimester (15–22 weeks' gestation)
  1. Calculates risk for trisomy 18 and 21 and NTDs
  2. Includes maternal serum and ultrasound

TABLE **9.2** **Comparison of Detection Rates for Trisomy 21 Among Screening Tests**

Screening Method	Detection Rate for Trisomy 21[a]
Maternal age	30%
Maternal age + 2nd-trimester quad screen	81%
Maternal age + fetal nuchal translucency at 11–13 + 6 weeks	70%
Maternal age + fetal nuchal translucency + fetal nasal bone + maternal serum at 11–13 + 6 weeks	90%

[a]False-positive rate of 5%.

FIGURE 9.5 Ultrasound image of first-trimester fetus with normal nuchal translucency measurement and nasal bone present.

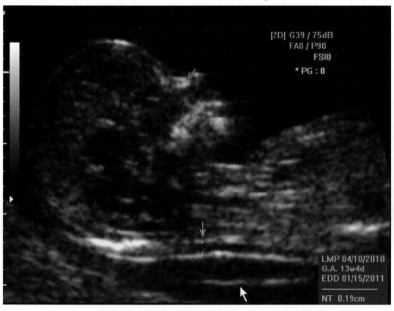

The *white arrow* is pointing to amnion; the green calipers are measuring nuchal translucency as indicated by the *green arrow*, and the *blue arrow* is pointing to nasal bone. (Courtesy of Dr. Britton D. Rink.)

3. Maternal serum analytes: α-fetoprotein (msAFP), unconjugated estriol, β-hCG, inhibin A (Table 9.3)
4. AFP independent marker for NTD risk assessment
5. Incidence 1–2 per 1,000 live births
   a. Role of folate in decreasing risk
   b. Sensitivity for detection 80%–90% with 3% false-positive rate
   c. "Gold standard" diagnostic test: amniocentesis to detect neural-specific acetylcholinesterase in amniotic fluid
6. Ultrasound
   a. Anatomic survey 18–22 weeks' gestation
   b. Diagnose birth defect
   c. Screen for genetic condition: 1 or more anomalies increases likelihood for underlying cause
   d. 2nd-trimester ultrasound identifies ~50% fetuses with trisomy 21
7. Fetal magnetic resonance imaging and X-ray used for evaluation of specific genetic conditions or birth defects (Figure 9.6)
8. Combined 1st- and 2nd-trimester screening
   a. Various methods (integrated or sequential) to include 1st-trimester maternal serum, ultrasound, and 2nd-trimester serum in combined risk assessment
   b. Increases sensitivity for detection of trisomy 21 up to 95%–97% with 5% fixed false-positive rate

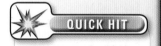

QUICK HIT

Women should take 0.4 mg folate daily to reduce risk for NTDs or 4 mg daily in women with previously affected pregnancies.

TABLE 9.3 Patterns of Analytes in Quad Screen

	Trisomy 21	Trisomy 18	Neural Tube Defects
Inhibin A	↑	N/A	N/A
Unconjugated estriol	↓	↓	N/A
α-Fetoprotein	↓	↓	↑
β-Human chorionic gonadotropin	↑	↓	N/A

FIGURE 9.6 Fetal magnetic resonance imaging.

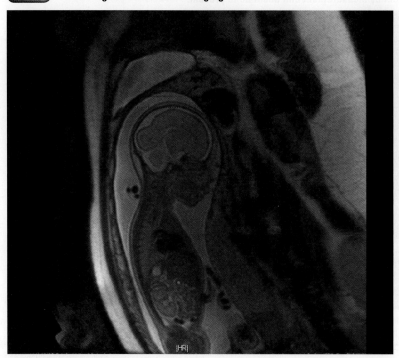

(Courtesy of Dr. Britton D. Rink.)

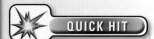

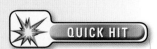

IV. Screening Based on Ethnicity or Family History *(Table 9.4)*

A. Some autosomal-recessive conditions occur at increased frequency in certain racial or ethnic backgrounds
B. CF screening
C. 3-Generation pedigree as screening tool
D. Carrier testing available for many genetic conditions

TABLE 9.4 Carrier Frequencies for Autosomal-Recessive Conditions Based on Ethnic Origin

Population	Condition	Carrier Frequency
African American	Sickle cell	1 in 10
	Cystic fibrosis	1 in 65
	β-Thalassemia	1 in 75
Ashkenazi Jewish	Gaucher disease	1 in 15
	Cystic fibrosis	1 in 25
	Tay-Sachs disease	1 in 30
	Familial dysautonomia	1 in 32
	Canavan disease	1 in 40
Asian	α-Thalassemia	1 in 20
	β-Thalassemia	1 in 50
European Caucasian	Cystic fibrosis	1 in 25
French Canadian, Cajun	Tay-Sachs disease	1 in 30
Hispanic	Cystic fibrosis	1 in 46
	β-Thalassemia	1 in 30 to 1 in 50
Mediterranean	β-Thalassemia	1 in 25
	Cystic fibrosis	1 in 25
	Sickle cell disease	1 in 40

FIGURE
9.7 Transcervical chorionic villus sampling under ultrasound guidance.

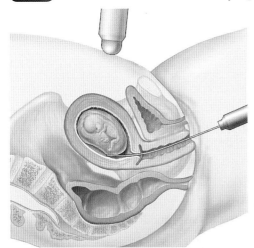

(LifeART image copyright © 2015. Lippincott Williams & Wilkins. All rights reserved.)

E. Genetic counseling recommended

F. Referral to medical genetics for comprehensive evaluation

V. Diagnostic Testing for Aneuploidy

A. 1st trimester: chorionic villus sampling (Figure 9.7)
1. Performed no earlier than 10 weeks' gestation
2. Miscarriage risk = 1 in 100
3. Transabdominal or transcervical approach using ultrasound guidance
4. Obtain placental tissue for karyotype analysis and DNA testing

B. 2nd and 3rd trimester: amniocentesis (Figure 9.8)
1. Performed no earlier than 15 weeks' gestation
2. Miscarriage risk = 1 in 300

FIGURE
9.8 Amniocentesis.

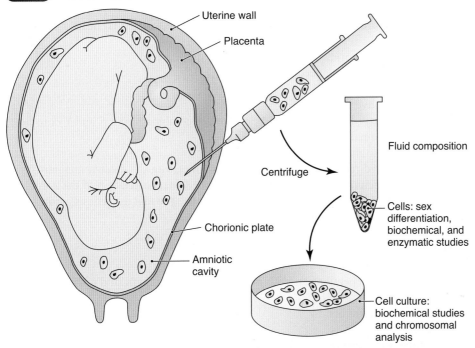

Under ultrasound guidance, a needle is inserted into the uterus through the abdominal wall, and a sample of amniotic fluid is withdrawn for chromosomal and biochemical studies. (From U.S. Department of Health, Education, and Welfare. *What Are the Facts About Genetic Disease?* Washington, DC: U.S. Department of Health, Education, and Welfare; 1977.)

3. Transabdominal approach under ultrasound guidance
4. Obtain fetal cells for karyotype analysis or DNA testing

C. 2nd and 3rd trimester: cordocentesis
1. Performed after 18–20 weeks' gestation
2. Fetal blood sample from umbilical cord
3. Risk for miscarriage and rupture of membranes = 1%–3%
4. Used to diagnose fetal anemia, infection, or chromosomal abnormalities

VI. Chromosomal Disorders

A. Over 20% of all conceptions expected to be aneuploidy
B. Recurrence risk for translocation aneuploidy depends on karyotype and parent of origin
C. Trisomy 21 (Down syndrome)
1. 1 in 800 live births
2. Mild to moderate mental retardation
3. Structural birth defects: congenital heart disease, duodenal atresia, renal abnormalities, short long bones
4. 95% result of nondisjunction, predominantly maternal
5. 3%–5% result of unbalanced translocation inherited from balanced carrier parents
6. 1% mosaic with 2 cell lines present, with 46 and 47 chromosomes
D. Trisomy 18 (Edward syndrome)
1. 1 in 8,000 live births
2. 95% conceptions result in miscarriage or stillbirth
3. 10% of live births survive at 1 month
4. Severe mental retardation
5. Other features: characteristic facial features, congenital heart defects, diaphragmatic hernia, renal malformations, intrauterine growth restriction
6. 80% result of nondisjunction, predominantly maternal
7. 20% result of unbalanced translocation
E. Trisomy 13 (Patau syndrome)
1. 1 in 20,000 live births
2. 95% conceptions result in miscarriage or stillbirth
3. 10% of live births survive at 1 month
4. Severe mental retardation
5. Other features: holoprosencephaly, cleft lip/palate, congenital heart defects, omphalocele, renal malformations, polydactyly
6. 80% result of nondisjunction, predominantly maternal
7. 20% result of unbalanced translocation
F. Turner syndrome
1. 1 in 3,000 live births
2. Most frequent karyotype = 45,X; remainder combination of X and Y chromosome abnormalities
3. Unrelated to maternal age
4. No increased recurrence risk for couple with previously affected pregnancy
5. Features include cystic hygroma and lymphedema, coarctation of the aorta and bicuspid aortic valve, renal malformations, gonadal dysgenesis, short stature

VII. Teratology

A. Exposure in pregnancy with harmful fetal effect
B. Fetal outcome dependent on both maternal and fetal genetic and environmental factors
C. Fetal effect determined by
1. Dose
2. Timing of exposure
a. Fetus most vulnerable during organogenesis (weeks 3–8)
b. 1st-trimester insult typically results in malformations or disruptions

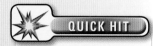

QUICK HIT

Chromosome errors account for about 50% of spontaneous miscarriage.

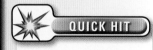

QUICK HIT

Recurrence risk for trisomy 13, 18, or 21 as a result of nondisjunction is ~1% or maternal age–related risk, whichever is greater.

    c. 2nd- and 3rd-trimester insult typically results in abnormalities of growth and cognition

D. Potential fetal effects: miscarriage, growth restriction, major and minor malformations, stillbirth, cognitive dysfunction, placental abruption

E. Drugs and chemical agents (Table 9.5)

    1. Very few medications with *absolute* contraindication in pregnancy

    2. Review risk *versus* benefit for specific agent

    3. Common exposures in pregnancy

        a. Tobacco: increased risk of miscarriage, fetal death, preterm birth, growth restriction, and placental abruption

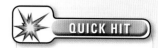

QUICK HIT

Females who were exposed in utero to maternal diethylstilbestrol (DES) have increased risk for vaginal clear cell adenocarcinoma.

TABLE 9.5 Summary of Selected Substances and Associated Teratogenicity

Drug	Effect
Serotonin reuptake inhibitors	Paroxetine: associated with cardiovascular abnormalities in some epidemiology studies, but data have not been consistent All: exposure in 3rd trimester associated with mild transient neonatal syndrome characterized by central nervous system, respiratory, and gastrointestinal symptoms
Angiotensin-converting enzyme inhibitors	1st-trimester exposure associated with congenital malformations, although data not consistent; 2nd- and 3rd-trimester exposure clearly associated with adverse outcomes including fetal hypotension and oligohydramnios or fetal anuria
β-Blockers: Propranolol Labetalol	 Associated with intrauterine growth restriction Generally considered safe in pregnancy
Calcium channel blockers	Generally considered safe in pregnancy
Methyldopa	Generally considered safe in pregnancy
Methotrexate	Miscarriage, stillbirth, growth restriction, craniofacial malformations, mental retardation
Coumadin	1st-trimester exposure associated with craniofacial anomalies Safe for breastfeeding
Heparin and Lovenox	Generally considered safe in pregnancy; does not cross the placenta
Valproate	Neural tube defect risk 1%–2%, facial clefts and other craniofacial malformations, limb defects, neurocognitive delay
Carbamazepine	Neural tube defects risk 1%, craniofacial malformations, neurocognitive delay
Phenytoin	Neonatal malformation syndrome present in up to 10% of exposed pregnancies including cardiac defects, facial clefts, and other craniofacial malformations; hypoplasia of distal phalanges involving nails; neurocognitive delay
Isotretinoin	Craniofacial malformations, cardiac defects, mental retardation
Alcohol	Fetal alcohol spectrum disorder: growth restriction, microcephaly, craniofacial malformations; cardiac defects, mental retardation, behavioral disorders
Lithium	Possible increase in cardiac defects including Ebstein anomaly
Benzodiazepines	No associated structural fetal anomalies; neonatal withdrawal
Opiates	No associated structural anomalies; neonatal withdrawal
Diethylstilbestrol	Uterine and cervical malformations, pregnancy loss, ectopic pregnancy, increased risk for vaginal clear cell adenocarcinoma
Cocaine	Growth restriction, placental abruption, preterm birth

Prenatal Diagnosis and Teratology

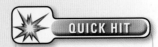

   b. Alcohol
      i. Fetal alcohol spectrum disorder: characterized by prenatal and/or postnatal growth deficiency, congenital heart disease, central nervous system dysfunction, and characteristic facial features
      ii. No clear dose–response threshold
   c. Hyperglycemia
      i. Poorly controlled pregestational diabetes associated with structural malformations
      ii. Increasing risk for malformation and miscarriage with increasing hemoglobin A1C (HbA1c)
   d. Radiation: fetal risks of anomalies, growth restriction, or miscarriage not increased with radiation exposure <5 rad

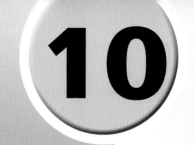

Normal Labor and Delivery

I. Maternal Changes Prior to Labor

A. **Braxton-Hicks contractions**
  1. Shorter and less intense than true labor
  2. Not associated with cervical dilation
B. **Lightening**
  1. Fetal head descends into maternal pelvis
  2. Associated with increased pelvic pressure
C. **Bloody show**
  1. Extrusion of mucus from endocervical glands
  2. Bleeding from small vessels
  3. Associated with cervical thinning (**effacement**)

II. Evaluation for Labor

A. Review of prenatal records
  1. Identify complications
  2. Confirm gestational age
  3. Review laboratory information
B. Focused history
  1. Timing and quality of contractions
  2. Status of membranes
  3. Presence of bleeding
  4. Presence of fetal movement
C. Exam
  1. Vital signs
  2. Auscultation of heart tones
  3. Abdominal exam
    a. Determine fetal **lie**: relation of fetal long axis to maternal long axis
    b. Determine fetal **presentation**: portion of fetus lowest in birth canal
    c. Determine fetal **position**: relation of fetal presenting part relative to maternal pelvis (Figure 10.1)
    d. **Leopold maneuvers** (Figure 10.2)
      i. Determine what fetal part is in uterine fundus
      ii. Determine what side fetal back is on
      iii. Identify descent of presenting part
      iv. Identify cephalic prominence
  4. Digital vaginal exam
    a. Cervical dilation expressed in centimeters
    b. Cervical effacement expressed as % of thinning
    c. Fetal station (Figure 10.3)
      i. Level of presenting part relative to ischial spines
      ii. Pelvic inlet to ischial spines: stations $-5, -4, -3, -2, -1$
      iii. Ischial spines: 0 station
      iv. Ischial spines to pelvic outlet: stations $+1, +2, +3, +4, +5$
      v. Fetal head is "engaged" at 0 station

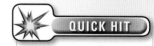

The initial examination of the patient's abdomen may be accomplished using Leopold maneuvers.

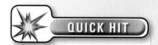

When the fetal head is at zero station, the greatest transverse dimension of the fetal head (biparietal diameter [BPD]) has passed through the pelvic inlet.

FIGURE 10.1 Fetal positions in vertex presentations.

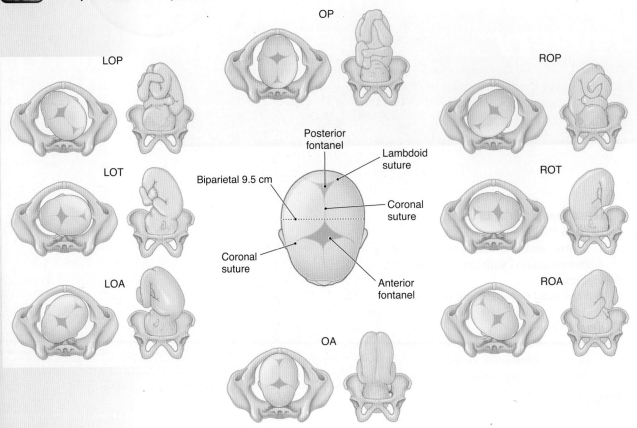

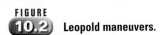

(From Beckmann CRB, Ling FW, et al. *Obstetrics and Gynecology*, 7th ed. Baltimore: Lippincott Williams & Wilkins; 2014.)

FIGURE 10.2 Leopold maneuvers.

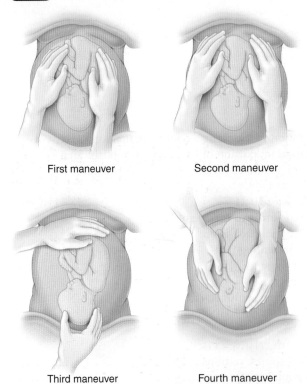

These maneuvers involve palpation of the maternal abdomen to determine fetal position. (From Beckmann CRB, Ling FW, et al. *Obstetrics and Gynecology*, 7th ed. Baltimore: Lippincott Williams & Wilkins; 2014.)

FIGURE 10.3 Station and engagement of the fetal head.

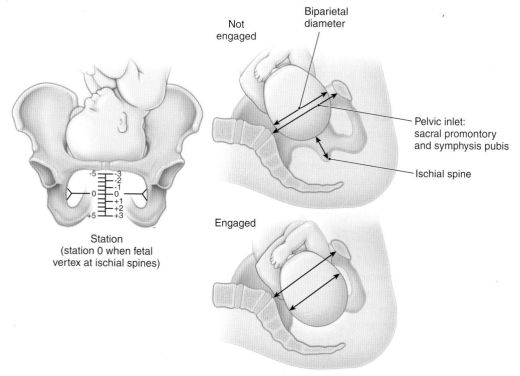

Note that the physician's hands are on the external abdomen. (From Beckmann CRB, Ling FW, et al. *Obstetrics and Gynecology*, 7th ed. Baltimore: Lippincott Williams & Wilkins; 2014.)

III. Stages of Labor

A. 1st stage
   1. Latent phase: cervical effacement and early dilation
   2. Active phase: advanced dilation beginning after 4 cm
B. 2nd stage: complete cervical dilation through delivery of infant
C. 3rd stage: after delivery of infant through delivery of placenta
D. 4th stage: 1st 2 hours postpartum
E. Length of stages varies by parity (Table 10.1)

TABLE 10.1	Mean Duration of the Various Phases and Stages of Labor With Their Distribution Characteristics			
Parity	**Latent Phase (hrs)**	**Active Phase (hrs)**	**Maximum Dilation (cm/hr)**	**2nd Stage (hrs)**
Nulliparous				
Mean	6.5	4.5	3.0	1.0
Upper limit[a]	20.0	12.0	1.0	3.0
Multiparous				
Mean	5.0	2.5	6.0	0.5
Upper limit[a]	13.5	5.0	1.5	1.0

[a]5th or 95th percentile.
(From Beckmann CRB, Ling FW, et al. *Obstetrics and Gynecology*, 7th ed. Baltimore: Lippincott Williams & Wilkins; 2014.)

IV. Cardinal Movements of Labor
  A. Engagement: descent of BPD below pelvic inlet
  B. Flexion: allows smaller diameters of fetal head to present to maternal pelvis
  C. Descent: occurs during late 1st stage and 2nd stage
  D. Internal rotation: usually from transverse to anterior or posterior
  E. Extension: fetal head reaches introitus
  F. External rotation: after delivery of head, it turns to align with shoulders
  G. Expulsion: delivery of body

V. Normal Labor and Delivery
  A. General management
    1. Ambulation and position
      a. Left lateral maternal position avoids compression of vena cava
      b. Dorsal lithotomy used for vaginal delivery
    2. Fluid management and oral intake
      a. Concern for aspiration with anesthesia
      b. Clear liquids or intravenous (IV) 1/2 normal saline or D5 1/2 normal saline
    3. Evaluation of fetal well-being
      a. Intermittent auscultation, handheld Doppler, or electronic fetal monitor
      b. Risk factors: vaginal bleeding, acute abdominal pain, temperature >100.4°F, preterm labor, hypertension, nonreassuring fetal pattern
      c. Frequency of evaluation
        i. Without risk factors
          (a) 1st stage: every 30 minutes
          (b) 2nd stage: every 15 minutes
        ii. With risk factors
          (a) 1st stage: every 15 minutes
          (b) 2nd stage: every 5 minutes
  B. Pain control
    1. 1st stage
      a. Pain from uterine contractions and cervical dilation
      b. Visceral afferents T10–L1
    2. 2nd stage
      a. Pain from descent of fetal head
      b. Somatic afferents S2–S4
    3. Anesthetics
      a. Epidural
        i. Continuous infusion for labor and delivery
        ii. Usually given early 1st stage of labor
      b. Spinal: single injection just prior to delivery
      c. Combined spinal–epidural
      d. Local block
        i. Pudendal block at time of delivery
        ii. Paracervical block during labor
        iii. Local infiltration at potential episiotomy site
      e. General anesthesia when emergent delivery needed
    4. Analgesics sometimes used in lieu of/prior to administration of anesthesia
  C. Management of labor
    1. 1st stage
      a. Serial exams assess cervical dilation, effacement, station, position, membrane status
      b. When membranes rupture, assess for meconium and cord prolapse
    2. 2nd stage
      a. Maternal expulsive efforts added to uterine contractile force
      b. Fetal head adjusts to maternal bony pelvis
        i. **Molding:** alteration in fetal cranial bones resulting in bony overlap
        ii. **Caput succedaneum:** edema of fetal scalp

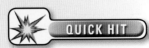

QUICK HIT

Alternative laboring positions (e.g., sitting or crouching on birthing chairs, birthing balls, and even in tubs of water) are advocated by some to provide more comfort and/or reduce the need for pain medications.

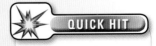

QUICK HIT

Molding and caput succedaneum are the most common causes of fetal descent overestimation.

Normal Labor and Delivery

    c. Crowning: fetal head distends vaginal opening
       i. Episiotomy: cutting vaginal opening to enlarge it
      ii. Modified Ritgen maneuver: perineal pressure used to facilitate extension and delivery of fetal head
  3. 3rd stage
    a. Signs of placental separation
       i. Uterus rises in abdomen
      ii. Umbilical cord lengthens
     iii. Gush of blood from vagina
     iv. Uterus becomes globular and firm
    b. Avoiding excessive traction on cord prevents complications
       i. Cord avulsion would require manual removal of placenta
      ii. Uterine inversion would require manual replacement of fundus
    c. Atony: absence of uterine muscle tone resulting in hemorrhage
       i. Risk factors: prolonged labor, overdistention of uterus, use of magnesium sulfate
      ii. Often associated with retained placental fragments
     iii. Treated with uterine massage and uterotonic medications
    d. Lacerations: vaginal, perineal, and cervical
  4. 4th stage: greatest risk for complications during 1st hour postpartum

VI. Labor Induction

  A. Benefits of delivery for either mother or baby outweigh those of continuing pregnancy
  B. **Bishop score:** scoring system used to predict success of induction (Table 10.2)
    1. Low scores: "unfavorable cervix"; would benefit from cervical ripening
      a. Medical ripening using prostaglandins
      b. Mechanical ripening using dilators or Foley bulb
      c. "Membrane sweeping" to free amniotic membranes from surrounding cervix
    2. High scores: "favorable cervix"
      a. Amniotomy
      b. IV Pitocin infusion

VII. Cesarean Delivery

  A. Maternal mortality rate is 2–4 times the rate associated with vaginal delivery
  B. Indications: placenta previa, placental abruption, umbilical cord prolapse, arrest of labor, nonreassuring fetal status, breech presentation
  C. Types
    1. Low transverse: incision in lower uterine segment
    2. Classical: vertical incision in upper contractile uterine segment

Normal Labor and Delivery

TABLE **10.2** **Bishop Score**				
	Points[a]			
Factor	**0**	**1**	**2**	**3**
Dilation (cm)	0	1–2	3–4	5 or greater
Effacement (%)	0–30	40–50	60–70	80 or greater
Station	−3	−2, −1	0	+1 or lower
Consistency	Firm	Medium	Soft	
Position	Posterior	Mid	Anterior	

[a]Used to predict need for cervical ripening and successful induction. Scores of ≤4 benefit from cervical ripening and have lower rates for successful elective induction.

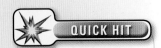

Elective repeat or maternal request Cesarean delivery should only be performed after 39 weeks' gestation or with documented fetal lung maturity.

D. Disadvantages
   1. Higher rate of hemorrhage and transfusion
   2. Higher rate of infection
   3. Longer, more painful recovery
   4. Increased risk of previa, accreta, and hysterectomy with subsequent pregnancy

VIII. Vaginal Birth After Cesarean Delivery

A. Risk of uterine rupture <1% with spontaneous labor
B. Candidate selection for trial of labor after Cesarean delivery (Box 10.1)
C. Facility requirements
   1. 24-hour blood bank
   2. Continuous external fetal monitoring
   3. In-house anesthesia
   4. Physician capable of performing Cesarean delivery
   5. 30-minute "decision-to-incision" window if Cesarean delivery is necessary

---

BOX 10.1

Clinical Considerations in Vaginal Birth After Cesarean Delivery

Criteria useful in identifying candidates for TOLAC
Patient
- One previous low transverse Cesarean delivery
- Clinically adequate pelvis
- No other uterine scars or previous ruptures
- Desires trial of labor

Facility/Physician
- Physician immediately available throughout active labor who is capable of performing a Cesarean delivery
- Availability of anesthesia, facility, and personnel for emergent Cesarean delivery

Circumstances under which a TOLAC should not be attempted
Patient
- Previous classical or T-shaped uterine incision or extensive transfundal uterine surgery
- Previous uterine rupture
- Medical or obstetric complications that precludes vaginal delivery

Facility/Physician
- Lack of anesthesia, facility, or personnel for an emergent Cesarean delivery

(Adapted from Beckmann CRB, Ling FW, et al. *Obstetrics and Gynecology*, 7th ed. Baltimore: Lippincott Williams & Wilkins; 2014.)

Normal Labor and Delivery

Intrapartum Fetal Surveillance

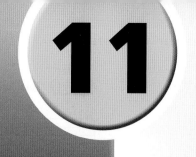

I. Pathophysiology

A. Uteroplacental unit
  1. Transports oxygen and nutrients to fetus
  2. Receives carbon dioxide and wastes from fetus
B. Uteroplacental insufficiency
  1. Compromised uteroplacental unit
    a. Fetal hypoxia
    b. Blood shunted to fetal heart, brain, and adrenal glands
    c. Observation of late decelerations of fetal heart rate (FHR)
    d. Metabolic acidosis
      i. Accumulation of lactic acid
      ii. Can lead to brain and cardiac damage
  2. May progress to fetal compromise or death if no intervention
C. Neonatal encephalopathy
  1. Abnormal neurologic function in term infant
    a. Difficulty initiating or maintaining respiration
    b. Depressed tone and reflexes
    c. Abnormal level of consciousness
    d. Seizures
  2. Hypoxic-ischemic encephalopathy (HIE)
    a. Subtype of neonatal encephalopathy
    b. Decreased oxygen and blood flow surrounding time of birth
    c. Incidence of HIE = 1.6/10,000
D. Cerebral palsy
  1. Central nervous system (CNS) disability
  2. Movement and posture control is aberrant
  3. Spastic quadriplegia possibly associated with decreased fetal blood supply

II. Intrapartum Fetal Heart Rate Monitoring

A. FHR patterns
  1. Baseline FHR
    a. Mean FHR over 10-minute period of time rounded to nearest 5 beat per minute (bpm) increment
    b. Minimum baseline duration: 2 minutes over 10 minutes
    c. Excludes periods of marked FHR variability
    d. Normal FHR baseline: 110–160 bpm
      i. Bradycardia: baseline <110 bpm
      ii. Tachycardia: baseline >160 bpm
  2. Baseline variability
    a. Fluctuation in FHR of >2 cycles per minute
    b. Quantified by visualizing amplitude from peak to trough (Figure 11.1)

Fetal heart rate variability.

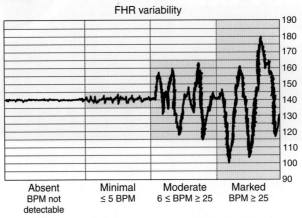

(From Beckmann CRB, Ling FW, et al. *Obstetrics and Gynecology*, 7th ed. Baltimore: Lippincott Williams & Wilkins; 2014.)

c. Etiologies for decreased FHR variability
   i. Fetal hypoxia or acidemia
   ii. Maternal narcotic use
   iii. Fetal anomaly (cardiac, CNS)
   iv. Prematurity
   v. Fetal sleep cycle
d. Moderate variability is reassuring
   i. Suggests sufficient fetal oxygenation
   ii. Normal fetal brain function

3. **Accelerations**
   a. Abrupt increase in FHR (30 seconds or less from onset to peak)
   b. Duration = time from onset to time of return to baseline
      i. Prolonged acceleration lasts 2–10 minutes
      ii. Considered baseline change if lasts >10 minutes
   c. Prior to 32 weeks: acceleration = 10 bpm above baseline and lasts for >10 seconds
   d. After 32 weeks: acceleration = 15 bpm above baseline and lasts for at least 15 seconds
   e. Associated with reassuring fetal status

4. **Decelerations** (Box 11.1)
   a. Definitions
      i. **Periodic decelerations**: associated with uterine contractions
      ii. **Episodic decelerations**: not associated with uterine contractions
      iii. **Recurrent decelerations**: occur with >50% of contractions during 20-minute period
      iv. **Intermittent decelerations**: occur with <50% of contractions during 20-minute period
   b. Early decelerations (Figure 11.2A)
      i. Caused by fetal head compression
      ii. Vagal nerve is stimulated, leading to acetylcholinesterase release at sinoatrial node
      iii. Considered physiologic
   c. Late decelerations (see Figure 11.2B)
      i. Nonreassuring, especially when recurrent or coupled with decreased FHR variability
      ii. Associated with uteroplacental insufficiency
         (a) Diminished uterine perfusion
         (b) Diminished placental function

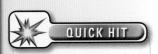

Normal FHR variability suggests adequate oxygenation and normal brain function.

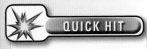

Accelerations in FHR may vary with gestational age.

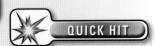

Early decelerations (onset of deceleration same as onset of contraction) are associated with fetal head compression.

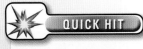

Late decelerations suggest uteroplacental insufficiency.

Intrapartum Fetal Surveillance

BOX 11.1

Characteristics of Decelerations

Late Deceleration

- Visually apparent, usually symmetric, *gradual* decrease, and return of the fetal heart rate (FHR) associated with a uterine contraction.
- A *gradual* FHR decrease is defined as from the onset to the FHR nadir of ≥30 seconds.
- The decrease in FHR is calculated from the onset to the nadir of the deceleration.
- The deceleration is delayed in timing, with the nadir of the deceleration occurring after the peak of the contraction.
- In most cases, the onset, nadir, and recovery of the deceleration occur after the beginning, peak, and ending of the contraction, respectively.

Early Deceleration

- Visually apparent, usually symmetric, *gradual* decrease, and return of the FHR associated with a uterine contraction.
- A *gradual* FHR decrease is defined as from the onset to the FHR nadir of ≥30 seconds.
- The decrease in FHR is calculated from the onset to the nadir of the deceleration.
- The nadir of the deceleration occurs at the same time as the peak of the contraction.
- In most cases, the onset, nadir, and recovery of the deceleration are coincident with the beginning, peak, and ending of the contraction, respectively.

Variable Deceleration

- Visually apparent *abrupt* decrease in FHR.
- An *abrupt* FHR decrease is defined as from the onset of the deceleration to the beginning of the FHR nadir of <30 seconds.
- The decrease in FHR is calculated from the onset to the nadir of the deceleration.
- The decrease in FHR is ≥15 bpm, lasts ≥15 seconds, and is <2 minutes in duration.
- When variable decelerations are associated with uterine contractions, their onset, depth, and duration commonly vary with successive contractions.

(From Macones GA, Hankins GDV, Spong CY, et al. The 2008 National Institute of Child Health and Human Development workshop report on electronic fetal monitoring: update on definitions, interpretation, and research guidelines. *J Obstet Gynecol Neonatal Nurs.* 2008;*37*[5]:510–515.)

FIGURE 11.2 (A–C) Fetal heart rate patterns.

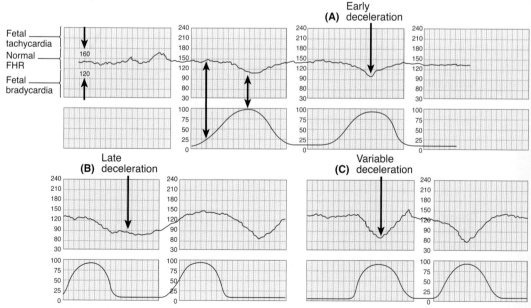

(From Beckmann CRB, Ling FW, et al. *Obstetrics and Gynecology*, 7th ed. Baltimore: Lippincott Williams & Wilkins; 2014.)

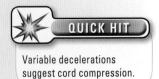

    d. Variable decelerations (see Figure 11.2C)
      i. Associated with umbilical cord compression
      ii. Associated with oligohydramnios
      iii. Most common periodic FHR pattern
      iv. Often resolve with maternal position changes
      v. Amnioinfusion can be used to manage oligohydramnios

B. FHR classification (see Box 11.2)
  1. Category I
    a. Predictive of normal fetal acid–base status
    b. Continue routine care
  2. Category II
    a. Not predictive of abnormal fetal acid–base status
    b. Warrants close surveillance and repeat assessment
  3. Category III
    a. Predictive of abnormal fetal acid–base status
    b. Requires evaluation and intervention to resolve

BOX 11.2

Three-Tier Fetal Heart Rate Interpretation System

Category I

Category I fetal heart rate (FHR) tracings include all *of the following:*
- Baseline rate: 110–160 bpm
- Baseline FHR variability: moderate
- Late or variable decelerations: absent
- Early decelerations: present or absent
- Accelerations: present or absent

Category II

Category II FHR tracings include all FHR tracings not categorized as category I or category III. Category II tracings may represent an appreciable fraction of those encountered in clinical care. Examples of category II FHR tracings include any of the following:

Baseline Rate
- Bradycardia not accompanied by absent baseline variability
- Tachycardia

Baseline FHR Variability
- Minimal baseline variability
- Absent baseline variability not accompanied by recurrent decelerations
- Marked baseline variability

Accelerations
- Absence of induced accelerations after fetal stimulation

Periodic or Episodic Decelerations
- Recurrent variable decelerations accompanied by minimal or moderate baseline variability
- Prolonged deceleration ≥2 minutes but <10 minutes
- Recurrent late decelerations with moderate baseline variability
- Variable decelerations with other characteristics, such as slow return to baseline, "overshoots," or "shoulders"

Category III

Category III FHR tracings include either:
- Absent baseline FHR variability and any of the following:
  - Recurrent late decelerations
  - Recurrent variable decelerations
  - Bradycardia
- Sinusoidal pattern

(From Macones GA, Hankins GDV, Spong CY, et al. The 2008 National Institute of Child Health and Human Development workshop report on electronic fetal monitoring: update on definitions, interpretation, and research guidelines. *J Obstet Gynecol Neonatal Nurs.* 2008;*37*[5]:510–515.)

C. Intrapartum fetal monitoring guidelines
   1. Low risk
      a. 1st stage (active phase): evaluate FHR every 30 minutes following contraction
      b. 2nd stage: evaluate FHR every 15 minutes
   2. High risk
      a. 1st stage (active phase): evaluate FHR every 15 minutes following contraction
      b. 2nd stage: evaluate FHR a minimum of every 5 minutes

III. Ancillary Tests

A. Fetal stimulation
   1. Scalp stimulation
   2. Evaluate for presence of acceleration
   3. Fetal acidosis unlikely if acceleration following stimulation
B. Fetal blood pH determination: use has decreased in recent years
C. Pulse oximetry
   1. Use has not decreased rate of Cesarean delivery
   2. Not used in clinical practice

IV. Management of Nonreassuring Fetal Heart Rate Pattern

A. Maternal position change
B. Administer oxygen by face mask
C. Evaluate maternal blood pressure and treat hypotension
D. Evaluate for uterine hyperstimulation
   1. Discontinue Pitocin
   2. Consider administration of terbutaline
E. Perform cervical examination
F. Proceed with delivery if persistent nonreassuring FHR

V. Meconium

A. Tarry, thick, black substance from fetal intestinal tract
B. Meconium aspiration syndrome
   1. Fetus inhales meconium-stained amniotic fluid
   2. Occurs in 6% of births with meconium present
   3. Upper airway suctioning should be performed after delivery

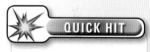

> **QUICK HIT**
>
> Persistent nonreassuring FHR suggests that delivery should be expedited.

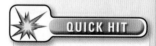

> **QUICK HIT**
>
> Passage of meconium in utero can be a sign of fetal stress.

Intrapartum Fetal Surveillance

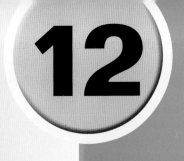

12 Immediate Care of Newborn

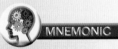

APGAR scoring system
Appearance (body color)
Pulse (heart rate)
Grimace (reflex/irritability)
Activity (muscle/grasp)
Respiration (breathing rate)

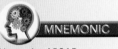

Alternative APGAR memory tool:
"Hurry, Rapidly Resuscitate
My Child"
Heart rate
Reflexes
Respirations
Muscle tone
Color

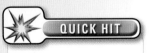

The 1-minute Apgar score
determines whether a new-
born requires increased
attention.

I. Initial Care of Well Newborn

A. Initial neonatal assessment
   1. Reassuring characteristics
      a. Full term
      b. Clear amniotic fluid; no meconium or purulent fluid
      c. Spontaneous breathing/crying
      d. Good muscle tone
   2. Postdelivery gestational age assessment: Ballard scoring system
      (Figure 12.1)
      a. Points (-1 to 5) assigned for neuromuscular and physical maturity
      b. Scale is -10 (20 weeks' estimated gestational age) to 50 (44 weeks'
         estimated gestational age)
   3. Assessment of newborn status: Apgar scoring system (Table 12.1)
      a. 5 signs (color, heart rate, reflex activity, muscle tone, respirations) assigned
         0, 1, or 2 points per category
      b. Scores assigned at 1 and 5 minutes and then every additional 5 minutes
         up to 20 minutes if initial 5-minute score <7
         i. Score 7–10: infant requires no active resuscitation
         ii. Score 4–6: mildly to moderately depressed infant
         iii. Score <4: severely depressed infant
      c. Rule of thumb
         i. 1-minute Apgar determines need for resuscitation
         ii. 5-minute Apgar used to evaluate effectiveness of that resuscitation or
             whether more management is needed

B. Routine care following delivery
   1. Maintenance of temperature
      a. Drying infant
      b. Skin-to-skin contact with mother
      c. Use of warm blankets
      d. Radiant warmers
   2. Vital sign assessment: temperature, pulse, respirations, core/peripheral color,
      tone, and alertness assessed every 30 minutes after birth until stable for
      2 hours
   3. Management of umbilical cord following clamping/cutting
      a. Left exposed to air to facilitate drying
      b. Application of topical antimicrobial agents
      c. Blackened, dried stump sloughs off 3–5 days postpartum

II. Transitional Care of Newborn

A. Indicators of potential neonatal instability
   1. Temperature instability
   2. Excessive lethargy or somnolence
   3. Refusal to feed

The Ballard score.

Neuromuscular maturity

	−1	0	1	2	3	4	5
Posture							
Square window (wrist)	>90°	90°	60°	45°	30°	0°	
Arm recoil		180°	140°–180°	110°–140°	90°–110°	<90°	
Popliteal angle	180°	160°	140°	120°	100°	90°	<90°
Scarf sign							
Heel to ear							

Physical maturity

Skin	Sticky friable, transparent	Gelatinous red, translucent	Smooth pink, visible veins	Superficial peeling or rash or both, few veins	Cracking pale areas, rare veins	Parchment deep cracking, no vessels	Leathery, cracked, wrinkled
Lanugo	None	Sparse	Abundant	Thinning	Bald areas	Mostly bald	
Plantar surface	Heel-toe 40–50 mm: −1 <40 mm: −2	<50 mm, no crease	Faint red marks	Anterior transverse crease only	Creases on anterior 2/3	Creases over entire sole	
Breast	Imperceptible	Barely perceptible	Flat areola, no bud	Stripped areola, 1–2 mm bud	Raised areola, 3–4 mm bud	Full areola, 5–10 mm bud	
Eye/ear	Lids fused loosely (−1) tightly (−2)	Lids open, pinna flat, stays folded	Slightly curved pinna, soft, slow recoil	Well curved pinna, soft but ready recoil	Formed and firm, instant recoil	Thick cartilage, ear stiff	
Genitals male	Scrotum flat, smooth	Scrotum empty, faint rugae	Testes in upper canal rare rugae	Testes descending, few rugae	Testes down, good rugae	Testes pendulous deep rugae	
Genitals female	Clitoris prominent, labia flat	Prominent clitoris, small labia minora	Prominent clitoris, enlarged minora	Majora and minora equally prominent	Majora large, minora small	Majora cover clitoris and minora	

A

Maturity rating

Score	Weeks
−10	20
-5	22
0	24
5	26
10	28
15	30
20	32
25	34
30	36
35	38
40	40
45	42
50	44

B

(A) The Ballard scoring system uses points assigned to observations about neuromuscular maturity and physical maturity. (B) The points are summed yielding a score used to arrive at an estimated age in weeks. (From American Academy of Pediatrics, American College of Obstetricians and Gynecologists. *Guidelines for Perinatal Care*, 6th ed. Washington, DC: American College of Obstetricians and Gynecologists; 2007:216–217. Original source: Ballard JL, Khoury JC, Wedig K, et al. New Ballard Score expanded to include extremely premature infants. *J Pediatr*. 1991;*119*[3]:417–423.)

Immediate Care of Newborn

TABLE 12.1	Apgar Scoring System		
Sign	**0**	**1**	**2**
Color	Blue or pale	Acrocyanotic	Completely pink
Heart rate	Absent	<100 bpm	>100 bpm
Reflex activity response to stimulation	No response	Grimace	Cry or active withdrawal
Muscle tone	Limp	Some flexion	Active motion
Respirations	Absent	Weak cry; hypoventilation	Good, crying

bpm, beats per minute.

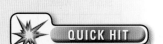

QUICK HIT

If the infant does not pass stool, rule out imperforate anus, meconium ileus, and Hirschsprung disease.

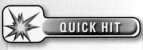

QUICK HIT

Vitamin D prophylaxis is given as a parenteral dose of vitamin K1 oxide following delivery and *should be given within the 1st hour of life.*

4. Abnormal cardiac/respiratory effort
5. Cyanosis
6. Delayed voiding
   a. Should occur within 24 hours of life
   b. If no voiding, work up for obstruction
7. Delayed/abnormal stools
   a. 90% of infants pass stool within 1st 24 hours of life
   b. Stool should appear greenish brown and tar-like for 1st few days of life until regular ingestion of milk
B. Prophylactic treatments
   1. Gonococcal ophthalmia neonatorum
      a. Bacterial conjunctivitis that manifests in 1st 5 days of life
      b. Contracted by infant during delivery
      c. Prophylactic antibiotic ointment (erythromycin or tetracycline) to both eyes following delivery
         i. Recommended regardless of route of delivery
         ii. Should be administered within 1st hour of life
   2. Vitamin K–dependent hemorrhagic disease of newborn
      a. Reasons for newborn vitamin K deficiency
         i. Low vitamin K stores at birth
         ii. Vitamin K passes poorly through placenta
         iii. Absence of gut flora important in production of vitamin K
      b. Sites of bleeding: umbilicus, mucous membranes, gastrointestinal tract, circumcision, venipunctures
C. Neonatal circumcision
   1. Definition: elective surgical removal of distal foreskin
   2. Procedure
      a. Usually performed within 48 hours of life; may be cultural/religious variations in timing and location of procedure
      b. Use of local anesthetic (ring block or dorsal penile nerve block)
      c. Use of specialized surgical devices (Gomco, Plastibell, Mogen clamps)
   3. Complications rare (infection, bleeding)
D. Neonatal jaundice (hyperbilirubinemia)
   1. Etiology
      a. Physiologic
         i. Typically presents days 3–4 of life and resolves by 2 weeks
         ii. Increased red blood cell (RBC) turnover due to fetal RBC destruction (shorter lifespan)
         iii. Decreased hepatic excretory function in the newborn
         iv. Breast milk jaundice: breast milk components may lead to uncoupling of bilirubin → reabsorption → jaundice
         v. Breast-nonfeeding jaundice: inadequate fluid and nutrient intake → increased enterohepatic circulation → jaundice

b. Pathologic
   i. Presentation within 24 hours of life or present beyond 2 weeks of life
   ii. Hemolytic disease of newborn
   iii. Structural defects (e.g., biliary atresia)
   iv. Genetic defects in bilirubin conversion and conjugation (e.g., Gilbert and Crigler-Najjar syndromes)
2. Assessment: identify those at high risk for hyperbilirubinemia and assess in 1 of 2 ways
   a. Total serum bilirubin or transcutaneous bilirubin: if jaundice within 24 hours of life
   b. Screen based on clinical risk factors that are predictive of severe hyperbilirubinemia (e.g., preterm *versus* term birth)
3. Complications: acute bilirubin encephalopathy (kernicterus)
   a. 1.5/100,000 live births in United States
   b. Associated with total serum bilirubin >30 mg/dL
4. Treatment of hyperbilirubinemia
   a. Phototherapy
   b. Exchange transfusion

III. Initial Care of the Newborn

A. Resuscitation
   1. Risk factors: prematurity, low birth weight, nonreassuring fetal testing, fetal anomalies, birth trauma, asphyxia
   2. Diagnosis of ill newborn
      a. Initial assessment (as outlined previously in normal newborn)
         i. Provide warmth: dry infant and remove wet towels
         ii. Provide gentle stimulation: rub back, flick soles of feet
         iii. Position infant and clear airway
         iv. Assess respiratory effort, pulse, tone, color
      b. Infants requiring additional resuscitation
         i. Respiratory effort: difficulty breathing (retractions), apnea
         ii. Pulse: <100 or absent
         iii. Color: cyanosis
         iv. Muscle tone: absent or lacking
   3. Resuscitation: "ABCs" (Figure 12.2)
      a. Airway: open airway, suction nose and mouth, position head in "sniffing position"
      b. Breathing
         i. Apnea → provide positive pressure ventilation
         ii. Consider maternal narcotic use: if administered during course of labor → administer naloxone (narcotic antagonist)
         iii. Consider endotracheal intubation (Figure 12.3A,B)
      c. Cardiovascular
         i. Pulse <100 → provide positive pressure ventilation
         ii. Pulse <60 despite positive pressure ventilation → chest compressions
         iii. Pulse <60 despite ventilation and chest compression → administer epinephrine
         iv. If evidence of hypovolemia, administer normal saline (10 mL/kg)
B. Umbilical cord blood gases
   1. Purpose
      a. Assessment of fetal acid–base status by measurement of pH, PO_2, PCO_2, HCO_3, and base deficit from cord blood obtained following delivery
      b. Most important assessment is umbilical artery blood gas
         i. Measure blood metabolized by fetus as it travels back to placenta
         ii. Obtaining arterial and venous pH (paired specimen) recommended to prevent debate of measurements

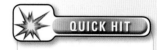

QUICK HIT

Ten percent of neonates require some resuscitative effort, and 1% require major resuscitation.

Immediate Care of Newborn

FIGURE 12.2 Algorithm for newborn resuscitation.

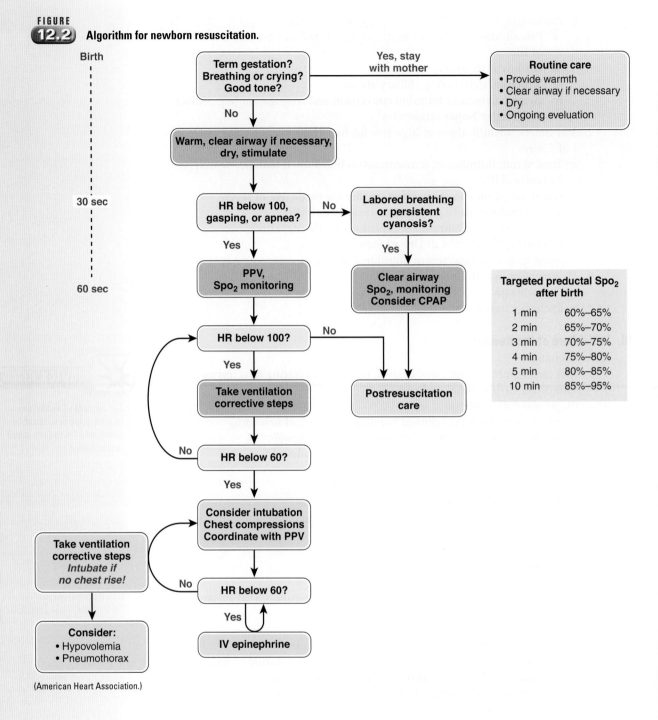

(American Heart Association.)

2. Indications
   a. Low 5-minute Apgar score
      i. Segment of umbilical cord is double-clamped, cut, and placed on delivery table
      ii. Send to lab depending on neonatal assessment
   b. Nonreassuring fetal heart rate tracing was indication for Cesarean delivery
   c. Intrauterine growth restriction
   d. Intrapartum fever or intra-amniotic infection
   e. Prematurity
   f. Multifetal gestation
3. Acidemia: pH <7.20 (Table 12.2)
4. Fetal asphyxia: metabolic acidosis (base deficit >12 mmol/L)
   a. Impaired blood gas exchange leading to progressive hypoxemia and hypercapnia

TABLE **12.2** Normal Umbilical Cord Blood Gas Values		
	Arterial	**Venous**
pH	7.25–7.30	7.30–7.40
Pco_2 (mm Hg)	50	40
Po_2 (mm Hg)	20	30
HCO_3 (mEq/L)	25	20

     b. 10% and 40% of neonates with base deficit of 12–16 mmol/L and >16 mmol/L respectively will have moderate to severe complications (encephalopathy, cardiovascular and respiratory complications)

C. Cord blood banking
   1. May be used for future autologous transplant
   2. Remote chance: 1/2,700

IV. Newborn Screening

A. Designed to detect infants with conditions that benefit from early diagnosis and intervention (e.g., phenylketonuria, hypothyroidism, galactosemia, hemoglobinopathies, cystic fibrosis)

B. Blood sample obtained at 24 hours of life (if obtained earlier, may require additional samples)

C. Individual states may include different tests as part of screen

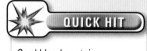

QUICK HIT

Cord blood contains hematopoietic stem cells.

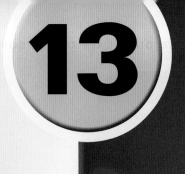
13 Abnormal Labor and Malpresentation

I. Definitions

A. Normal labor: uterine contractions that lead to cervical change—both dilation and effacement
1. 1st stage: from onset of labor to complete dilation (10 cm) and effacement
   a. Latent phase: initial phase of slow cervical dilation and effacement (usually until 3–4 cm of dilation, although this is controversial)
   b. Active phase: more rapid cervical dilation and fetal descent
2. 2nd stage: from complete dilation to delivery of fetus
3. 3rd stage: delivery of placenta
B. Abnormal labor (**labor dystocia**): literally "difficult labor"
1. Any abnormal progression of labor in cervical dilation or fetal descent
2. Diagnostic criteria requiring intervention are variable, making management challenging
3. Leading indication for Cesarean delivery in United States

II. Labor Dystocia: Assessing 3 Ps

A. Power: strength of uterine contractions or maternal pushing effort
1. Methods to monitor contractions
   a. Palpation: assess frequency and subjective intensity
   b. External tocodynamometry: external strain gauge used to assess frequency and duration
   c. Intrauterine pressure catheter (IUPC): assess frequency, duration, and measures uterine pressure in mm Hg
2. "Optimal" contractions determined by frequency and intensity
   a. Optimal frequency: at least 3 contractions in 10 minutes
   b. Optimal intensity (measured by IUPC): 50–60 mm Hg per contraction or Montevideo unit (MVU) >200 mm Hg
3. More is not always better: time between contractions allows fetus to receive unrestricted blood flow from placenta, which reduces risk of fetal heart rate (FHR) abnormalities
B. Passenger: assess fetal weight, lie, presentation, and position
1. Fetal weight
   a. Weight >4,000–4,500 g increases risk for labor dystocia and shoulder dystocia
   b. Difficult to predict: estimated fetal weight (EFW) by ultrasound at term can be +/− 500–1,000 g
2. Fetal lie: relationship between long axis of mother and long axis of fetus; transverse lie requires Cesarean delivery
3. Fetal presentation
   a. Cephalic: vertex, brow, face, chin
   b. Breech: frank, complete, incomplete, single/double footling (Figure 13.1A–C)
   c. Shoulder: usually requires Cesarean delivery
   d. Compound: most commonly hand next to head

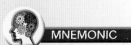

The 3 Ps
Power: contractions and maternal pushing effort
Passenger: fetal factors
Passage: maternal pelvis

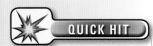

To calculate MVUs, add the total intensity of contractions from baseline (mm Hg) over 10 minutes.

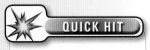

Brow presentation (1:3,000 deliveries) usually converts to vertex or face, but, if not, it can lead to labor dystocia. **Face presentation** (1:600 deliveries) requires Cesarean delivery unless the mentum (fetal chin) is anterior (toward the maternal abdomen).

FIGURE 13.1 Breech presentation.

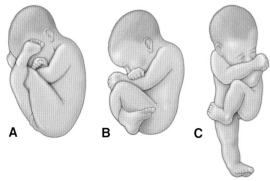

(A) Frank breech. (B) Complete breech. (C) Single footling breech. (From Beckmann CRB, Ling FW, et al. *Obstetrics and Gynecology*, 7th ed. Baltimore: Lippincott Williams & Wilkins; 2014.)

4. Fetal position: determined by relationship of fetal occiput (in vertex) or sacrum (in breech) to maternal abdomen (Figure 13.2)
   a. Occiput anterior: occiput is closest to maternal abdomen (most common position)
   b. Occiput posterior: occiput is closest to maternal back; increased risk of longer labors and disorders of fetal descent
   c. Occiput transverse: occiput is either to maternal left or right

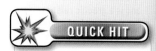

QUICK HIT

Fetal anomalies such as fetal hydrops or soft tissue tumors can lead to labor dystocia. Usually, ultrasound can detect these anomalies to plan a mode of delivery.

FIGURE 13.2 Fetal position in the cephalic presentation.

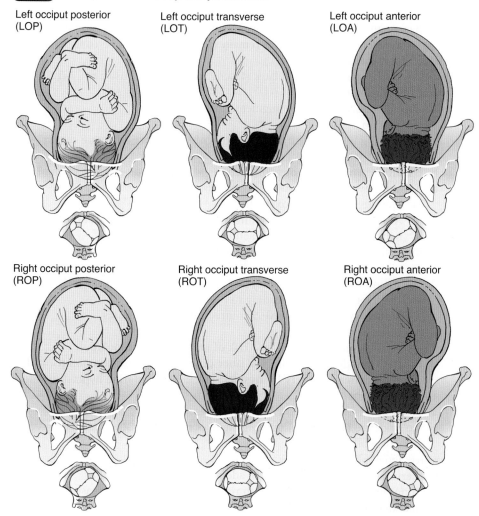

Left occiput posterior (LOP)

Left occiput transverse (LOT)

Left occiput anterior (LOA)

Right occiput posterior (ROP)

Right occiput transverse (ROT)

Right occiput anterior (ROA)

Klossner NJ, Hatfield N. *Introductory Maternity and Pediatric Nursing.* Philadelphia: Lippincott Williams & Wilkins; 2005.

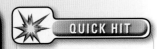

QUICK HIT

Risks associated with labor dystocia include infection (chorioamnionitis) related to prolonged labor, operative vaginal delivery, and Cesarean delivery.

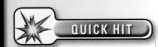

QUICK HIT

The **Friedman curve** is used to describe "normal" labor and is a graphic relationship between cervical dilation, fetal descent, and time.

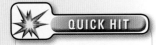

QUICK HIT

Amniotomy and oxytocin used in combination early in active labor may decrease length of labor by 2 hours with no change to the Cesarean delivery rate.

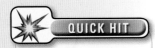

QUICK HIT

Continuous labor support *decreases* need for pain medications, oxytocin, operative/Cesarean deliveries, and low fetal Apgar scores and *increases* maternal satisfaction.

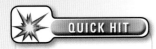

QUICK HIT

Cesarean delivery is indicated for nonreassuring maternal or fetal indications. Operative vaginal deliveries *cannot* be performed in the first stage of labor.

C. Passage: includes both bony structures and soft tissue of maternal pelvis
  1. Cephalopelvic disproportion (CPD): seen with small maternal pelvis
    a. Prevents presenting part from descending into pelvis
    b. Usually determined retrospectively in labor when fetal descent is inadequate
  2. Clinical pelvimetry: uses specific landmarks during pelvic exam to characterize maternal pelvis
    a. Poor predictor of successful vaginal births
    b. May be helpful if pelvis is found to be "completely contracted"
  3. Radiographic and computed tomography measurements of minimal use for CPD

III. Diagnosis and Management of Labor Dystocia

A. Categories of labor abnormalities
  1. Protraction disorders: slow progress either in latent or active labor
  2. Arrest disorders: cessation of labor; only used in active phase
B. Management of labor dystocia is to assess 3Ps
  1. Power: adequate uterine contractions?
  2. Passenger: evidence of fetal malpresentation or CPD? FHR reassuring?
  3. Passage: any maternal factors inhibiting labor?
C. Management options: observation, augmentation, operative vaginal or Cesarean delivery

IV. First-Stage Labor Disorders

A. Protracted or prolonged latent phase: >20 hours in nulliparous patients or >14 hours in multiparous patients
  1. Often diagnosed in patients who may really be in "false labor"
  2. Does not predict abnormalities with active phase of labor; not considered dangerous for either mother or fetus
  3. Management: observation or intravenous sedation; patient will stop contracting *or* progress to active labor *or* remain in latent labor and be considered for labor augmentation
B. Protracted active phase: cervix dilates <1 cm/hr for nulliparous or <1.2–1.5 cm/hr for multiparous patients
  1. Management: observation *or* augmentation
  2. Augmentation
    a. Stimulating uterine contractions sufficient to produce adequate cervical dilation or fetal descent
    b. Usually when spontaneous contractions <3/hr or intensity is <25 mmHg
    c. **Amniotomy:** artificially rupturing membranes
      i. May negate need for oxytocin
      ii. Allows fetal head to be dilating force and release prostaglandins, which help increase force of contractions
      iii. Risks: FHR changes from cord compression, cord prolapse, chorioamnionitis (if labor is prolonged after rupture)
    d. Oxytocin: to increase frequency and strength of contractions while avoiding uterine hyperstimulation leading to FHR changes
      i. Titrate oxytocin to achieve 5 contractions in 10 minutes
      ii. Different regimens
        (a) Low-dose oxytocin = ↓ risk of uterine hyperstimulation
        (b) High-dose oxytocin = ↓ labor time, risk of chorioamnionitis, and Cesarean delivery for dystocia *but* ↑ risk of uterine hyperstimulation
  3. Continuous labor support
    a. From nurses, midwives, or lay individuals
    b. No evidence that level of training changes benefits or that there are any risks to mother and fetus
C. Arrested active phase
  1. No cervical change after 2 hours of adequate uterine contractions
  2. Waiting up to 4 or more hours with reassuring fetal status increases rate of vaginal delivery without fetal complications

V. Second-Stage Labor Disorders

A. Protracted 2nd stage
1. In nullipara = >3 hours with epidural *or* >2 hours without epidural
2. In multipara = >2 hours with epidural *or* >1 hour without epidural *or* fetus descends <1 cm/hr without epidural

B. Arrested 2nd stage: no fetal descent after 1 hour of pushing

C. Management of 2nd-stage disorders
1. If insufficient uterine contractions and CPD ruled out with reassuring fetal heart tones, start or increase oxytocin
2. Facilitate maternal pushing with position change from dorsal lithotomy to knee–chest, sitting, squatting, or birth chair
3. Increase tone of pelvic floor muscles by decreasing rate of epidural anesthesia
4. If fetal position is occiput posterior, consider manual rotation to assist fetal descent
5. Operative vaginal or Cesarean delivery

D. **Shoulder dystocia**: entrapment of anterior fetal shoulder by bony pelvis (symphysis) after delivery of head
1. Cannot be predicted or prevented
2. Certain conditions do increase risk: multiparity, postterm fetus, previous history of macrosomia, or shoulder dystocia
3. Interventions aimed at dislodging fetal shoulder without excessive traction
   a. **McRoberts maneuver**
      i. Maternal hips hyperflexed to increase anteroposterior (AP) diameter; usually accompanied by downward suprapubic pressure
      ii. Fundal pressure is *contraindicated* and can worsen dystocia
   b. Fetal maneuvers
      i. Rotating impacted shoulder
      ii. Delivering posterior arm
      iii. Manually fracturing clavicle
   c. Zavanelli maneuver: fetus pushed back into uterus prior to Cesarean delivery
4. Brachial plexus injuries occur in 4%–40% of shoulder dystocia cases
   a. Possibly related to traction on fetal head in attempt to deliver shoulder
   b. <10% associated with permanent injury

VI. Operative Vaginal Deliveries

A. Application of direct traction on fetal head = 10%–15% of all deliveries
B. Capability for immediate Cesarean delivery if operative vaginal delivery fails (associated with worse fetal outcome)
C. Risk of intracranial hemorrhage similar for vacuum or forceps
D. Classification: based on fetal station at time of vacuum or forceps delivery
1. Outlet delivery: +4 station = scalp visible at introitus without separating labia
   a. Fetal skull on pelvic floor and fetal head at or on perineum
   b. Sagittal suture is in AP diameter or right or left of midline <45°

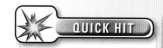

QUICK HIT

Time in second stage is not an absolute indication for Cesarean delivery if fetal heart tones are reassuring and CPD has been ruled out.

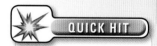

QUICK HIT

"Turtle sign" occurs when the delivered head retracts against the perineum and may be a sign of shoulder dystocia.

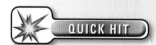

QUICK HIT

Fetal station is the relationship between the leading part of the fetal head and the maternal ischial spine (Figure 13.3).

FIGURE 13.3 Fetal station: relation of leading fetal part to maternal ischial spine.

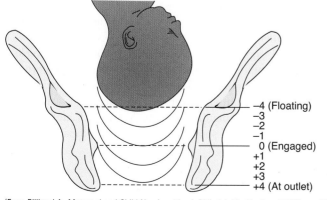

(From Pillitteri A. *Maternal and Child Nursing*, 4th ed. Philadelphia: Lippincott Williams & Wilkins; 2003.)

2. Low delivery: +2 station = leading point is *not* on pelvic floor; includes rotation both < and >45°
   3. Midpelvis delivery: between 0 and +2 station = performed under rare conditions while preparations are made for immediate Cesarean delivery
E. Criteria for operative delivery
   1. Fetal position known and fetal head at appropriate station
   2. Cervix fully dilated and membranes ruptured
   3. Fetus <34 weeks = vacuum avoided due to risk of intraventricular hemorrhage
   4. Contraindicated for fetus with bone demineralization (osteogenesis imperfecta) or bleeding disorders (hemophilia or von Willebrand disease)
F. Indications for operative delivery
   1. Prolonged or arrested 2nd stage
   2. Risk of deterioration of fetal well-being
   3. Shortening 2nd stage for maternal benefit
G. Forceps delivery: provides direct traction on fetal skull in conjunction with maternal effort; occasionally used to rotate fetus
   1. Different forceps used depending on molding of fetal head or presenting part
   2. Maternal complications: perineal trauma, hematoma, pelvic floor injury
   3. Fetal complications: musculoskeletal, brain, spine injury; facial bruising; corneal abrasions due to incorrect placement
H. Vacuum delivery: soft cup vacuum applies traction to fetal skull using mechanical pump
   1. Maternal complications: fewer compared to forceps delivery
   2. Fetal complications
      a. Intracranial hemorrhage, subgaleal hematoma, scalp laceration, hyperbilirubinemia, retinal hemorrhage, and cephalohematoma
      b. Overall rate = 5%
   3. Avoid excessive torque or rocking motion during operative delivery

VII. Breech Presentation

A. 2% of singleton deliveries at term
B. Diagnosed through Leopold maneuvers, pelvic examination, and ultrasound
C. Increased risk of fetal and maternal morbidity and mortality regardless of mode of delivery for breech compared to cephalic presentations
D. External cephalic version (ECV): pressure on maternal abdomen to turn fetus into vertex position prior to delivery
   1. Usually performed ~36–37 weeks since spontaneous version usually occurs by this gestational age and reversion after ECV to breech decreases closer to term
   2. Criteria: normal fetus, adequate fluid, reassuring fetal heart tracing, unengaged presenting part, and no previous uterine surgeries
      a. May be more successful in parous patients
      b. May require tocolytic agent during ECV attempt
   3. Risks: rupture of membrane, placental abruption, cord accident, and uterine rupture
   4. Success rate = ~50%
E. Term vaginal breech delivery: most term breech presentations in United States undergo Cesarean delivery
   1. Vaginal breech delivery given greater consideration when patient presents late in labor when other criteria met
   2. Suggested criteria for planned vaginal breech: normal labor curve, >37 weeks, frank or complete breech presentation, no fetal anomalies, adequate maternal pelvis, EFW = 2,500–4,000 g, documented flexion of fetal head by ultrasound, adequate amniotic fluid, and availability of anesthesia and neonatal team
   3. Appropriate consent documented: women must be made aware of higher risk of perinatal/neonatal mortality and short-term morbidity compared to Cesarean delivery

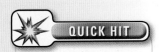

QUICK HIT

Risk of breech presentation increases with multiples, polyhydramnios, hydro-cephaly, anencephaly, aneuploidy, uterine anomalies, and uterine tumors.

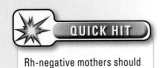

QUICK HIT

Rh-negative mothers should get RhoGAM after ECV.

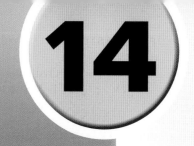

Postpartum Care/ Complications

I. Physiology of Puerperium

A. Uterine involution
1. Weight ~1,000 g immediately after delivery
2. Contraction of smooth muscle of arterial walls and compression of vasculature by uterine musculature maintains hemostasis
3. Palpable at umbilicus or below within 24 hours of delivery
4. Returns to pelvis by 2 weeks' postpartum
5. Nonpregnancy size (60–70 g) by 6–8 weeks

B. Lochia (normal postpartum vaginal discharge)
1. 1st 3 days: remaining decidua differentiates
   a. Superficial layer (becomes necrotic and sloughs)
   b. Basal layer (regenerates new endometrium)
2. Initially heavy, decreases rapidly over 1st few days
3. May last several weeks (15% continue 6–8 weeks)
4. Total volume: ~200–500 mL
   a. **Lochia rubra:** menses-like bleeding 1st several days
   b. **Lochia serosa:** lighter discharge (watery pink-brown) with less blood over next 2–3 weeks
   c. **Lochia alba:** whitish discharge may persist several weeks
   d. Breastfeeding: release of oxytocin causes more rapid uterine involution and shorter duration of lochia due to uterine contraction
5. Occasionally increased lochia 1–2 weeks postpartum due to eschar sloughing from placental site
6. Endometrium reestablished by 3rd week postpartum

C. Cervix/vulva/vagina
1. Cervix
   a. By 1 week postpartum, cervix admits only 1 finger (<1 cm dilation)
   b. Round nulliparous cervical shape replaced by transverse, "fish-mouth"–shaped external os
2. Vulvar/vaginal tissue
   a. Return to normal over 1st several days
   b. Vaginal mucosa may demonstrate hypoestrogenic effect during lactation
   c. Fascial stretching/trauma from childbirth may result in pelvic muscle relaxation, which may not return to pregravid state.
   d. Pelvic floor muscles gradually regain tone; **Kegel exercises** (repetitive contractions of pelvic floor muscles) may strengthen tone

D. Hormonal changes
1. Human chorionic gonadotropin returns to nonpregnant levels 2–4 weeks after term delivery
2. Estrogen falls immediately after delivery in all patients; begins to rise by 2 weeks' postpartum if not breastfeeding
3. Prolactin
   a. Not breastfeeding: returns to normal levels in 3 weeks
   b. Breastfeeding: remains elevated

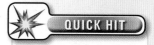

QUICK HIT

Foul-smelling lochia indicates possible endometritis, requiring antibiotics.

E. Ovulation
1. Nonlactating women
   a. Average ovulation 45–95 days (as early as 25)
   b. 70% resume menstruation by 12 weeks
2. Lactating women
   a. Variable (likelihood of ovulation increases as frequency and duration of breastfeeding decreases)
   b. Likely related to prolactin-induced inhibition of pulsatile gonadotropin-releasing hormone release
F. Skin changes
1. **Striae gravidarum** (due to loss of elastic fibers of skin): silvery initially, lightens over time
2. **Diastasis recti** (separated rectus muscles): improves over time but may persist
3. **Chloasma** (facial pigmentation): resolves with time
4. **Telogen effluvium** (hair loss commonly 1–5 months' postpartum): temporary
G. Cardiovascular changes
1. Plasma volume decreases 1,000 mL
   a. Primarily due to blood loss
   b. Also shift of extravascular fluid to intravascular space
2. Increased cardiac output persists 1st few hours
3. Tachycardia of labor persists 1 hour postpartum then decreases
4. 5-kg weight loss (due to diuresis and loss of extravascular fluid)
5. Normal cardiovascular changes can contribute to decompensation in patients with heart disease
6. Cardiovascular changes return to normal 2–3 weeks' postpartum
H. Other hematologic
1. Leukocytosis of labor may persist several days
2. Mitigates usefulness of early postpartum white blood cell count for identification of infection
3. Some postpartum autotransfusion of red blood cells to intravascular spaces by uterine contraction
I. Renal
1. Glomerular filtration rate remains elevated for several weeks
2. Drugs with renal excretion may require dosage increase
3. Ureter and renal pelvis dilation regresses by 6–8 weeks
4. Periurethral edema after vaginal delivery may cause urinary retention
5. Stress urinary incontinence
   a. Experienced by 7%
   b. Usually resolved by 3 months

II. Management of Immediate Postpartum Period
A. Hospital stay
1. Duration for uncomplicated delivery
   a. Vaginal delivery up to 48 hours
   b. Cesarean delivery up to 96 hours
2. Shortened stay appropriate if
   a. Normal vital signs
   b. Appropriate lochia
   c. Normal physical, laboratory, and emotional evaluation
   d. Mother able to adequately perform self-care and newborn care
   e. Adequate postdischarge support
3. Rooming-in recommended
   a. Appropriate if healthy infant–mother dyad
   b. Focuses new family's preparation to care for newborn
   c. Facilitates lactation assistance/consultation if breastfeeding
   d. Minimizes interventions and separation of infant from family
4. Patients and newborns discharged early: need for contact with health care provider within 48 hours of discharge

B. Postpartum concerns
  1. Fever
    a. Incidence 5%
    b. Differential diagnosis
      i. Urinary tract infection
      ii. Wound infection (episiotomy, laceration, or Cesarean)
      iii. Mastitis/breast abscess
      iv. Endometritis
      v. Septic pelvic thrombophlebitis
      vi. Drug reaction
      vii. Other unrelated infections
  2. Bleeding
    a. Uterine palpation/massage performed frequently to identify atony
    b. Peripad count
    c. Pulse and blood pressure monitoring for several hours
    d. Increased bleeding 8–14 days' postpartum
      i. Possibly related to separation of placental site eschar
      ii. Self-limited
      iii. Therapy not required
    e. Delayed postpartum hemorrhage
      i. Incidence 1%
      ii. Treatment
        (a) Oxytocic therapy
        (b) Suction uterine evacuation can be effective even if no retained placental tissue
C. Analgesia
  1. Vaginal delivery: topical analgesic (e.g., lidocaine cream): for perineum/episiotomy
  2. Cesarean delivery
    a. Spinal or epidural opiates
    b. Patient-controlled epidural
    c. Patient-controlled intravenous (IV) analgesia
    d. Oral analgesics (with potential side effects of opiates)
      i. Respiratory depression
      ii. Decreased intestinal motility
      iii. Infant sedation if breastfeeding
      iv. Suck alteration if breastfeeding
D. Ambulation
  1. Early ambulation with assistance encouraged
  2. Reduction of complications
    a. Urinary retention
    b. Deep venous thrombosis (DVT)
      i. More common in postpartum women
      ii. Increased risk with Cesarean
      iii. Highest risk 2 weeks' postpartum (returns to baseline by 4 weeks)
      iv. A leading cause of maternal mortality
      v. Cesarean birth: DVT prophylaxis (pneumatic compression devices) recommended until full ambulation
    c. Pulmonary embolus (PE)
E. Breast care
  1. Engorgement
    a. Typically starts days 3–5; more common in postpartum women
    b. Abates gradually with time
    c. May cause difficulty with infant latch
    d. Well-fitting bra, ice packs/cold (after feeding), and analgesics as needed for pain
  2. Plugged duct (**galactocele**)
    a. Localized tender "lump"
    b. Due to inadequate drainage of portion of breast
    c. Improve drainage (warm compresses prior to feeding, frequent feeding, massage)

3. **Mastitis** (breast infection): 10% of nursing mothers
   a. Unilateral, sudden onset, localized pain, erythema, fever
   b. Culture indications
      i. Concern regarding hospital-acquired organism
      ii. Premature/ill infant
      iii. Recurrent or persistent infection
      iv. High rate of resistant organisms in community
      v. Allergy to typical treatment antibiotics
      vi. Failure to respond after 24 hours of therapy
   c. Most common organisms
      i. *Staphylococcus aureus*
      ii. Groups A and B streptococci
      iii. *Haemophilus* species
      iv. *Escherichia coli*
   d. Treatment
      i. Continue breastfeeding (other drainage if breastfeeding not feasible)
      ii. Antibiotics to cover penicillinase-resistant *S. aureus*
         (a) Dicloxacillin, cephalexin
         (b) For penicillin allergic: erythromycin/azithromycin
         (c) For suspected methicillin-resistant *S. aureus* (MRSA): vancomycin, or trimethoprim–sulfamethoxazole (if infant age >1 month)
      iii. Removal of predisposing factors if any
4. Breast abscess (occurs in ~3% of mastitis patients)
   a. Similar symptoms as mastitis + **fluctuant mass**
   b. More common if mastitis treatment delayed or antibiotic therapy inadequate
   c. Milk cultures performed in all cases (over 50% + MRSA)
   d. Antibiotics
   e. Ultrasound-guided aspiration (drainage catheter may be used in larger abscesses)
   f. Incision and drainage if conservative management fails

F. Immunizations
   1. Breastfeeding *not* contraindication
   2. Rubella nonimmune: rubella vaccine should be given prior to hospital discharge
   3. If >2 years since last tetanus booster: tetanus, diphtheria, acellular pertussis (Tdap) vaccine recommended
   4. If woman D negative (not isoimmunized)
      a. Infant Rh status determined
      b. 300 mcg anti-D immune globulin to mothers of D+ infant
      c. Within 72 hours of delivery recommended
      d. Dosage may need to be increased for greater than average feto–maternal hemorrhage such as
         i. Placental abruption
         ii. Placenta previa
         iii. Manual placental removal
   5. Influenza vaccine: nonimmunized women during appropriate seasons
   6. Hepatitis B surface antigen immunization: for all newborns >2,000 g

G. Bowel and bladder function
   1. Normal not to stool 1st 1–2 days postpartum
   2. Stool softener (especially with 3rd or 4th degree episiotomy, extension, or laceration)
   3. Hemorrhoids: up to 35%
      a. Sitz baths
      b. Stool softener
      c. Local topical analgesics
      d. Reassurance
   4. Urinary retention
      a. Cause: periurethral edema or pudendal nerve injury with vaginal delivery
      b. Risk factors: nulliparity, instrumented vaginal delivery, prolonged 1st-or 2nd-stage labor, Cesarean

      c. Pharmacologic intervention ineffective

      d. Indwelling catheter × 24 hours or intermittent catheterization recommended if catheterization required >2 × in 24 hours

      e. Resolves within 1 week

H. Perineal care

  1. 1st 24–72 hours: ice (minimize swelling), oral analgesics (nonsteroidal anti-inflammatory drugs [NSAIDS]), local anesthetics (witch hazel, benzocaine spray)

  2. Severe unresponsive pain requires examination of vulva, vagina, rectum for hematoma

  3. Episiotomy/laceration

      a. Infection: <1%; broad-spectrum antibiotics recommended

      b. **Dehiscence** (rupture of incision): rare; repair individualized based on extent of wound

I. Contraception

  1. Discussion prior to discharge

  2. 15% nonnursing women fertile by 6 weeks' postpartum

  3. Reversible contraception

      a. Estrogen-containing contraceptives

         i. Discouraged by many until after 2 weeks' postpartum to minimize thrombotic risk

        ii. May have adverse effect on milk production prior to well-established milk supply

       iii. Lowest available estrogen products may be preferable during lactation

      b. Progesterone-only contraceptives

         i. Mini-pill, depot-medroxyprogesterone acetate injection, implantable rods

        ii. Not harmful to milk supply during established lactation

      c. Intrauterine contraceptive device

         i. Insertion 4–6 weeks' postpartum reduces risk of expulsion relative to earlier insertion

        ii. Does not adversely impact milk supply

       iii. Long-term reversible contraception

  4. Postpartum sterilization

      a. Counseling/informed consent (during prenatal care and hospital), risks *versus* benefits, alternatives, and regret discussed

      b. Cesarean delivery: convenience of same procedure

      c. Vaginal delivery: following delivery, but should not interfere with initial bonding between mother and newborn or extend hospital stay

         i. After assessment of maternal/neonatal well-being

        ii. Postpone in face of obstetric and/or maternal complications

       iii. Postpartum periumbilical minilaparotomy performed prior to significant uterine involution (12–24 hours' postpartum)

J. Sexual activity

  1. Risk of hemorrhage/infection: minimal 2 weeks'+ postpartum

  2. Earlier intercourse associated with increased risk dyspareunia

  3. During breastfeeding or while using progesterone-only contraceptives, water-soluble lubrication often needed due to low estrogen levels

  4. Potential temporary alteration in libido

  5. Most resume intercourse by 6–8 weeks' postpartum

K. Patient education

  1. Overall health care of infant and mother discussed

  2. Infant feeding method reviewed

  3. Discussion of high-risk behaviors: alcohol, tobacco, drugs

  4. Mental state assessment (depression)

  5. Contraception

  6. Infant safety (child restraints)

  7. Preexisting medical conditions reviewed

  8. Follow-up care (mother and infant) planned

L. Weight loss
 1. ~50% women retain >10 lb 6 months' postpartum; 25% retain >20 lb
 2. Average 2-lb weight retention 1 year postpartum
 3. Risk factors for postpartum weight retention (PPWR)
   a. Excessive weight gain in pregnancy
   b. Ethnicity (African)
   c. Obesity
   d. Quitting tobacco
   e. Increased parity
   f. Young age
 4. Excessive weight gain during pregnancy and higher PPWR: risk factors for later life obesity
 5. Optimal strategy for postpartum weight reduction unclear
 6. Diet/exercise/lifestyle (limited data in lactating women)
   a. Weight loss up to 4.5 lb per month unlikely to decrease milk volume; infant weight gain should be monitored
   b. Intakes <1,800 kcal/day not recommended

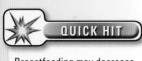

QUICK HIT

Breastfeeding may decrease PPWR. The caloric expenditure of exclusive breastfeeding is ~600 kcal/day.

M. Breastfeeding
 1. Breast milk ideal infant nutrition
   a. Exclusive breastfeeding 1st 6 months
   b. Continued breastfeeding with complementary foods beyond 6 months and as long as mutually desired
 2. Infant effects
   a. Decreased otitis (50%); respiratory infections (72%)
   b. Decreased diarrheal illnesses (64%)
   c. Reduced diabetes (19%–27% type 1 and 39% type 2)
   d. Decreased obesity (24%)
   e. Reduced sudden infant death syndrome (SIDS): 36%
   f. Reduced childhood malignancy (19% acute lymphoblastic leukemia; 15% acute myeloid leukemia)
   g. Reduction in childhood asthma/atopic disease
   h. Fewer hospitalizations 1st year of life
   i. Improved cognitive function
   j. Reduced necrotizing enterocolitis for premature infants
 3. Maternal effects
   a. Reduced breast and ovarian cancer
   b. Reduced risk of type 2 diabetes
   c. Increased caloric expenditure/reduction in PPWR
   d. Decreased postpartum bleeding/more rapid uterine involution
   e. Lactational amenorrhea
 4. Societal cost benefits: related to reduction of pediatric diseases
 5. Breastfeeding contraindications
   a. Maternal conditions
     i. Human immunodeficiency virus (HIV)
     ii. Untreated tuberculosis: mother should not be in direct contact with infant (expressed milk may be given to infant)
     iii. Chemotherapy
     iv. Radioactive isotope treatment (i.e., I131)
     v. Active illegal drug use (those on successful methadone maintenance may breastfeed)
     vi. Medications: rarely (e.g., cabergoline, bromocriptine)
   b. Infant conditions: galactosemia
 6. Medication use during lactation
   a. Adequate source of information recommended
   b. Unnecessary medications, herbal products to be avoided
   c. Safer alternatives with more information specific to lactation to be considered
   d. Infant risk evaluation (premature infants, neonates <30 days, infant with other medical conditions such as jaundice or taking medications may require special consideration)

e. Potential resources
    i. *Medications and Mother's Milk* by Thomas Hale, RPh, PhD
    ii. LactMed: http://toxnet.nlm.nih.gov

7. Hormones
  a. Drop in estrogen/placental hormones major factor in removing inhibition to action of prolactin
  b. Infant suckling
    i. Oxytocin released from neurohypophysis
    ii. Prolactin released
  c. Oxytocin effects
    i. Contraction of myoepithelial cells emptying alveolar lumen causing milk flow (milk ejection)
    ii. Uterine contractions

8. Milk
  a. Initial colostrum (1st 5 days)
    i. Higher mineral/protein content
    ii. Lower fat/sugar content
    iii. Secretory immunoglobulin A (some protection from enteric pathogens)
  b. Transitional milk
  c. Mature milk (by 2–4 weeks)
    i. Water primary component
    ii. Higher fat content (3.6%)
    iii. Dynamic composition
    iv. Varies over time (higher fat in morning)
    v. Immune properties (antibodies, lactoferrin, lysozyme, oligosaccharides)
  d. Composition
    i. Contains all vitamins except vitamin K (which is administered to newborn to prevent hemorrhagic disease)
    ii. Restricted infant exposure to ultraviolet light (vitamin D supplement recommended)
    iii. B12 supplement recommended for infants if mother is vegan, malnourished, history of gastric bypass

9. Nipple care
  a. Correct latch and assessment to minimize trauma
  b. Water-based lanolin cream applied for comfort if needed
  c. **Fissuring**: evaluation needed by lactation expert to assess latch

N. Depression
1. Postpartum blues
  a. Incidence 70%–80%
  b. Mild, intermittent feeling of sadness, anxiety, or anger
  c. Onset days 2–4; abates by 1–2 weeks
  d. Treatment: supportive care

2. Postpartum depression
  a. Incidence 10%–15%
  b. Treatment: usually requires medication or counseling
  c. More pronounced feelings of sadness, anxiety, despair
  d. Interferes with daily functioning
  e. Worsens over weeks
  f. Cause unknown
  g. More common in women with
    i. Personal history of depression/anxiety
    ii. Family history
    iii. Acute stressors
    iv. Child with difficult health issues
    v. Depression in pregnancy (strong predictor)

3. Psychosis
  a. Incidence: rare
  b. Severe symptoms

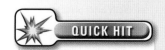

QUICK HIT

Psychosis is a medical emergency! A referral for therapy (often inpatient) is required.

c. More common in women with preexisting psychiatric disorders
   i. Bipolar disorder
   ii. Schizophrenia
O. Thyroid disease
   1. 8% within 6 months
   2. Increased risk: type 1 diabetes (2 times), antithyroid peroxidase antibodies (5 times)
   3. May be hyperthyroidism, hypothyroidism, or both hyperthyroidism followed by hypothyroidism
   4. Laboratory evaluation if symptomatic
P. Postpartum visit (routine visit 4–6 weeks' postpartum); early visit (1–2 weeks) if Cesarean delivery, medical issues requiring attention, or women with risk of mood disturbance
   1. Infant feeding status (review amount of breastfeeding if not exclusive)
   2. Address breastfeeding difficulties
   3. Infant health/newborn interaction
   4. Presence/resolution of lochia or return of menses
   5. Resumption of sexual activities
   6. Contraception
   7. Vaccinations (Tdap, influenza if not previously given)
   8. Postpartum weight (relative to prepregnancy weight) addressed including exercise and goals for postpartum weight reduction
   9. Plans for return to work/infant care
   10. Mood (depression screening)

III. Postpartum Hemorrhage (PPH)

A. >50% occur within 24 hours' postpartum
B. Serious sequelae
   1. Adult respiratory distress syndrome
   2. Coagulopathy
   3. Shock
   4. Loss of fertility
   5. Pituitary necrosis (Sheehan syndrome)
   6. Death
C. Definitions
   1. Average normal blood loss
      a. Vaginal delivery: >500 mL
      b. Cesarean delivery: >1,000 mL
      c. Measurements are subjective and likely inaccurate
   2. Objective criteria more useful
      a. 10% drop in hematocrit
      b. Need for transfusion
      c. Signs/symptoms of blood loss
D. Detection of blood loss
   1. 10%–15% loss (500 mL for average patient): no signs/symptoms
   2. 20%: tachycardia, tachypnea, delayed capillary refill, orthostatic changes, narrowed pulse pressure (due to elevated diastolic pressure from vasoconstriction to maintain systolic pressure)
   3. 30%+: tachycardia/tachypnea worsen, overt hypotension
   4. 40%–50% profound blood loss: oliguria, shock, coma, and death
E. Source of bleeding
   1. Identification as soon as possible
   2. Most likely causes
      a. Uterine atony (80%)
      b. Retained placenta
      c. Genital tract trauma (e.g., laceration)
      d. Coagulation disorder
      e. Hematoma
      f. Ruptured uterus
      g. Inverted uterus

MNEMONIC

10 Bs of Postpartum Visit
Blues
Breast/**b**reastfeeding
Belly
Bottom (episiotomy/tears)
Bladder
Boinking (intercourse)
Baby
Birth control
Bowels
Bleeding

QUICK HIT

Sheehan syndrome may present as an inability to breastfeed.

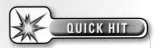

QUICK HIT

Usually, the uterus contracts promptly after placental delivery, constricting spiral arteries of the placental bed and limiting bleeding (i.e., muscular contraction *not coagulation* normally prevents bleeding from the placental site).

F. Risk factors
   1. Prolonged labor
   2. Augmented labor
   3. Rapid labor
   4. History of prior hemorrhage
   5. Episiotomy (especially mediolateral)
   6. Preeclampsia
   7. Overdistended uterus (macrosomia, multiple gestation, polyhydramnios)
   8. Operative delivery
   9. Ethnicity (Asian, Hispanic)
   10. Intra-amniotic infection
G. General management
   1. Management facilitated if high-risk patients identified and preparations made occur prior to bleeding
   2. Planning
      a. Before delivery
         i. Baseline hematocrit
         ii. Blood type and screen (crossmatch for high risk)
         iii. IV access
         iv. Baseline coagulation tests and platelets if indicated
         v. Assessment of risk factors
      b. Delivery room
         i. Excess umbilical cord traction avoided
         ii. Judicious use of forceps/vacuum
         iii. Inspection of placenta for complete removal
         iv. Active management of 3rd stage
         v. Visualization of cervix/vagina
         vi. Removal of clots from uterus/vagina prior to transfer to recovery
      c. After delivery
         i. Observation of patient for excessive bleeding
         ii. Continuation of uterotonics
         iii. Frequent palpation/massage of uterus
         iv. Vital signs frequently monitored
H. Uterine atony
   1. Prevention
      a. Active management of 3rd stage reduces PPH by 70%
      b. 3rd stage management
         i. Infusion of oxytocin (20 units/1 L normal saline infused 200–500 mL/hr) after delivery of infant or anterior shoulder
         ii. Gentle cord traction
         iii. Uterine massage
         iv. Immediate breastfeeding may be beneficial
   2. Management
      a. Manipulative: bimanual massage often successful while preparing other treatments
      b. Medical/uterotonic agents
         i. Oxytocin: normal infusion rate increased
         ii. Methylergonovine maleate
            (a) Given intramuscularly (IM)
            (b) Potential hypertension side effect
            (c) Extreme caution with cardiac disease
         iii. Misoprostol (prostaglandin E1 analogue)
         iv. Dinoprostone (prostaglandin E2 analogue): given by vaginal or rectal suppository
         v. 15-methyl prostaglandin F2α
            (a) Given IM or into uterus directly
            (b) Use in asthmatics avoided
         vi. Surgical management: indicated if massage and uterotonic agents fail to result in uterine contraction

c. Surgical management
  i. Uterine packing or placement of uterine compression balloon
  ii. Uterine compression sutures (B-Lynch stitch)
  iii. Sequential arterial ligation (ascending or descending uterine branches, utero-ovarian, internal iliacs)
  iv. Selective arterial embolization
  v. Hysterectomy
  vi. Good success noted with surgical compression: decreasing need for hysterectomy and iliac artery ligation (both have high morbidity)

I. Lacerations
  1. Risk factors
    a. Instrumented delivery
    b. Manipulative delivery (i.e., breech extraction)
    c. Precipitous delivery
    d. Macrosomia
    e. Fetal presentations other than occiput anterior
  2. Cervix
    a. Minor lacerations common (expectant management)
    b. Extensive lacerations with active bleeding require repair
  3. Vagina/perineum
    a. Not common cause of substantial bleeding
    b. Steady blood loss may occur and repair indicated with bleeding
    c. Periurethral lacerations may have associated edema and urinary retention requiring catheter for 12–24 hours

J. Retained placenta
  1. Normal process of separation is cleavage between zona basalis and zona spongiosa facilitated by uterine contractions
  2. Retained placenta occurs from incomplete separation or expulsion
  3. Predisposing factors
    a. Prior Cesarean delivery
    b. Uterine leiomyomata
    c. Prior uterine curettage
    d. **Succenturiate (accessory) placental lobe**
  4. Retained placental tissue prevents uterine contractions, leading to atony and hemorrhage
  5. Placental inspection: routinely performed to identify missing cotyledons
  6. If retained placenta suspected: manual removal using 2 fingers in uterine cavity often successful
  7. If not successful or uncertain diagnosis: ultrasound of uterus can assist with diagnosis
  8. Uterine curettage (with either large sharp or suction curette) can be performed
  9. Special situations: abnormal placental adherence
    a. **Placenta accreta**: abnormal placental adherence to uterine wall
    b. **Placenta increta**: penetration into uterine muscle
    c. **Placenta percreta**: complete invasion through thickness of uterine muscle
    d. If all or portion of placenta retained: hysterectomy often required
    e. If only small portion: curettage may be attempted

K. Other causes
  1. Hematomas
    a. Anywhere from vulva to upper vagina: requires careful inspection
    b. May/may not interrupt vaginal mucosa
    c. Vulvar/vaginal hematomas: exquisite pain
      i. <5 cm and not enlarging may be followed frequently to ensure no expansion
        (a) Vitals and urine output monitored
        (b) Ice packs may help
      ii. >5 cm and enlarging hematomas: surgical evacuation
        (a) Episiotomy site hematomas: suture removal, identification of bleeding source and ligation if found

(b) If not at episiotomy site: surgical drainage at most dependent end, bleeding site identified/sutured/closed

(c) Drains/vaginal packs used to prevent reaccumulation

2. Bleeding disorders
   a. Congenital or acquired
   b. Obstetric conditions associated with disseminated intravascular coagulopathy
      i. Placental abruption
      ii. Amniotic fluid embolism
      iii. Sepsis
      iv. Severe preeclampsia
      v. Intrauterine fetal demise
      vi. Profuse hemorrhage
   c. Treatment involves correction of coagulation defect with appropriate factor replacement
   d. When assessing PPH: specimen should be collected to assess if blood is clotting (red top tube)

3. Amniotic fluid embolism
   a. Rare, sudden, often fatal complication (mortality 30%–50%)
   b. Caused by entry of amniotic fluid into maternal circulation
   c. Biochemical mediators involved with sequence
      i. Respiratory distress
      ii. Cyanosis
      iii. Cardiovascular collapse
      iv. Hemorrhage
      v. Coma
   d. Severe coagulopathy often
   e. Treatment: supportive care

4. Uterine inversion
   a. Rare condition: uterus inverts (inside out), fundus extends through cervix into/past vagina
   b. Severe, sudden hemorrhage
   c. Treatment
      i. Manual uterine replacement (often requires uterine relaxant such as terbutaline, magnesium, halogenated general anesthetic, or nitroglycerin)
      ii. Surgery: if manual replacement with relaxant agent unsuccessful

5. Uterine rupture
   a. Frank opening between uterine cavity and abdominal cavity
   b. Significant maternal and fetal morbidity/mortality
   c. Associated factors
      i. Prior Cesarean delivery scar
         (a) Rupture more common with classical incision
         (b) Less common with low transverse incision
      ii. Prior other uterine surgery
      iii. Trauma
      iv. Congenital malformations (small uterine horn)
      v. Abnormal labor
      vi. Operative delivery
      vii. Placenta accreta
      viii. Spontaneous labor with prior Cesarean delivery
   d. Repair of rupture required with reconstruction of uterine defect
   e. Hysterectomy if life-threatening situation regardless of desire for future fertility
   f. Early identification of uterine rupture
      i. Maternal hemodynamic changes
      ii. Acute abdominal pain
      iii. Change in abdominal contour
      iv. Nonreassuring fetal heart rate pattern
      v. Loss of fetal station

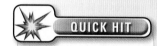

QUICK HIT

Uterine inversion is often caused by excess traction placed on the umbilical cord without appropriate corresponding pressure placed on the uterine fundus.

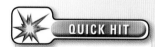

QUICK HIT

Uterine rupture should not be confused with uterine *dehiscence*, which is a "window" covered by visceral peritoneum with less clinical significance.

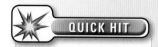

QUICK HIT

Trial of labor after cesarean (TOLAC) is acceptable with a low transverse incision but is contraindicated with classical incision due to the high incidence of uterine rupture.

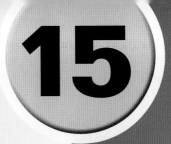

15

Ectopic Pregnancy

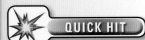
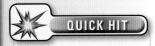

QUICK HIT

An ectopic pregnancy occurs when a blastocyst implants *anywhere* other than in the endometrial lining.

QUICK HIT

Since 1980, morbidity has reduced by 56.6% with better diagnosis and treatment.

I. **Epidemiology/Morbidity and Mortality**
   A. Leading cause of maternal death in 1st trimester
   B. Reduction in subsequent fertility
   C. 1%–2% of all pregnancies in United States
      1. Higher incidence among nonwhite women
      2. Higher incidence among women age >35 years
   D. Earlier diagnosis leads to reduction in complications
      1. Increased maternal survival
      2. Increased future reproductive capacity

II. **Etiology**
   A. Risk factors (Box 15.1)
      1. Mechanical: impaired passage of fertilized ovum through tube
      2. Functional: slow passage of fertilized ovum through tube
      3. Assisted reproductive technology (ART): possibly related to tubal factors that cause infertility
      4. Half of ectopic pregnancies have *no* risk factors
   B. Anatomy (Figure 15.1)
      1. 98% occur in fallopian tube
         a. Ampullary (most frequent)
         b. Isthmic
         c. Interstitial (least frequent)
      2. Other sites (more common with ART)
         a. Abdominal
         b. Ovarian
         c. Cervical
         d. **Heterotopic** (simultaneous intrauterine pregnancy [IUP] and ectopic)

BOX 15.1

Risk Factors for Ectopic Pregnancy

- History of sexually transmitted infections or pelvic inflammatory disease
- Prior ectopic pregnancy
- Previous tubal surgery
- Prior pelvic or abdominal surgery resulting in adhesions
- Endometriosis
- Current use of exogenous hormones including progesterone or estrogen
- In vitro fertilization and other assisted reproduction
- Diethylstilbestrol-exposed patients with congenital abnormalities
- Congenital abnormalities of the fallopian tubes
- Use of an intrauterine device for birth control

(From Callahan TL, Caughey AB. *Blueprints Obstetrics & Gynecology*, 5th ed. Baltimore: Lippincott Williams & Wilkins; 2009.)

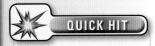

Ectopic Pregnancy

FIGURE 15.1 Incidence of types of ectopic pregnancies by location.

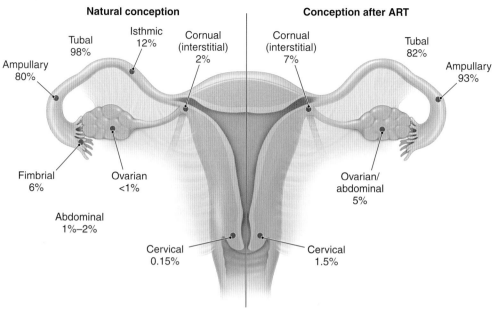

(Beckmann CRB, Ling FW, et al. *Obstetrics and Gynecology*, 7th ed. Baltimore: Lippincott Williams & Wilkins; 2014.)

III. Clinical Presentation

A. Signs and symptoms

1. Classic triad: amenorrhea, pain, and irregular vaginal bleeding
2. Ruptured ectopic
   a. Acute abdominal exam
   b. Hypotension, tachycardia (when hypovolemia becomes significant)
3. Unruptured ectopic
   a. Nonspecific abdominal pain
   b. Palpable mass possible
   c. Asymptomatic

IV. Differential Diagnosis

A. Evaluation

1. History
2. Physical
3. Labs
   a. Type and screen
      i. Type and crossmatch, if necessary
      ii. RhoGAM if indicated
   b. Complete blood count (CBC)
   c. Quantitative β-human chorionic gonadotropin (β-hCG)
      i. Often markedly reduced compared to IUP at same gestational age
      ii. 1,500–2,000 = discriminatory zone [DZ] (level at which sonogram should visualize IUP)
      iii. Repeat in 48 hours if patient stable and diagnosis uncertain (Figure 15.2)
   d. Progesterone
      i. <5 ng/mL suggests *nonviable* pregnancy
      ii. 5–20 ng/mL inconclusive
      iii. >20 ng/mL suggestive of IUP
4. Ultrasound
   a. Abdominal sonogram
      i. Difficult to diagnose ectopic pregnancy
      ii. Cannot detect IUP until 5–6 weeks' gestation

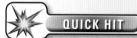

The classic triad of ectopic pregnancy presentation is amenorrhea, pain, and irregular vaginal bleeding.

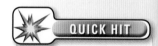

First-trimester bleeding occurs in 20% of normal pregnancies.

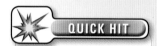

A pregnancy test is key because ectopic pregnancy can mimic both obstetric and gynecologic conditions (Table 15.1).

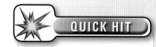

The initial CBC reading may not be indicative of *acute* blood loss, so vital signs must be carefully monitored.

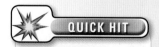

Distinguishing a failed IUP from an unruptured ectopic pregnancy is often difficult.

Ectopic Pregnancy

Ectopic Pregnancy

TABLE 15.1 Differential Diagnosis for Acute Pain/Suspected Ectopic Pregnancy	
If Pregnancy Test +	**If Pregnancy Test −**
Normal pregnancy	**Pelvic infection**
Abortion/miscarriage	**Ovarian cyst/torsion**
Threatened	**Appendicitis**
Incomplete	**Pyelonephritis**
Inevitable	**Nephrolithiasis**
Complete	**Gastroenteritis**
Corpus luteum cyst	**Endometriosis**
Ruptured	**Ovarian mass**
Nonruptured	Neoplasm
Torsion	Tubo-ovarian abscess
Ectopic pregnancy	**Pedunculated fibroid**

(Beckmann CRB, Ling FW, et al. *Obstetrics and Gynecology*, 7th ed. Baltimore: Lippincott Williams & Wilkins; 2014.)

    b. Transvaginal sonogram (TVUS)
       i. Detects IUP as early as 1 week after missed menses
       ii. IUP should be visible if β-hCG >1,500 mIU/mL
  5. Other
    a. **Culdocentesis**
       i. 16–18-gauge needle passed through posterior fornix
       ii. Old blood or nonclotting bloody fluid is indicative of hemoperitoneum, but not necessarily ectopic
       iii. Infrequently used
    b. Dilation and curettage (see Figure 15.2)
       i. If chorionic villi obtained, identifies abnormal IUP rather than ectopic (heterotopic pregnancy also possible, but unlikely)
       ii. Performed if β-hCG rise is abnormal and no intact IUP or ectopic seen on TVUS
    c. Diagnostic laparoscopy
       i. Definitive diagnosis can be made by visualizing tube
       ii. Treatment can be accomplished surgically at time of diagnosis

V. Management
  A. Medical (Table 15.2)
    1. Methotrexate
      a. Chemotherapy agent
      b. Folic acid antagonist
      c. Single and variable dose regimens (see Table 15.2)
      d. Contraindications (Table 15.3)
    2. Medical treatment versus salpingostomy: comparable rates of successful treatment, future tubal patency, and subsequent IUP
  B. Surgical
    1. Laparoscopy usual route
      a. Salpingostomy (open the tube and remove gestation)
      b. Salpingectomy (remove segment or entire tube)
    2. Laparotomy in select populations
      a. Emergent/unstable patient
      b. Patient is poor candidate for laparoscopy (e.g., due to complicated surgical history)
  C. Expectant management
    1. Possible, but infrequently done
    2. Appropriate patient selection mandatory
    3. Spontaneous resolution can be seen in women with falling β-hCG

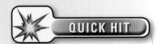

Medical treatment has similar success rates, future tubal patency rates, and subsequent IUP rates as salpingostomy.

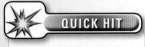

Rupture can still occur if β-hCG is falling.

FIGURE 15.2 Algorithm for nonsurgical diagnosis and treatment of ectopic pregnancy.

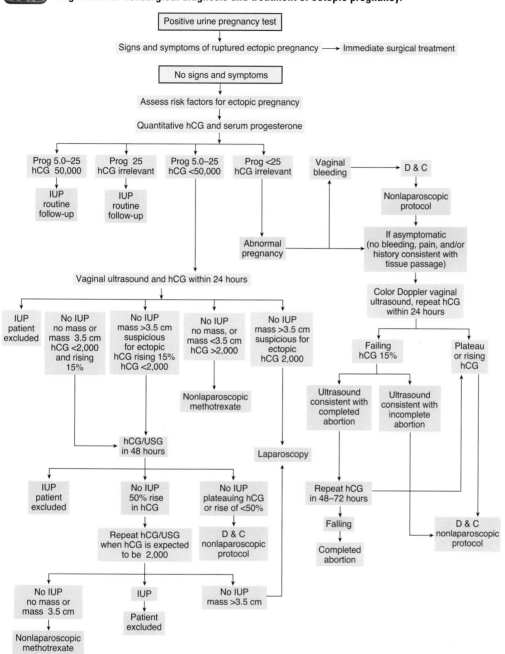

(Beckmann CRB, Ling FW, et al. *Obstetrics and Gynecology*, 5th ed. Philadelphia: Lippincott Williams & Wilkins; 2006.)

TABLE 15.2 Methotrexate Regimens	
Single Dose (most common)	**Multidose**
50 mg/m² IM Serum β-hCG levels days 1 (day of injection), 4, and 7 >15% decline from day 4 to 7 initial success Follow weekly β-hCG levels until undetectable If failure to decline or plateau, consider repeat dose or surgical management	1 mg/kg IM or IV/day on days 1, 3, 5, and 7 PLUS **Leucovorin** 0.1 mg/kg po on days 2, 4, 6, and 8 Serum β-hCG levels on days 1, 3, 5, and 7 >15% decline in levels STOPS treatment and weekly β-hCG levels are monitored IF <15% decline then repeat MTX and leucovorin dose Follow weekly levels until undetectable If failure to decline, repeat dose or surgical management

β-hCG, β-human chorionic gonadotropin; IM, intramuscular; IV, intravenous; MTX, methotrexate.
(Modified from Beckmann CRB, Ling FW, et al. *Obstetrics and Gynecology*, 7th ed. Baltimore: Lippincott Williams & Wilkins; 2014.)

Ectopic Pregnancy

TABLE 15.3 **Methotrexate Contraindications**	
Absolute	**Relative**[a]
Poorly compliant β-hCG >5,000	Fetal cardiac activity
Clinically unstable patient	Ectopic size >3.5 cm
Suspected ruptured ectopic	
Hematologic, renal, or hepatic dysfunction	
Serum abnormalities	
Immunodeficiency	
Active pulmonary disease	
Peptic ulcer disease	
Breastfeeding	
Heterotopic pregnancy	
Allergy or sensitivity to MTX	

β-hCG, β-human chorionic gonadotropin.
[a]Associated with methotrexate (MTX) treatment failure.
(Modified from Beckmann CRB, Ling FW, et al. *Obstetrics and Gynecology*, 7th ed. Baltimore: Lippincott Williams & Wilkins; 2014.)

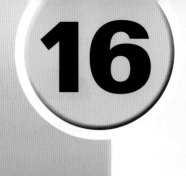

16

Common Medical and Surgical Problems in Pregnancy

I. Anemia in Pregnancy

A. Definitions
1. "Physiologic" decrease of hematocrit (Hct) during pregnancy is due to hemodilution, with relatively greater increase in plasma volume than red blood cell (RBC) volume
2. Hct <30% or hemoglobin (Hgb) <10 g/dL
3. Correction of anemia improves ability to respond to acute peripartum blood loss
4. Severe anemia (Hgb <6 g/dL) may impair fetal oxygenation
B. Iron-deficiency anemia
1. Responsible for 90% of cases of anemia in pregnancy
a. All pregnant women should be screened
b. 30 mg of elemental iron daily recommended for *all* pregnant women
c. Treatment includes additional supplementation of elemental iron, with vitamin C supplementation to enhance absorption
2. Laboratory abnormalities
a. Low **mean corpuscular volume** and low **mean corpuscular Hgb concentration**
b. Low serum iron and ferritin, elevated **total iron-binding capacity**
C. Megaloblastic anemia
1. Folate deficiency
a. Associated with fetal neural tube defects (NTDs)
b. Folate intake and supplementation preconception and 1st trimester
i. Routine: 0.4 mg daily
ii. Prior NTD-affected pregnancy or taking anticonvulsants: 4 mg daily
2. Vitamin B12 deficiency
a. May be due to long-term vegetarian diet, tropical sprue, malabsorption related to bariatric surgery
b. May be associated with placental abruption, preeclampsia, intrauterine growth restriction (IUGR), and prematurity
D. Hemoglobinopathies (Table 16.1)
1. Defining normal Hgb
a. 4 polypeptide chains, each attached to heme molecule
b. Adult Hgbs include 2 α-globin chains and 2 additional chains
i. With 2 β-globin chains = HgbA
ii. With 2 γ-globin chains = HgbF
iii. With 2 δ-globin chains = HgbA$_2$
c. Normal Hgb comprises 96%–97% HgbA, 2%–3% HgbA$_2$, and <1% HgbF
2. **Thalassemias:** caused by missing/defective polypeptide genes
a. α-Thalassemia (Table 16.2)
i. Normal human has 4 copies of α-globin gene
ii. Missing or nonfunctional copies of α-globin gene cause α-thalassemia

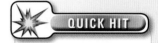

QUICK HIT

To screen for anemia as a result of hemodilution and fetal demand, a complete blood count (CBC) is obtained at ~28 weeks, with third trimester labs.

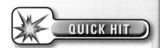

QUICK HIT

Supplementation with 30 mg of elemental iron daily is recommended for *all* pregnant women.

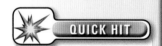

QUICK HIT

Prenatal vitamin formulations provide 60–65 mg of elemental iron and 1 mg of folic acid, enough to provide the recommended supplementation for the average pregnant woman.

Common Medical and Surgical Problems

TABLE **16.1**	Hemoglobinopathies			
Condition	**Globin Abnormality**	**Genetics**	**Phenotype**	**Risk Groups**
Sickle cell	HgbS or HgbC	Autosomal recessive	Sickle cell trait: HgbAS Sickle cell disease: HgbSS or HgbSC	African, Mediterranean, Turkish, Arabian, East Indian heritage; African American (1/200 have sickle trait; 1/600 have sickle cell disease)
α-Thalassemia	Normal hemoglobin; production of α-globin chains is decreased	Autosomal recessive	Severity depends on amount of globin produced	Asian, African, East Indian, Mediterranean heritage
β-Thalassemia	Normal hemoglobin; production of β-globin chains is decreased	Autosomal recessive	**Homozygous:** β-thalassemia major (Cooley anemia); no HgbA is produced = severe disease **Heterozygous:** β-thalassemia minor; one normal and one abnormal β-globin allele = mild to moderate disease	Mediterranean, Middle Eastern, African, East Indian, and Asian heritage
Sickle cell/ β-thalassemia	One globin is HgbS and one globin codes for β-thalassemia	Autosomal recessive in 1/1,700 pregnancies	Severity of disease depends on the β-allele (no HgbA production = severe disease; moderate production = milder disease)	Same as for sickle cell and β-thalassemia

Hgb, hemoglobin.
(From Beckmann CRB, Ling FW, et al. *Obstetrics and Gynecology*, 7th ed. Baltimore: Lippincott Williams & Wilkins; 2014.)

   b. β-Thalassemia (Table 16.3)
      i. Mutations in β-globin gene cause absent (β^0) or defective (β^+) protein
      ii. Phenotype varies
         (a) Homozygotes: β-thalassemia major (severe disease)
         (b) Heterozygotes: β-thalassemia minor (asymptomatic to clinically anemic)

TABLE **16.2**	Variants of α-Thalassemia
Number of Functional α-Globin Genes	**Phenotypic Expression**
4	Normal
3	Asymptomatic
2	Mild anemia
1	Hemolytic anemia
0 = Hgb Barts	Hydrops fetalis and intrauterine death

Hgb, hemoglobin.

TABLE **16.3** Variants of β-Thalassemia		
Type	**Genotype**	**Phenotypic Expression**
β-Thalassemia minor	β^0/β	Asymptomatic or mild microcytic anemia Resistance to falciparum malaria
β-Thalassemia trait	β^+/β	Mild or no anemia
Cooley anemia = thalassemia major	β^0/β^0 or β^+/β^+	Severity depends on amount of globin produced and manifests at ages 6–9 months, when HgbF changes to HgbA β^0/β^0 causes severe anemia β/β^+ associated with splenomegaly, increased hematopoiesis, severe iron overload

Hgb, hemoglobin.

3. Sickle cell disorders
   a. Point mutations in β-globin genes
      i. Form HgbS instead of HgbA
      ii. Causes structural abnormalities in RBCs
   b. Sickle cell disease
      i. Homozygous, HgbSS
      ii. Abnormally shaped cells can cause vaso-occlusive crises
      iii. Functional asplenia increases risk of infections
   c. Sickle cell trait
      i. Heterozygous, HgbAS
      ii. Asymptomatic
      iii. Increased risk for urinary tract infections (UTIs)
   d. Other sickle cell disorders occur in presence of HgbS and 1 other abnormality of β-globin structure (e.g., **sickle β-thalassemia**)
4. Carrier screening should be offered to women at highest risk
   a. CBC for women of Mediterranean or Southeast Asian descent
   b. CBC and Hg electrophoresis for women of African descent
   c. Maternal hemoglobinopathies (except sickle trait) increase risks of preterm labor, IUGR, and low birth weight
   d. Genetic counseling offered if both parents are carriers

II. Diabetes Mellitus
A. Placental hormones affect glucose metabolism in pregnancy
   1. Human placental lactogen (hPL) acts as anti-insulin
   2. Insulinase degrades insulin
B. Poor glucose control increases risks of pregnancy complications
   1. Spontaneous abortion, especially for pregestational diabetics
   2. Intrauterine fetal demise and stillbirth
   3. Infection, especially UTIs and pyelonephritis
   4. Fetal macrosomia, shoulder dystocia
   5. IUGR
   6. **Polyhydramnios** = increase in amniotic fluid volume >2,000 mL
      a. Increased risk of placental abruption and preterm labor
      b. Increased risk of postpartum uterine atony
   7. Neonatal hypoglycemia related to maternal glucose levels at delivery
   8. Respiratory distress syndrome
C. Pregestational diabetes
   1. 6-fold increase in risk of congenital anomalies over baseline, resulting in 6%–10% of infants of diabetic mothers having major congenital anomaly
      a. Cardiac, central nervous system, gastrointestinal, and genitourinary anomalies more common

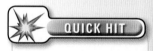

QUICK HIT

Maternal hemoglobinopathies (except sickle cell trait) increase risks for preterm labor, IUGR, and low birth weight.

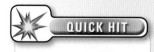

QUICK HIT

Neonatal hypoglycemia correlates with maternal glucose levels at delivery.

Common Medical and Surgical Problems

   b. **Sacral agenesis/caudal regression** (abnormal development of lower fetal spine): unique to diabetes

2. Antepartum testing
   a. Early ultrasound for viability and dating
   b. Anatomy screen at 18–20 weeks
   c. Fetal echocardiogram (echo): 19–22 weeks
   d. Fetal kick counts: beginning at 28 weeks
   e. Serial growth ultrasounds: starting at 28 weeks
   f. Weekly or twice weekly nonstress tests: starting at 32–34 weeks

3. Maternal complications
   a. **Diabetic ketoacidosis (DKA)** can occur at lower glucose levels and more rapidly than in nonpregnant women
   b. Symptomatic hypoglycemia, especially with nausea and vomiting in early pregnancy
   c. 2-fold increased risk of pregnancy-induced hypertension or preeclampsia
   d. Progression of diabetic nephropathy to end-stage renal disease
   e. Worsening of diabetic retinopathy

4. Management
   a. Optimal glucose control before and during pregnancy
   b. Combination of diet, exercise, and insulin therapy

D. **Gestational diabetes mellitus (GDM)**

1. Diagnosis
   a. Screen with 50-g 1-hour glucose tolerance test at 24–28 weeks
   b. Abnormal result (glucose ≥130 or 140) requires further testing with fasting 100-g 3-hour glucose tolerance test
   c. A1: can be managed with dietary changes alone
   d. A2: requires pharmacologic therapy to maintain euglycemia

2. Antepartum testing
   a. For well-controlled, diet-controlled GDM: insufficient evidence to recommend any specific testing regimen
   b. For poorly controlled GDM or patients requiring insulin: should be tested as for pregestational diabetes, starting at 32–34 weeks

3. Management
   a. Diabetic counseling
   b. Home monitoring of fasting and 1- or 2-hour postprandial glucose (Table 16.4)
   c. Exercise and proper diet
   d. Pharmacologic control when diet alone is not enough
      i. Oral hypoglycemics, especially glyburide and metformin
      ii. Insulin therapy, as combination of rapid-acting and intermediate-acting insulins
      iii. Home glucose logs frequently monitored and therapy adjusted as needed

E. Labor and delivery

1. Labor induction
   a. Well-controlled, uncomplicated GDMA2 or PGDM: at 39 weeks
   b. Well-controlled GDMA1: no specific recommendations
2. Estimated fetal weight ≥4,500 g: elective Cesarean delivery may be offered
3. Insulin drip intrapartum to maintain glucose at 100 mg/dL

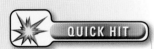

QUICK HIT

DKA can occur at lower glucose levels and more rapidly in pregnant women than in nonpregnant women.

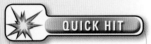

QUICK HIT

Maternal mortality is rare with DKA, but fetal mortality rates can range from 10% to 30%.

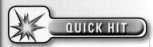

QUICK HIT

Insulin requirements will increase throughout pregnancy, most markedly between 28 and 32 weeks of gestation, due to increased production of hPL (anti-insulin).

TABLE **16.4** Goal Blood Glucose Values in Pregnancy	
Fasting	60–90 mg/dL
1-hour postprandial	<140 mg/dL
2-hour postprandial	<120 mg/dL

F. Postpartum care
1. GDM: no further insulin
   a. Glucose tolerance screening at 2–4 months' postpartum
   b. 3%–5% will remain diabetic after delivery
   c. 50% will develop type 2 diabetes later in life
2. Pregestational diabetes: start insulin at prepregnancy dose or at 50% of predelivery dose and adjust as needed

III. Thyroid Disease
A. Physiologic changes in pregnancy
1. Increased thyroid-binding globulin
2. Transient increase in free thyroxine (T_4) and free T_4 index (FTI) in 1st trimester
B. Hyperthyroidism, including Graves disease
1. Treated with propylthiouracil (PTU) and methimazole (MMI)
   a. Some recommend PTU in 1st trimester, then switch to MMI in 2nd and 3rd trimesters
   b. Goal to maintain high–normal levels of free T_4 and FTI
   c. May cause transient neonatal hypothyroidism
   d. Iodine 131 thyroid ablation is contraindicated in pregnancy
2. Thyrotoxicosis
   a. May present with tachycardia, exophthalmos, thyromegaly, heat intolerance, pretibial myxedema, and weight loss
   b. Symptoms can be managed with β-blockers
3. Thyroid storm
   a. Symptoms include fever >103°F, severe tachycardia, widened pulse pressure, and changes in mentation
   b. Rare, but carries high risk of maternal heart failure
   c. May be precipitated by infection, surgery, labor, or delivery
4. Hyperemesis gravidarum may be associated with elevated human chorionic gonadotropin (hCG) and hyperthyroidism (usually transient and rarely clinically overt)
C. Hypothyroidism
1. Treat as for nonpregnant women
2. Adjust levothyroxine doses every 4 weeks until TSH stabilizes, then check TSH once per trimester
3. Fetal complications: IUGR, cretinism, and stillbirth
D. Postpartum thyroiditis
1. Occurs in 5% of women who have no prior history of thyroid disease
2. May manifest as hypothyroidism, thyrotoxicosis, or thyrotoxicosis followed by hypothyroidism

IV. Urinary Tract Disorders
A. Asymptomatic bacteriuria: should be treated because more likely during pregnancy to lead to cystitis and pyelonephritis
B. Recurrent UTIs or pyelonephritis warrant suppressive antimicrobial therapy
C. Pyelonephritis
1. More common in pregnancy due to pressure on bladder by enlarging uterus and increase in size of ureters related to smooth muscle relaxation
2. Presents with fever, costovertebral angle (CVA) tenderness, malaise, and dehydration
3. Treatment: intravenous (IV) hydration and IV antibiotics
4. Prophylaxis for remainder of pregnancy with nitrofurantoin or cephalexin, especially if pyelonephritis is recurrent
D. Urinary calculi
1. Presents with CVA tenderness, malaise, microhematuria
2. Renal colic not seen as frequently in pregnant women compared with nonpregnant women

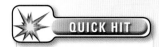

Approximately half of women with gestational diabetes will develop type 2 diabetes later in life. This risk is lower in women who achieve a normal body weight after delivery.

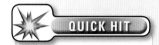

Screening for thyroid disease in pregnancy is indicated primarily in women with a history of thyroid disease or with symptoms and should be performed by measuring thyroid-stimulating hormone (TSH), free T_4, and FTI.

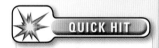

Iodine 131 thyroid ablation is *contraindicated* in pregnancy.

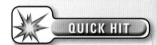

Thyrotoxicosis symptoms in pregnancy can be managed with β-blockers.

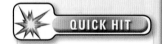

A urine culture is obtained at the onset of prenatal care, and patients with asymptomatic bacteriuria should be treated with antibiotics.

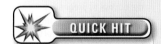

Acute cystitis occurs in ~1% of pregnancies and can manifest with dysuria, urinary frequency, and/or urgency. The treatment is the same as for asymptomatic bacteriuria.

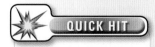

Sepsis occurs in 2%–3% of patients with pyelonephritis, and acute respiratory distress syndrome can occur.

Common Medical and Surgical Problems

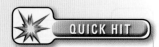

Pregnancy outcome is related to the degree of serum creatinine elevation and the presence of hypertension.

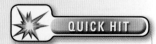

Due to the 40% increase in cardiac output during pregnancy, the risks to mother and fetus are often profound for women with preexisting cardiac disease.

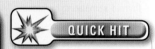

The most likely time of **decompensation** during pregnancy is at 32–34 weeks, when the blood volume increase peaks. However, most *deaths* related to cardiac disease in pregnancy occur after delivery, due to autotransfusion of blood that was going to the uterus.

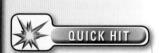

Primary pulmonary hypertension, uncorrected tetralogy of Fallot, Eisenmenger syndrome, and Marfan syndrome with significant aortic root dilation are associated with much worse prognoses (frequently death) through the course of pregnancy. Patients with these disorders are strongly advised *not* to become pregnant.

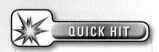

Effects of pregnancy on asthma are variable—about 1/3 of patients worsen, 1/3 improve, and 1/3 remain unchanged.

Common Medical and Surgical Problems

E. Preexisting renal disease
  1. Patients with moderate to severe renal impairment (serum creatinine ≥1.5 mg/dL) have increased risk of deterioration of renal function
  2. May have preexisting hypertension or develop hypertensive disorders of pregnancy
  3. Increased incidence of IUGR

V. Cardiac Disease
A. Prognosis worsens as severity of heart failure (New York Heart Association Classification) increases (Table 16.5)
B. General management principles
  1. Avoidance of conditions that increase heart's workload, such as anemia, infection, strenuous activity, significant weight gain
  2. Serial evaluation of maternal cardiac status and fetal growth
  3. Vaginal delivery preferable, due to increased cardiac stress of Cesarean delivery
  4. Epidural analgesia recommended
C. Fetal complications
  1. Increased risk of low birth weight and prematurity
  2. Congenital cardiac defects more common in fetuses of women with congenital heart defects; fetal echo is recommended
D. Rheumatic heart disease
  1. ~90% of patients have mitral stenosis, and mechanical obstruction worsens with increased cardiac output of pregnancy
  2. Severity of valvular lesion correlates with risks of thromboembolic disease, subacute bacterial endocarditis, cardiac failure, and pulmonary edema
E. Peripartum cardiomyopathy occurs in last month of pregnancy or within 6 months of delivery
  1. Treat as for cardiac failure outside of pregnancy, but avoid angiotensin-converting enzyme inhibitors in pregnancy (fetal and neonatal risks)
  2. Mortality is high, but prognosis improves if cardiac size returns to normal
  3. Diagnosis of exclusion

TABLE **16.5** New York Heart Association Functional Classification of Heart Disease	
Class	**Description**
I	No cardiac decompensation
II	No symptoms of cardiac decompensation at rest; minor limitations of physical activity
III	No symptoms of cardiac decompensation at rest; marked limitations of physical activity
IV	Symptoms of cardiac decompensation at rest; increased discomfort with any physical activity

(From Beckmann CRB, Ling FW, et al. *Obstetrics and Gynecology*, 7th ed. Baltimore: Lippincott Williams & Wilkins; 2014.)

VI. Asthma
A. Routine evaluation of pulmonary function performed
  1. Persistent asthma treated with inhaled corticosteroids
  2. Inhaled albuterol used for rescue therapy
  3. Severe exacerbations treated same as nonpregnant patient
B. Moderate to severe asthma: associated with increased risk of low birth weight and prematurity and should be treated aggressively

VII. Surgical Conditions in Pregnancy

A. General surgical principles in pregnancy
   1. Not all surgical emergencies are obstetrically or gynecologically related
   2. Risks and benefits of radiographic studies must be weighed; shielding of abdomen when possible
      a. Iodinated contrast avoided when possible (category B), but if iodinated contrast is used, newborn thyroid function to be checked in 1st week of life
      b. Magnetic resonance imaging in pregnancy: no known harmful effects, but gadolinium associated with IUGR and congenital anomalies in animal testing
   3. Patient positioned in lateral decubitus position if possible, to relieve pressure on inferior vena cava and reduce supine hypotension
   4. Optimal timing for surgery during pregnancy is 2nd trimester
   5. Fetal heart rate monitoring: depending on gestational age

B. Appendicitis: most common surgical complication of pregnancy
   1. Location of pain may differ due to upward displacement of appendix by gravid uterus
   2. Leukocytosis may be masked by normal leukocytosis of pregnancy
   3. Surgical management can be open or laparoscopic
   4. When diagnosed and treated early (i.e., before appendiceal rupture and generalized peritonitis), fetal and maternal outcomes are good

C. Cholelithiasis
   1. Increased risk in pregnancy due to reduced motility of gallbladder and increased cholesterol saturation in bile
   2. Asymptomatic cholelithiasis: manage expectantly
   3. Cholecystitis with common bile duct obstruction, ascending cholangitis, pancreatitis, or acute abdomen: requires immediate surgical management

D. Ovarian torsion
   1. 25% of cases occur in pregnancy
   2. Operative management is indicated

E. Adnexal masses
   1. Most masses are benign and resolve spontaneously
   2. Persistent cysts >6 cm, or contain solid elements may require surgery
   3. If surgical excision required, best done in 2nd trimester

VIII. Trauma in Pregnancy

A. Evaluation and management
   1. 1st priority: maternal stabilization and identification of fetal heart tones
   2. Electronic fetal monitoring (EFM): once secondary survey is done
      a. EFM for 2–6 hours following minor trauma
      b. EFM for at least 24 hours for moderate or major trauma or if signs of uterine tenderness, irritability or contractions, vaginal bleeding, rupture of membranes, or nonreassuring fetal status

B. Pregnancy-related consequences of trauma
   1. Maternal injury and death
      a. With cardiopulmonary arrest in 3rd trimester, emergent Cesarean delivery considered after 4 minutes of failed resuscitation
      b. Delivery within 5 minutes of cardiopulmonary arrest has best fetal outcomes
      c. Fetal survival unlikely if maternal vital signs have been absent for 10–15 minutes
   2. Feto–maternal hemorrhage
      a. Extent can be assessed using **Kleihauer-Betke test** (see Chapter 21)
      b. RhoGAM administered to Rh– mother
   3. In cases of placental abruption, uterine rupture, or fetal distress, Cesarean delivery may be considered if patient stable, depending on gestational age
   4. Preterm labor or premature rupture of membranes or direct fetal injury may also occur

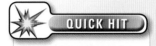

QUICK HIT

Appendicitis is the most common surgical complication of pregnancy.

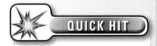

QUICK HIT

Appendicitis is often associated with right upper quadrant (RUQ) pain in pregnancy due to the upward displacement of the appendix outside of the pelvis by the uterus.

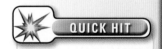

QUICK HIT

Pregnancy carries increased risk of gallstone disease due to reduced motility of the gallbladder and increased cholesterol saturation in bile.

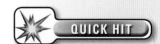

QUICK HIT

The most common cause of trauma in pregnancy is motor vehicle accidents, which is associated with placental abruption. The second most common cause is physical violence against women, most frequently intimate partner violence.

Common Medical and Surgical Problems

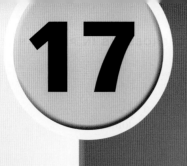

17 Infectious Diseases in Pregnancy

I. Group B *Streptococcus* (GBS)

  A. Epidemiology
   1. Asymptomatic lower genital tract colonization in 30% of pregnant women
   2. 50% exposed infants become colonized
      a. Only 1%–2% infants become infected without maternal treatment
   3. Incidence
      a. Early-onset GBS infection in 0.28/1,000 live births
      b. Late-onset GBS infection in 0.3–0.4/1,000 live births
   4. Case fatality
      a. Early onset: 2%–3% term, 20% preterm
      b. Late onset: 1%–2% term, 5%–6% preterm
  B. Pathophysiology
   1. 2 manifestations of neonatal clinical infection
      a. Early-onset infection
         i. <7 days
         ii. Vertical transmission
         iii. Sepsis, pneumonia, or meningitis
      b. Late-onset infection
         i. 7–90 days
         ii. Vertical transmission, nosocomial, or community-acquired infection
   2. Risk factors for early-onset infection
      a. Maternal genitourinary (GU) or gastrointestinal colonization
      b. Delivery <37 weeks' gestation
      c. Premature rupture of membranes (PROM)
      d. Rupture of membranes >18 hours
      e. Chorioamnionitis
      f. GBS bacteriuria
      g. Prior infant with GBS disease
   3. Maternal infection
      a. Urinary tract infection
      b. Chorioamnionitis
      c. Endometritis
      d. Bacteremia
  C. Screening (Table 17.1)
   1. Universal screening recommended between 35 and 37 weeks' gestation
   2. Swab both lower vagina and rectum
  D. Diagnosis
   1. Clinical criteria in neonate: lethargy, irritability, respiratory distress, temperature instability, hypotension
   2. Chest X-ray with diffuse alveolar infiltrates
   3. Blood culture GBS positive

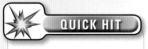

QUICK HIT

All women who are GBS positive by rectovaginal culture should receive antibiotic prophylaxis in labor or with rupture of membranes.

TABLE **17.1**	**Screening Recommendations for Sexually Transmitted Diseases in Pregnancy**
First prenatal visit	
HIV	All women
Hepatitis B	All women
Hepatitis C	All women
HSV	Inquire about history, no routine screening
Chlamydia	All women
Gonorrhea	All women
Third trimester	
HIV	High risk or previously undocumented
Syphilis	High risk
Chlamydia	High risk
Gonorrhea	High risk
Group B *Streptococcus*	All women at 35–37 weeks' gestation
Delivery/postpartum stay	
HIV	High risk or if previously undocumented Perform rapid HIV testing
Syphilis	High risk or if previously undocumented
Hepatitis B	High risk or if previously undocumented
HSV	With prior history of new diagnosis in pregnancy, inquire about prodromal symptoms and carefully examine lower genital tract before delivery

HIV, human immunodeficiency virus; HSV, herpes simplex virus.

E. Treatment
  1. Maternal prophylaxis in labor
    a. GBS positive by antepartum culture within 5 weeks of delivery
    b. GBS status unknown, treat if
      i. Preterm labor (<37 weeks' gestation)
      ii. Preterm PROM (<37 weeks' gestation)
      iii. Rupture of membranes ≥18 hours
      iv. Maternal fever during labor (≥100.4°F [38°C])
    c. GBS bacteriuria in current pregnancy
    d. Previous birth of infant with early-onset GBS disease
  2. Penicillin: drug of choice for labor prophylaxis
    a. Alternatives: cefazolin, clindamycin, erythromycin, vancomycin
    b. *Must* perform antibiotic sensitivities if using clindamycin or erythromycin
  3. Antimicrobial therapy to infant for GBS disease

II. Herpes Simplex Virus (HSV)
  A. Epidemiology
    1. 1/3 female population positive for HSV-1 or HSV-2
    2. Most genital infections from HSV-2 but HSV-1 infections rising
  B. Pathophysiology
    1. Double-stranded DNA virus
    2. 2 serotypes
      a. HSV-1
        i. Primary cause of herpes labialis, gingivostomatitis, keratoconjunctivitis

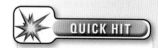

QUICK HIT

Routine prophylaxis is *not* recommended for a woman undergoing planned Cesarean section without labor or rupture of membranes.

Infectious Diseases in Pregnancy

Infectious Diseases in Pregnancy

ii. Rising cause of *genital infections*

iii. Infrequently causes *genital recurrences*

   b. HSV-2

     i. Primary cause of *genital infections*

     ii. Common cause of *genital recurrences*

3. Types of HSV infection

   a. Primary: no evidence of prior infection

   b. Nonprimary 1st episode: history of heterologous infection

     i. 1st HSV-2 infection

     ii. Prior HSV-1 infection

   c. Recurrent disease: clinical/serologic evidence of prior same herpes infection

4. Transmission

   a. Maternal: direct oral or sexual contact

   b. Fetal: vertical

5. Risk of infection

   a. Primary infection at time of delivery = 50% risk neonatal infection

   b. Recurrent infection at time of delivery = 3% risk neonatal infection

C. Screening (see Table 17.1)

  1. Routine type-specific serologic screening *not* recommended

  2. May consider selective screening in high-risk population

D. Diagnosis

  1. Polymerase chain reaction (PCR) preferred test in acute setting

  2. Serologic testing for HSV-1 and HSV-2 for confirmation

  3. Culture vesicle base

   a. Limited sensitivity with recurrent disease

   b. Sensitivity decreases as lesion crusts over

E. Treatment

  1. Acyclovir and related compounds *safe* in pregnancy

  2. Prophylaxis *should* be offered at 36 weeks

   a. Decreases risk of viral shedding

   b. Decreases need for Cesarean delivery

III. Human Immunodeficiency Virus/Acquired Immunodeficiency Syndrome (HIV/AIDS)

A. Epidemiology

  1. 50% HIV-infected patients are women

  2. 27% patients with AIDS are women

  3. 70% female transmission through heterosexual contact; 30% intravenous (IV) drug use

  4. 1% population with AIDS age <13 years old; most acquired perinatally

B. Pathophysiology

  1. Single-stranded RNA, enveloped retrovirus

  2. Transmission

   a. Maternal: direct sexual contact

   b. Fetal: vertical

   c. Infant: breastfeeding

  3. Seroconversion usually within 2–8 weeks of infection

  4. CD4 count gradually decreases until immunodeficiency occurs

   a. Usual latency from untreated HIV to AIDS = 11 years

   b. Host now more susceptible to other infections

  5. Perinatal transmission

   a. 25% risk without prophylactic therapy

   b. 8% risk with zidovudine monotherapy

   c. 1%–2% risk with combination antiretroviral therapy and undetectable viral load

C. Screening (see Table 17.1)

  1. Universal, voluntary opt-out screening is standard

  2. 3rd trimester repeat screening for at-risk populations

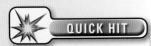

QUICK HIT

Risks of neonatal HSV infection: localized (skin, eye, mouth), disseminated (especially liver), and central nervous system (CNS) (encephalitis).

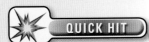

QUICK HIT

Infants with localized infection do well, whereas infants with disseminated disease do poorly.

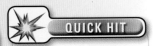

QUICK HIT

With labor onset, Cesarean delivery is recommended if prodromal symptoms are reported *or* a herpetic lesion is found on exam.

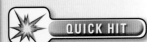

QUICK HIT

HIV infection has *no* direct effect on pregnancy course or outcome; likewise, pregnancy does *not* affect the course of HIV.

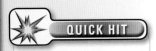

QUICK HIT

HIV and pregnancy can affect infections (e.g., candidiasis, cytomegalovirus [CMV], toxoplasmosis, HSV), which can result in preterm labor or perinatal infection.

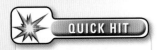

QUICK HIT

The risk of transmission increases with a higher viral load and lower CD4 count.

D. Diagnosis
  1. Enzyme-linked immunosorbent assay (ELISA)
     a. Screening test
     b. Antigen–antibody reaction
     c. More sensitive, less specific
  2. Western blot
     a. Diagnostic test
     b. Identifies antibodies to specific virus antigens
     c. More specific, less sensitive
  3. Combination of ELISA and Western blot 99% sensitive and specific for HIV
  4. Rapid HIV testing standard during labor if no documented prenatal testing
E. Treatment
  1. Combination antiretroviral antepartum, intrapartum, and to neonate
  2. Risk factors for increased transmission
     a. Chorioamnionitis
     b. Prolonged rupture of membranes
     c. Invasive fetal monitoring
     d. Mode of delivery
  3. Cesarean delivery before labor onset or rupture of membranes decreases perinatal transmission
     a. Only if viral load >1,000 copies/mL
     b. Recommended at 38 weeks

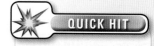

> **QUICK HIT**
>
> Breastfeeding is *usually* contraindicated in HIV-positive women; however, breastfeeding with concomitant administration of antiretroviral medications to the mother is acceptable in some developing regions.

IV. Syphilis

A. Epidemiology
  1. 1.5 cases per 100,000 women
  2. 80% women with syphilis are of reproductive age
B. Pathophysiology
  1. Systemic disease caused by spirochete *Treponema pallidum*
  2. Transmission
     a. Maternal: direct sexual contact
     b. Fetal: vertical or transplacental
  3. Maternal stages of infection
     a. Primary syphilis: painless ulcer (chancre) 6 weeks after exposure
     b. Secondary syphilis
        i. Early
           (a) 1–3 months later
           (b) Adenopathy, maculopapular rash on palms/soles/mucous membranes, genital condyloma lata
        ii. Latent
           (a) Asymptomatic
           (b) May last years
     c. Tertiary syphilis: cardiac, neurologic, ophthalmic, auditory, or gummatous lesions
  4. Fetal effects
     a. Spontaneous abortion, stillbirth, and neonatal death more frequent if untreated
     b. Congenital syphilis
        i. More frequent in primary or secondary (nonlatent) phase
        ii. Some asymptomatic
        iii. Early signs: maculopapular rash, snuffles, oropharynx mucous patches, hepatosplenomegaly, jaundice, adenopathy, chorioretinitis
        iv. Late signs: Hutchinson teeth, mulberry molars, saddle nose, saber shins
C. Screening (see Table 17.1)
  1. Universal screening at initial prenatal visit
  2. Rapid plasma reagin (RPR)

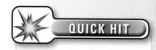

> **QUICK HIT**
>
> Most infections are detected during the latent phase with routine serologic testing.

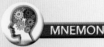

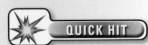

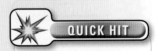

Penicillin is the drug of choice for maternal syphilis because it crosses the placenta.

If the mother is allergic to penicillin, perform allergy testing and desensitize her.

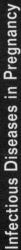

Infectious Diseases in Pregnancy

D. Diagnosis
1. RPR
   a. Screening test
   b. False positives with systemic lupus erythematosus, Lyme disease, HIV
2. Treponemal-specific antibody test (FTA-Abs)
   a. Confirmatory diagnostic test
   b. Remains positive for lifetime
E. Treatment
1. Penicillin
2. Jarisch-Herxheimer reaction
   a. Acute febrile reaction within 24 hours of treatment
   b. Due to treponemal lipopolysaccharide release from dying spirochetes
   c. May cause preterm labor or fetal distress
3. Follow posttreatment titers for 1 year: 4-fold increase in serologic titer or persistent/recurrent symptoms indicates need for retreatment

V. *Neisseria gonorrhoeae*
A. Epidemiology
1. Incidence in pregnancy 1%–7%
2. Perinatal transmission occurs in 30%–40% cases
B. Pathophysiology
1. Gram-negative diplococci
2. Transmission
   a. Maternal: direct sexual contact
   b. Fetal: vertical
3. Cervicitis, urethritis, pharyngitis, and disseminated disease
4. Rare cause of pelvic inflammatory disease after 1st few weeks of pregnancy given cervical mucus plug and protective fetal membranes
5. Neonatal gonococcal ophthalmia
   a. Purulent conjunctivitis, eyelid edema
   b. Progresses to scarring, visual impairment without treatment
C. Screening (see Table 17.1)
1. Screen *all* pregnant women at 1st prenatal visit
2. Rescreen high-risk women in 3rd trimester
D. Diagnosis
1. Nucleic acid amplification tests (DNA or RNA)—endocervical or urine
2. Culture rarely used because less sensitive than PCR
E. Treatment
1. Antibiotic therapy (ceftriaxone + azithromycin)
2. Routine prophylactic ophthalmic antibiotic ointment for *all* neonates

VI. *Chlamydia trachomatis*
A. Epidemiology
1. Incidence in pregnancy 2%–13%
2. Perinatal transmission with symptoms varies
   a. Conjunctivitis 20%–50%
   b. Pneumonia 5%–30%
B. Pathophysiology
1. Transmission
   a. Maternal: direct sexual contact
   b. Fetal: vertical
2. Asymptomatic, urethritis, mucopurulent cervicitis
3. Rare cause of pelvic inflammatory disease after 1st few weeks of pregnancy given cervical mucus plug and protective fetal membranes
4. Neonatal chlamydial conjunctivitis and pneumonia
C. Screening (see Table 17.1)
1. Screen *all* pregnant women at 1st prenatal visit
2. Rescreen high-risk women in 3rd trimester

D. Diagnosis
1. Nucleic acid amplification tests (DNA or RNA)—endocervical or urine
2. Culture rarely used because less sensitive than PCR
E. Treatment
1. Antibiotic therapy (azithromycin or amoxicillin)
2. Routine prophylaxis against chlamydial conjunctivitis *not* effective
3. Repeat testing 3 weeks after treatment necessary to confirm cure

VII. Cytomegalovirus (CMV)

A. Epidemiology
1. 1%–3% incidence primary CMV infection in pregnancy
2. 50%–85% adults have serologic evidence of prior CMV by age 40 years
3. CMV transmitted to fetus in 30% of primary maternal infections
   a. Most infants asymptomatic at birth
   b. 5%–20% infants overtly symptomatic at birth
      i. 5% mortality rate among symptomatic
      ii. 50%–60% survivors develop severe neurologic morbidity
B. Pathophysiology
1. Double-stranded DNA herpes virus
2. Transmission
   a. Maternal: direct contact via saliva, semen, cervical secretions, breast milk, blood, urine
   b. Maternal: household contacts and daycare centers high risk
   c. Fetal: vertical or transplacental
   d. Infant: breastfeeding
3. Maternal infection
   a. Asymptomatic in up to 90% of cases
   b. Short mononucleosis-like febrile illness
4. Congenital infection
   a. Almost exclusively associated with *primary* maternal infection
   b. Only 2% neonates infected after *recurrent* maternal infection
   c. Signs and symptoms
      i. Intrauterine growth restriction (IUGR)
      ii. Jaundice
      iii. Petechiae
      iv. Hepatosplenomegaly
      v. Thrombocytopenia
      vi. Microcephaly
      vii. Chorioretinitis
      viii. Nonimmune hydrops/ascites
   d. Of neonates with symptoms at birth, 80%–90% develop
      i. Hearing loss
      ii. Vision impairment
      iii. Mental retardation
C. Screening: routine screening *not* recommended
D. Diagnosis
1. Maternal culture of GU tract
2. Confirm with maternal serology
   a. 4-fold rise in immunoglobulin (Ig) G over 2 weeks *or*
   b. IgM level ≥30% IgG level
3. Neonatal infection suspected with ultrasonography
   a. Abdominal and liver calcifications
   b. IUGR
   c. Echogenic bowel
   d. Hepatosplenomegaly
   e. Periventricular calcifications
   f. Ventriculomegaly
   g. Hydrops and ascites
4. Neonatal infection confirmed with amniotic fluid PCR

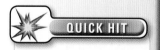

QUICK HIT

The risk of neonatal CMV infection is higher if transmission occurs in the third trimester, but infection is more severe if transmission occurs in the first trimester.

Infectious Diseases in Pregnancy

E. Treatment
1. *No* effective therapy
2. Prevention is key with good hygiene

VIII. Hepatitis A Virus (HAV)
A. Epidemiology
1. 50% of hepatitis in United States
2. 30% of adult women are immune
3. Incidence in pregnancy <1 in 1,000
4. High-risk individuals include IV drug abusers, travelers to endemic areas, those with liver disease
B. Pathophysiology
1. RNA picornavirus
2. Transmission
   a. Maternal: fecal–oral contamination
   b. *No* direct fetal infection
3. Maternal infection: fever, malaise, nausea, vomiting, abdominal discomfort, jaundice
C. Screening: routine screening *not* recommended
D. Diagnosis: serologic testing with IgM
E. Treatment
1. Supportive therapy
2. Preexposure vaccination
3. Vaccination safety in pregnancy not established but theoretically safe as vaccine contains inactivated viral protein (Table 17.2)

IX. Hepatitis B Virus (HBV)
A. Epidemiology
1. 40% of hepatitis cases
   a. Acute infection occurs 1–2/1,000 pregnancies
   b. Chronic infection in 5–15/1,000 pregnancies
2. Chronic infection depends on age at acquisition
   a. 90% in infancy
   b. 60% in children
   c. 10%–15% in adults
B. Pathophysiology
1. DNA virus
2. Transmission
   a. Maternal: parenteral exposure or direct sexual contact
   b. Fetal: vertical or transplacental
3. Maternal infection
   a. 50% asymptomatic
   b. 50% abdominal pain, jaundice
      i. Rarely acute liver failure
      ii. 15%–20% chronic carriers develop cirrhosis or carcinoma
4. Congenital infection
   a. Risk of transplacental infection increases later in pregnancy
   b. HBeAg (HBV "e" antigen) increases risk of vertical transmission up to 90%
C. Screening: screen *all* patients at 1st prenatal visit (see Table 17.1)
D. Diagnosis
1. Serologic testing for HBV surface antigen
2. Serologic testing for IgM to core antigen
3. HBeAg portends more serious disease
   a. Higher viral load
   b. Active replication
E. Treatment
1. Exposed individuals receive HBV immunoglobulin (HBIG) and vaccine series—even if pregnant (see Table 17.2)

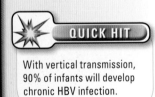

QUICK HIT

With vertical transmission, 90% of infants will develop chronic HBV infection.

TABLE 17.2 Immunizations During Pregnancy

Immuno-biological Agent	Risk From Disease to Pregnant Woman	Risk From Disease to Fetus or Neonate	Type of Immunizing Agent	Risk From Immunizing Agent to Fetus	Indications for Immunization During Pregnancy	Dose Schedule	Comments
Live Virus Vaccines							
Measles	Significant morbidity, low mortality; not altered by pregnancy	Significant increase in abortion rate; may cause malformations	Live attenuated virus vaccine	None confirmed	Contraindicated	Single dose SC; preferably as measles-mumps-rubella	Vaccination of susceptible women should be part of post-partum care
Mumps	Low morbidity and mortality; not altered by pregnancy	Probable increased rate of abortion in 1st trimester	Live attenuated virus vaccine	None confirmed	Contraindicated	Single dose SC; preferably as measles-mumps-rubella	Vaccination of susceptible women should be part of post-partum care
Poliomyelitis	No increased incidence in pregnancy but may be more severe if it does occur	Anoxic fetal damage reported; 50% mortality in neonatal disease	Live attenuated (OPV) and e-IPV vaccine	None confirmed	Not routinely recommended for women in United States, except persons at increased risk of exposure	*Primary:* 2 doses e-IPV SC at 4–8 weeks intervals and a 3rd dose 6–12 months after 2nd dose *Immediate protection:* 1 dose OPV orally	Vaccine indicated for susceptible women traveling in endemic areas or in other high-risk situations
Rubella	Low morbidity and mortality; not altered in pregnancy	High rate of abortion and congenital rubella syndrome	Live attenuated virus vaccine	None confirmed	Contraindicated	Single dose SC, preferably as measles-mumps-rubella	Teratogenicity of vaccine is theoretic, not confirmed to date; vaccination of susceptible women should be part of post-partum care
Yellow fever	Significant morbidity and mortality; not altered by pregnancy	Unknown	Live attenuated virus vaccine	Unknown	Contraindicated except if exposure is unavoidable	Single dose SC	Postponement of travel preferable to vaccination, if possible
Inactivated Virus Vaccines							
Influenza	Possible increase in morbidity and mortality during epidemic of new antigenic strain	Possible increased abortion rate; no malformations confirmed	Inactivated virus vaccine	None confirmed	Women with serious underlying diseases; public health authorities to be consulted for current recommendation	1 dose IM every year	
Rabies	Near 100% fatality; not altered by pregnancy	Determined by maternal disease	Killed virus vaccine	Unknown	Indications for prophylaxis not altered by pregnancy; each case considered individually	Public health authorities to be consulted for indications, dosage, and route of administration	

Infectious Diseases in Pregnancy

(continued)

TABLE 17.2 Immunizations During Pregnancy *(Continued)*

Immuno-biological Agent	Risk From Disease to Pregnant Woman	Risk From Disease to Fetus or Neonate	Type of Immunizing Agent	Risk From Immunizing Agent to Fetus	Indications for Immunization During Pregnancy	Dose Schedule	Comments
Hepatitis B	Possible increased severity during 3rd trimester	Possible increase in abortion rate and prematurity; neonatal hepatitis can occur; high risk of newborn carrier state	Recombinant vaccine	None reported	Pre- and post-exposure for women at risk of infection	3- or 4-dose series IM	Used with hepatitis B Ig for some exposures; exposed newborn needs vaccination as soon as possible
Inactivated Bacterial Vaccines							
Cholera	Significant morbidity and mortality; more severe during 3rd trimester	Increased risk of fetal death during 3rd-trimester maternal illness	Killed bacterial vaccine	None confirmed	Indications not altered by pregnancy; vaccination recommended only in unusual outbreak situations	Single dose SC or IM, depending on manufacturer's recommendations when indicated	
Plague	Significant morbidity and mortality; not altered by pregnancy	Increased risk of fetal death during 3rd-trimester maternal illness	Killed bacterial vaccine	None reported	Selective vaccination of exposed persons	Public health authorities to be consulted for indications, dosage, and route of administration	
Pneumococcus	No increased risk during pregnancy; no increase in severity of disease	Unknown	Polyvalent polysaccharide vaccine	No data available on use during pregnancy	Indications not altered by pregnancy; vaccine used only for individuals	In adults, 1 SC or IM dose only; consider repeat dose in 6 years for high-risk individuals	
Typhoid	Significant morbidity and mortality; not altered by pregnancy	Unknown	Killed or live attenuated oral bacterial vaccine	None confirmed	Not recommended routinely except for close, continued exposure or travel to endemic areas	Killed: *Primary:* 2 injections SC at least 4 weeks apart *Booster:* Single dose SC or ID (depending on type of product used) every 3 years Oral: *Primary:* 4 doses on alternate days *Booster:* Schedule not yet determined	
Toxoids							
Tetanus-diphtheria	Severe morbidity; tetanus mortality 30%; diphtheria mortality 10%; unaltered by pregnancy	Neonatal mortality 60%	Combined tetanus-diphtheria toxoids preferred: adult tetanus-diphtheria formulation	None confirmed	Lack of primary series, or no booster within past 10 years	*Primary:* 2 doses IM at 1- to 2-month interval with a 3rd dose 6–12 months after the 2nd *Booster:* Single dose IM every 10 years, after completion of primary series	

TABLE 17.2 Immunizations During Pregnancy (Continued)

Immuno-biological Agent	Risk From Disease to Pregnant Woman	Risk From Disease to Fetus or Neonate	Type of Immunizing Agent	Risk From Immunizing Agent to Fetus	Indications for Immunization During Pregnancy	Dose Schedule	Comments
Specific Immune Globulins							
Hepatitis B	Possible increased severity during 3rd trimester	Possible increase in abortion rate and prematurity; neonatal hepatitis can occur; high risk of carriage in newborn	Hepatitis B Ig	None reported	Postexposure prophylaxis	Depends on exposure; consult Advisory Committee on Immunization Practices recommendations	Usually given with hepatitis B virus vaccine; exposed newborn needs immediate postexposure prophylaxis
Rabies	Near 100% fatality; not altered by pregnancy	Determined by maternal disease	Rabies Ig	None reported	Postexposure prophylaxis	Half dose at injury site; half dose in deltoid	Used in conjunction with killed rabies virus vaccine
Tetanus	Severe morbidity; mortality 21%	Neonatal tetanus mortality 60%	Tetanus Ig	None reported	Postexposure prophylaxis	1 dose IM	Used in conjunction with tetanus toxoid
Varicella	Possible increase in severe varicella pneumonia	Can cause congenital varicella with increased mortality in neonatal period; very rarely causes congenital defects	Varicella-zoster Ig	None reported	Can be considered for healthy pregnant women exposed to varicella to protect against maternal, not congenital, infection	1 dose IM within 96 hours of exposure	Indicated also for newborns of mothers who developed varicella within 4 days before or days after delivery; ~90%–95% of adults are immune to varicella; not indicated for prevention of congenital varicella
Standard Immune Globulins							
Hepatitis A	Possible increased severity during 3rd trimester	Probably increase in abortion rate and prematurity; possible transmission to neonate at delivery if mother is incubating the virus or is acutely ill at that time	Standard Ig	None reported	Postexposure prophylaxis	0.02 mL/kg IM in 1 dose of Ig	Ig should be given as soon as possible and within 2 weeks of exposure; infants born to mothers who are incubating the virus or are acutely ill at delivery should receive 1 dose of 0.5 mL as soon as possible after birth
Measles	Significant morbidity; low mortality; not altered by pregnancy	Significant increase in abortion rate; may cause malformations	Standard Ig	None reported	Postexposure prophylaxis	0.25 mL/kg IM in 1 dose of Ig up to 15 mL	Unclear if it prevents abortion; must be given within 6 days of exposure

e-IPV, enhanced-potency inactivated poliovirus vaccine; ID, intradermally; Ig, immunoglobulin; IM, intramuscularly; OPV, oral polio vaccine; SC, subcutaneously.

Infectious Diseases in Pregnancy

      2. HBsAg-negative women at risk should receive vaccine in pregnancy

      3. Infants born to HBV moms receive HBIG and vaccine within 12 hours of delivery

      4. Breastfeeding *not* contraindicated if therapy started appropriately

X. Hepatitis C Virus (HCV)

A. Epidemiology
1. 50% infected individuals develop chronic infection
2. Incidence of vertical transmission <10%

B. Pathophysiology
1. Single-stranded RNA virus
2. Transmission
    a. Maternal: direct blood-to-blood contact (IV drug abuse) or sexual contact
    b. Fetal: vertical
3. Maternal infection
    a. Many asymptomatic
    b. Mild clinical syndrome: fever, malaise
4. Congenital infection
    a. 2%–12% of infected pregnancies
       i. With increasing viral load, increased risk of vertical transmission
       ii. Coinfection with HIV increases vertical transmission
       iii. Prolonged rupture of membranes and invasive fetal monitoring may increase risk of fetal infection
    b. Breastfeeding is not contraindicated but may not be advisable if nipples cracked or bleeding

C. Screening (see Table 17.1)
1. Routine screening *not* recommended
2. Screen high-risk individuals
    a. IV drug abuse
    b. HIV+

D. Diagnosis
1. Serologic testing for anti-HCV antibody
2. Confirm with HCV-RNA for viral load

E. Treatment
1. No treatment in pregnancy
2. No postexposure prophylaxis

XI. Parvovirus B-19

A. Epidemiology: 60% of adolescents and adults demonstrate serologic immunity

B. Pathophysiology
1. Causes erythema infectiosum ("fifth" disease)
2. Transmission
    a. Maternal: close contact
    b. Fetal: transplacental
3. Maternal infection
    a. Fever, malaise, arthralgia
    b. "Slapped cheek" macular facial rash
4. Congenital infection
    a. Transplacental infection in 25%–50% of infected pregnancies
    b. Adverse fetal outcome <5% of infected pregnancies
    c. Signs and symptoms
       i. IUGR
       ii. Fetal hydrops/ascites
       iii. Placentomegaly

C. Screening for exposed or symptomatic individuals (see Table 17.1)

D. Diagnosis
1. IgM antibody or 4-fold increase in IgG
2. Stable IgG suggests prior infection

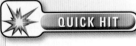
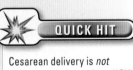

QUICK HIT

Cesarean delivery is *not* recommended to reduce HCV transmission.

      3. Neonatal infection suspected with ultrasonographic findings
        a. Growth restriction
        b. Placentomegaly
        c. Hydrops/ascites
   E. Treatment
      1. No treatment for maternal disease
      2. Follow with serial ultrasounds
      3. Hydrops may warrant cordocentesis and fetal blood transfusion

XII. Varicella

   A. Epidemiology
      1. Most adults are immune
      2. Introduction of vaccine in 1995 has reduced clinical disease
   B. Pathophysiology
      1. Member of *Herpesvirus*
        a. Causes chicken pox
        b. Recurrence from latency causes herpes zoster (shingles)
      2. Transmission
        a. Maternal: aerosolized droplets or direct contact with active lesions
        b. Fetal: vertical or transplacental
      3. Maternal infection
        a. Vesicular rash, fever, malaise
        b. In pregnancy, mothers at increased risk of varicella pneumonia
      4. Congenital infection
        a. Infection in 1st half of pregnancy
          i. IUGR
          ii. Limb hypoplasia
          iii. Scarring
          iv. Muscular atrophy
          v. Microcephaly
          vi. Encephalitis
          vii. Chorioretinitis
        b. Most serious fetal consequences if infection around delivery
   C. Screening for exposed individuals (see Table 17.2)
   D. Diagnosis
      1. Serologic testing for IgM and IgG
      2. Pathognomonic rash
      3. Neonatal infection suspected with ultrasonographic findings
   E. Treatment
      1. No curative therapy
      2. Varicella-zoster immunoglobulin (VZIG) within 72 hours of exposure
      3. Acyclovir within 24 hours of rash appearance
      4. VZIG to newborns of recently infected mothers
      5. IV acyclovir for varicella pneumonia
      6. Vaccine and prevention mainstay of therapy (see Table 17.2)
        a. Postpartum vaccine for nonimmune mothers
        b. Vaccine prior to pregnancy in nonimmune patients
        c. Contraceptive practice for 1 month after vaccine

XIII. *Toxoplasma gondii*

   A. Epidemiology: 15% of adults demonstrate immunity
   B. Pathophysiology
      1. Intracellular parasite
      2. Transmission
        a. Maternal: contaminated cat feces or consumption of undercooked meats
        b. Fetal: transplacental
      3. Maternal infection
        a. Many asymptomatic
        b. Self-limited: mild fevers and malaise

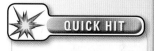

QUICK HIT

If maternal symptoms occur 5 days before to 2 days after delivery, the risk of severe neonatal infection is high.

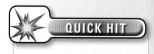

QUICK HIT

Live varicella vaccine is *not* recommended in pregnancy.

Infectious Diseases in Pregnancy

4. Congenital infection
   a. More common in 3rd trimester (50%)
   b. Less common in 1st trimester (20%)
      i. Mental retardation
      ii. Blindness
      iii. Hearing impairment
      iv. Epilepsy
      v. Microcephaly
      vi. Chorioretinitis
      vii. Hydrocephaly
C. Screening: routine screening is *not* recommended
D. Diagnosis
   1. Serologic testing with IgM and IgG
      a. IgM positive suggests recent infection
      b. IgM may remain positive for prolonged periods
      c. IgG positive suggests prior infection
   2. Neonatal infection suspected if ultrasonographic findings
      a. Microcephaly
      b. Ventriculomegaly
      c. IUGR
      d. Intracranial calcifications
      e. Hydrops/ascites
E. Treatment
   1. Spiramycin may help prevent vertical transmission but little value for fetal infection
   2. Pyrimethamine and sulfadiazine may reduce risk of congenital infection and sequelae
   3. Reduce exposure by cooking meat thoroughly
   4. Avoid caring for cats unless kept indoors and fed processed foods
   5. Prior to treatment, confirm diagnosis using qualified reference laboratory

XIV. Human Papillomavirus (HPV)

A. Epidemiology: >50% of reproductive age women exposed
B. Pathophysiology
   1. Double-stranded DNA virus
   2. Transmission
      a. Maternal: direct sexual contact
      b. Fetal: direct contact during delivery
   3. Maternal infection
      a. Many asymptomatic
      b. Low-risk HPVs (6, 11) cause warty growth
      c. High-risk HPVs cause dysplasia leading to abnormal Pap smears
   4. Congenital infection
      a. Limited potential effect on fetus
      b. Rare laryngeal papillomatosis from low-risk HPV
C. Screening (see Table 17.1)
   1. No direct screening recommended
   2. Indirect screening with Pap smear in all pregnancies
D. Diagnosis
   1. Indirectly from cytology or histopathology
   2. PCR testing
E. Treatment
   1. No direct viral therapy
   2. Treatment of warts permissible in pregnancy
      a. Excision
      b. Cryotherapy
      c. Laser
      d. Cautery
      e. Trichloroacetic acid

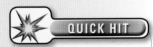

Fetal toxoplasma infection is more severe if disease is acquired in the first trimester.

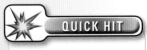

Podophyllin, 5-fluorouracil, and imiquimod are *not* recommended in pregnancy.

Infectious Diseases in Pregnancy

3. Colposcopy and ectocervical biopsy safe in pregnancy; endocervical curettage discouraged in pregnancy
4. HPV vaccine *not* recommended in pregnancy (see Table 17.2)
    a. Interrupt vaccine series if pregnant; resume postpartum
    b. No recognized adverse effects from vaccine in pregnancy
5. Route of delivery *not* dictated by HPV unless significant warty growth increases risk of obstruction or bleeding

XV. Rubella

A. Epidemiology: most reproductive age women immune from widespread vaccination
B. Pathophysiology
    1. RNA virus
    2. Cause of "German measles"
    3. Transmission
        a. Maternal: close contact aerosolized droplets
        b. Fetal: transplacental
    3. Maternal infection: mild fevers and reticular rash
    4. Congenital infection
        a. 20% risk of spontaneous abortion with 1st trimester infection
        b. Congenital rubella syndrome
            i. Congenital heart defect
            ii. Mental retardation
            iii. Deafness
            iv. Cataracts
C. Screening: screen *all* women at 1st prenatal visit (see Table 17.1)
D. Diagnosis
    1. Serologic testing for IgM and IgG
    2. Neonatal infection suspected if ultrasonographic findings
        a. Cardiac defects
        b. Hydrops/ascites
        c. IUGR
E. Treatment
    1. No treatment available
    2. Immunization and screening mainstay of therapy (see Table 17.2)
        a. Postpartum vaccine for nonimmune mothers
        b. Contraception for 1–3 months after vaccine

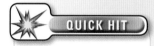

QUICK HIT

Risk of rubella infection is highest if acquired in the first trimester; risk decreases with increasing gestational age.

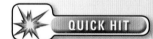

QUICK HIT

Live rubella vaccine is *not* recommended in pregnancy.

Infectious Diseases in Pregnancy

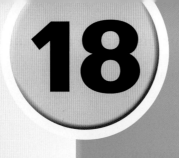

18 Hypertension in Pregnancy

I. Classification

A. **Chronic hypertension**
   1. Onset before pregnancy or prior to 20 weeks' gestational age
   2. Types of hypertension
      a. Mild: systolic ≥140–180 mm Hg or diastolic ≥90–110 mm Hg or both
      b. Severe: systolic ≥180 mm Hg or diastolic ≥100 mm Hg or both
   3. Major risk factors for development of superimposed preeclampsia: in chronic hypertension, preeclampsia is diagnosed by
      a. Acute-onset proteinuria
      b. Worsening of hypertension

B. **Gestational hypertension**
   1. Onset after 20 weeks' gestational age *without* proteinuria
   2. Resolves during postpartum period
   3. Complicates 30% of multifetal pregnancies
   4. 25% of women will eventually develop preeclampsia

C. **Preeclampsia**
   1. Development of hypertension after 20 weeks' gestation *with* proteinuria
   2. Diagnostic criteria
      a. Systolic ≥140 mm Hg or diastolic ≥90 mm Hg
      b. Proteinuria: urinary protein of 300 mg or higher on 24-hour specimen
   3. Risk factors
      a. Nulliparity
      b. Multifetal gestation
      c. Advanced maternal age (maternal age >35 years)
      d. History of preeclampsia in prior pregnancy
      e. Pregestational diabetes
      f. Vascular and connective tissue disorders
      g. Nephropathy
      h. Antiphospholipid syndrome
      i. Obesity
      j. African American
   4. Types
      a. Severe
         i. Systolic ≥160 mm Hg or diastolic ≥110 mm Hg
            (a) 2 occasions 6 hours apart
            (b) Patient should be on bed rest
         ii. Heavy proteinuria
            (a) 5 g on 24-hour urine
            (b) 3+ on dipstick at least 4 hours apart
         iii. Oliguria (<500 mL in 24 hours)
         iv. Neurologic symptoms (headache, scotomas)
         v. Pulmonary edema/hypoxia/cyanosis
         vi. Epigastric or right upper quadrant (RUQ) pain

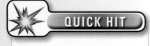

QUICK HIT

Onset of preeclampsia at <20 weeks' gestation is associated with gestational trophoblastic disease.

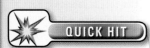

QUICK HIT

Proteinuria plus systolic heart rate ≥140 mm Hg or diastolic ≥90 mm Hg is diagnostic of preeclampsia.

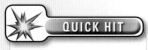

QUICK HIT

RUQ pain in preeclampsia is likely caused by subcapsular hematoma or stretching of the Glisson capsule.

    vii. Hepatic dysfunction (elevated liver enzymes)
    viii. Thrombocytopenia
    ix. Intrauterine growth restriction (IUGR)
  b. Mild: diagnosed when severe disease is ruled out
D. **Eclampsia**
  1. Grand mal seizures in presence of preeclampsia
  2. Can occur in mild or severe disease
  3. Neurologic causes should be ruled out
E. **HELLP** syndrome

II. Preeclampsia Pathophysiology (*Figure 18.1*)

A. Generalized maternal vasospasm potentially mediated by
  1. Vascular changes
    a. Lack of decrease in spiral arteriole musculature prevents creation of low-resistance, low-pressure system
    b. Endothelial damage
  2. Hemostatic changes
    a. Increased platelet activation and endothelial fibronectin
    b. Decreased antithrombin III and α_2-antiplasmin levels promote microthrombi development
  3. Changes in prostanoids
    a. Prostacyclin (PGI_2) dominates thromboxane A2 (TXA_2) in normal pregnancy
      i. Promotes vasodilation
      ii. Decreases platelet aggregation
    b. TXA_2 dominates PGI_2 in preeclampsia
      i. TXA_2 promotes vasoconstriction and platelet aggregation
      ii. Result is overall vessel constriction
  4. Changes in endothelium-derived factors
    a. Nitric oxide (potent vasodilator): decreased in preeclampsia
    b. May be 1st step of vasoconstriction in preeclampsia
  5. Altered lipid peroxides, free radicals, and antioxidants
    a. Elevated lipid peroxide and free radicals increase vascular injury
    b. Decreased levels of protective antioxidants
B. Systemic effects of vasospasm
  1. Cardiovascular
    a. Elevated blood pressure
    b. Increased cardiac output
  2. Hematologic
    a. Plasma volume contraction
      i. Increased risk of hypovolemic shock if hemorrhage occurs
      ii. Hematocrit elevated
      iii. Disseminated intravascular coagulation can occur
        (a) Results from microangiopathic hemolytic anemia
        (b) Can be worsened by hepatocellular dysfunction causing worsening coagulopathy
      iv. **Third spacing** of fluid (evidenced by pitting edema)
        (a) Results from increased blood pressure
        (b) Results from decreased oncotic pressure
  3. Renal effects
    a. Glomerular endotheliosis (atherosclerotic-like changes in renal vessels) causes
      i. Decreased glomerular filtration rate indicated by increasing serum creatinine
      ii. Proteinuria
    b. Decreased uric acid filtration
  4. Neurologic effects
    a. Hyperreflexia/hypersensitivity
    b. Grand mal seizures

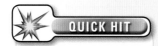

QUICK HIT

Most cases of eclampsia occur within 24 hours of delivery.

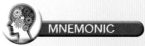

MNEMONIC

HELLP Syndrome
Hemolysis (microangiopathic)
Elevated **l**iver enzymes: hallmark of hepatocellular dysfunction
Low **p**latelet counts (thrombocytopenia)

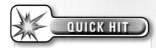

QUICK HIT

HELLP syndrome and eclampsia are both indications for delivery due to the risks of maternal morbidity if the pregnancy is continued.

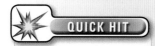

QUICK HIT

The actual cause of the pathophysiology in preeclampsia is unknown but is thought to be directly related to the placenta and the fetus insofar as delivery generally cures the disease.

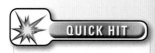

QUICK HIT

Supplementation with aspirin or calcium does not prevent preeclampsia.

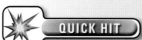
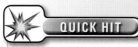

QUICK HIT

The decreased uric acid filtration in preeclampsia may serve as the hallmark of evolving disease.

Hypertension in Pregnancy

FIGURE 18.1 **Proposed pathways and markers implicated in the development of preeclampsia and eclampsia.**

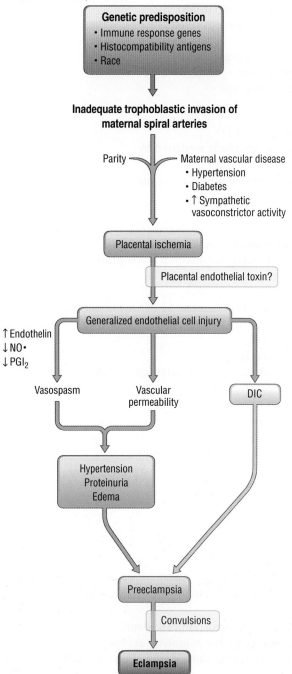

DIC, disseminated intravascular coagulation; NO•, nitric oxide; PGI$_2$, prostacyclin. (Beckmann CRB, Ling FW, et al. *Obstetrics and Gynecology*, 7th ed. Baltimore: Lippincott Williams & Wilkins; 2014.)

5. Pulmonary effects: pulmonary edema has several possible causes
   a. Decreased oncotic pressure
   b. Pulmonary capillary leak
   c. Left heart failure
   d. Iatrogenic fluid overload
6. Fetal effects: vasospasm decreases placental perfusion causing
   a. IUGR
   b. Oligohydramnios
   c. Increase perinatal mortality
   d. Increased placental abruption
   e. Increased incidence of nonreassuring fetal status in labor (results from inability of placenta to oxygenate fetus during contractions)

III. Evaluation

   A. History
      1. Directed at signs and symptoms
      2. Review current obstetric data (labs, previous blood pressures)
      3. Neurologic symptoms especially indicative of vasospasm
      4. RUQ pain can indicate liver involvement
      5. New or worsening seizures

   B. Blood pressure evaluation
      1. Correct size cuff
      2. Position matters
        a. Will be lowest in lateral position
        b. Will be highest when standing
        c. Generally declines in 2nd trimester
        d. Rises to prepregnancy levels in 3rd trimester

   C. Edema and weight gain
      1. Can be normal in pregnancy
      2. Look for rapid rise in weight over short period (indicative of fluid retention)
      3. Evaluate for edema that
        a. Does not improve with rest
        b. Involves upper extremities, face, sacral region

   D. Abdominal exam
      1. Fundal height is 1st step in evaluation of fetal size
      2. Fetal ultrasound is indicated in hypertensive diseases to
        a. Follow fetal growth
        b. Assess amniotic fluid index
      3. Tenderness over liver is seen with capsular distension

   E. Neurologic exam: deep tendon reflexes to evaluate for hyperreflexia/clonus

   F. Laboratory studies: aimed at evaluation of the involved organ systems (Table 18.1)

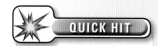

QUICK HIT

Clonus is a particularly worrisome finding and is often indicative of severe disease.

TABLE 18.1 Laboratory Assessment of Pregnant Hypertensive Patients

Test or Procedure	Rationale
Maternal studies	
Complete blood count	Increasing hematocrit may signify worsening vasoconstriction and decreased intravascular volume Decreasing hematocrit may signify hemolysis
Platelet count	Thrombocytopenia is associated with worsening disease
Coagulation profile (PT, PTT)	Coagulopathy is associated with worsening disease
Liver function studies	Hepatocellular dysfunction is associated with worsening disease

Serum creatinine
  Uric acid
  24-hour urine
  Creatinine clearance
  Total urinary protein
	Decreased renal function is associated with worsening disease

Fetal studies (To assess for pregnancy-associated hypertension effects on the fetus)	
Ultrasound examination	
Fetal weight and growth	IUGR
Amniotic fluid volume	Oligohydramnios
NST and/or biophysical profile	Placental status (indirect assessment)

IUGR, intrauterine growth restriction; NST, nonstress test; PT, prothrombin time; PTT, partial thromboplastin time.

Hypertension in Pregnancy

IV. Management

A. Chronic hypertension
   1. Blood pressure is closely monitored as outpatient
   2. Medications are indicated for severe blood pressures only
      a. Purpose is to reduce risk of cerebrovascular accident
      b. Does not improve course of pregnancy (Table 18.2)
   3. Monitor for evidence of superimposed preeclampsia
      a. Physical exam
      b. Laboratory studies
   4. Fetal assessment
      a. Serial ultrasound to assess growth
      b. Nonstress test (NST) at least weekly usually beginning at 28–32 weeks

B. Gestational hypertension
   1. Managed as outpatient similar to chronic hypertension
   2. Antihypertensives generally not utilized (severe range of blood pressure often hallmark of impending preeclampsia)
   3. Stable patients with mild blood pressures generally delivered by 39 weeks

C. Preeclampsia
   1. General considerations
      a. Care is individualized based on
         i. Maturity of fetus
         ii. Severity of disease
   2. Mild preeclampsia
      a. Bed rest and close observation
         i. Often initially done in hospital
         ii. Home management acceptable when severe disease has been ruled out
      b. Maternal assessment
         i. Daily blood pressure evaluation
         ii. At least weekly laboratory assessment (see Table 18.1)
      c. Fetal assessment
         i. Twice weekly NST or biophysical profile
         ii. Weekly fluid assessment

TABLE **18.2** **Antihypertensive Medications Used in Pregnancy**

Medication	Mechanism of Action	Effects
Thiazide	Decreased plasma volume and CO	CO decreased; RBF decreased; maternal depletion; neonatal thrombocytopenia
Methyldopa	False neurotransmission, CNS effect	CO unchanged; RBF unchanged; fever, maternal lethargy, hepatitis, and hemolytic anemia
Hydralazine	Direct peripheral vasodilation	CO increased; RBF unchanged or increased; maternal flushing, headache, tachycardia, lupus-like syndrome
Propranolol	β-Adrenergic blocker	CO decreased; RBF decreased; maternal increased uterine tone with possible decrease in placental perfusion; neonatal depressed respirations
Labetalol	α- and β-Adrenergic blocker	CO unchanged; RBF unchanged; maternal tremulousness, flushing, headache; neonatal depressed respirations; contraindicated in women with asthma and heart failure
Nifedipine	Calcium channel blocker	CO unchanged; RBF unchanged; maternal orthostatic hypotension and headache (also a tocolytic); no neonatal effects known

CNS, central nervous system; CO, cardiac output; RBF, renal blood flow.

     iii Serial ultrasound for growth every 2–4 weeks

     iv. Daily fetal movement counts

3. Severe preeclampsia

  a. Hospitalization necessary

  b. Maternal assessment

     i. Hospitalization for remainder of pregnancy

     ii. Daily laboratory studies

  c. Fetal assessment

     i. Daily NST

     ii. Continue serial ultrasound for growth and fluid assessment

  d. Delivery in severe preeclampsia

     i. Recommended upon diagnosis at 34 weeks or beyond; maternal risks generally outweigh any fetal benefit

     ii. Recommended with worsening status at any gestational age; administration of glucocorticoids for fetal lung maturity

4. Indications for delivery

  a. Worsening fetal status

     i. Abnormal NST

     ii. Development of IUGR

     iii. Development of oligohydramnios

  b. Worsening of maternal status

     i. Uncontrolled hypertension

     ii. Evidence of end-organ compromise

     iii. Development of HELLP syndrome

     iv. Eclampsia

  c. Induction of labor is recommended if feasible; Cesarean delivery for usual obstetric reasons

5. Medical therapy in preeclampsia

  a. Antihypertensives

     i. Prevention of maternal cerebrovascular accident

     ii. Will not prevent worsening of disease

     iii. May mask development of severe disease

     iv. Goal is to keep blood pressure in mild hypertensive range

  b. Magnesium therapy

     i. Prevent and treat eclampsia

       (a) Mild preeclampsia: start when induction is initiated

       (b) Severe preeclampsia: institute at time of diagnosis

       (c) Continue therapy for 24 hours after delivery

     ii. Better than traditional anticonvulsants (phenytoin, diazepam)

     iii. Prevents 98% of eclamptic convulsions

     iv. Therapeutic level is 4–6 mg/dL

     v. Routes of administration

       (a) Intravenous (IV) most commonly used

         (i) Loading bolus of 6 g

         (ii) Maintenance of 2 g/hr with normal renal function

       (b) Intramuscular (IM) used when IV cannot be established

         (i) Loading dose 5 g IM to each buttock

         (ii) Maintenance 5 g IM every 4 hours

     vi. Toxicity treatment (Table 18.3)

       (a) 10% calcium gluconate

       (b) Oxygen supplementation

       (c) Intubation if respiratory collapse

6. After care

  a. Diuresis generally seen in 24–48 hours; occurs as vasospasm reverses itself

  b. Laboratory studies generally normalize; irreversible renal or liver impairment can occur, but rare

  c. Blood pressure may require ongoing treatment even after discharge

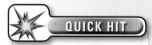

QUICK HIT

Attempts to return blood pressure to a normal range can adversely affect the health of the fetus due to decrease in placental perfusion.

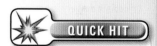

QUICK HIT

About 25% of eclamptic seizures occur prior to onset of labor, 50% occur during labor, and 25% occur in the first 24 hours after delivery.

Hypertension in Pregnancy

TABLE **18.3** **Magnesium Toxicity**	
Serum Concentration (mg/dL)	**Manifestation**
1.5–3	Normal concentration
4–6	Therapeutic levels
5–10	Electrocardiogram changes
8–12	Loss of patellar reflex
9–12	Feeling of warmth, flushing
10–12	Somnolence; slurred speech
15–17	Muscle paralysis; respiratory difficulty
30	Cardiac arrest

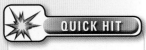

QUICK HIT

Eclampsia can result from either mild or severe preeclampsia.

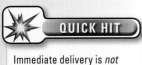

QUICK HIT

Immediate delivery is *not* indicated in eclampsia.

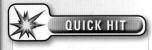

QUICK HIT

Always rule out HELLP syndrome when considering gallbladder disease or viral or GI illness in a pregnant patient.

D. Eclampsia
1. Life-threatening obstetric complication of preeclampsia
2. Maternal risks during seizure
    a. Musculoskeletal injury (biting tongue, bruising of extremities)
    b. Hypoxia
    c. Aspiration
3. Therapy is aimed at cause and limiting injury
    a. Initiate magnesium sulfate bolus
    b. Give additional 2-g bolus in those already on magnesium therapy
        i. Consider laboratory assessment of magnesium level
        ii. Monitor urine output closely as magnesium is cleared renally
    c. Protect against injury (padded bed rails, oral airway)
    d. Consider telemetry monitoring of maternal status
    e. Judicious use of antihypertensive therapy
4. Fetal effects: seizure may often cause heart rate abnormalities
    a. Often related to uterine tachysystole
    b. Generally self-limiting (<20 minutes)
    c. Immediate delivery is *not* indicated
        i Stabilize mother and baby before induction is started
        ii Cesarean delivery is not indicated for eclampsia alone
E. HELLP syndrome
1. More common in multiparous patients
2. Blood pressures are often in mild range
3. Symptoms
    a. RUQ pain
    b. Nausea and vomiting
    c. General malaise
4. Should not be mistaken for
    a. Gallbladder disease
    b. Viral illness
    c. Indigestion/other gastrointestinal (GI) illness
5. Treatment
    a. Individualized based on
        i. Severity of laboratory abnormalities
        ii. Fetal status and gestational age
        iii. Maternal symptoms
    b. Correction of coagulopathy if present
        i. Transfuse platelets if <20,000/mm³
        ii. Transfusion may be warranted earlier if Cesarean delivery planned

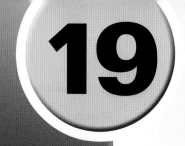

Multifetal Gestation

I. Types of Twins

A. **Dizygotic** (*fraternal* twins): 2 separate ova fertilized by 2 separate sperm

B. **Monozygotic** (*identical* twins): 1 ova fertilized by 1 sperm that divides after fertilization

C. Determination of zygosity by chorionicity (Table 19.1 and Figure 19.1)

1. Monochorionic (~23% of twins) = monozygotic
2. Dichorionic (~77% of twins)
   a. Discordant fetal sex (~33% of dichorionic twins) = dizygotic
   b. Concordant fetal sex (~67% of dichorionic twins)
      i. Discordant blood types (~57% of same-sex dichorionic twins) = dizygotic
      ii. Concordant blood types (~43% of same-sex dichorionic twins); need specialized genetic testing (human leukocyte antigen [HLA] typing or molecular DNA analysis for determination; usually not clinically important)

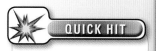

QUICK HIT

Dizygotic twins are *always* diamniotic (two sacs) and dichorionic (two placentas).

II. Rates

A. Rate of dizygotic twinning: 1:89

1. **Hellin law:** natural rate of twins = 89^1, triplets = 89^2, quadruplets = 89^3 (and so on)
2. Blacks > Whites > Asians
3. ↑ With assisted reproduction technology (ART)
   a. Twins rate ↑ 65% since 1980 (due to ART)
   b. Triplets and higher order multiples rate ↑ 500%
      i. 43% due to ART
      ii. 38% from ovulation induction
4. Patient's family history (genetic propensity to ovulate >1 egg)
5. ↑ With increasing maternal age and parity

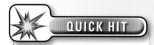

QUICK HIT

With monozygotic twins, the timing of division determines **chorionicity**.

TABLE 19.1 Chorionicity of Monozygotic Gestations Based on Timing of Division		
Timing of Division (Days After Fertilization)	**Chorionicity**	**Rate Among Monozygotic Twins**
0–3	Diamniotic dichorionic (two sacs, two placentas)	30%
4–8	Diamniotic monochorionic (two sacs, one placenta)	69%
9–12	Monoamniotic monochorionic (one sac, one placenta)	1%
13+	Monoamniotic monochorionic conjoined (one sac, one placenta)	0.5%

FIGURE 19.1 Chorionicity in twin pregnancies.

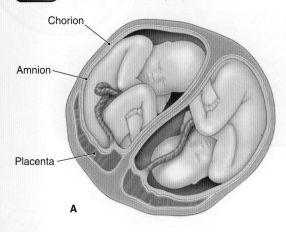
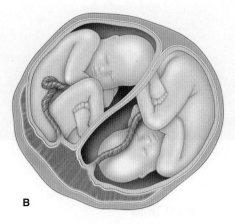

A

B

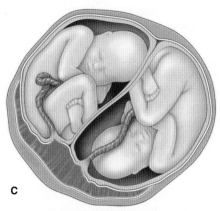
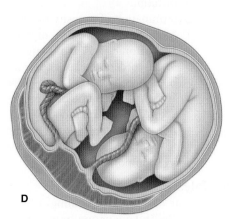

C

D

(A) Two placentas, two amnions, two chorions: diamniotic dichorionic. (B) One placenta, two amnions, two chorions: diamniotic/dichorionic. (C) One placenta, two amnions, one chorion: diamniotic/monochorionic. (D) One placenta, one amnion, one chorion: monoamniotic/ monochorionic. (Based on American College of Obstetricians and Gynecologists. *Having Twins*. Patient Education Pamphlet AP092. Washington, DC: American College of Obstetricians and Gynecologists; 2004.)

B. Rate of monozygotic twinning: 1:250
1. Stable across races
2. Not impacted by family history
3. Slight increase with ART

III. Risks

A. Maternal
1. Antepartum complications
   a. Preterm premature rupture of membranes (PPROM) (6 times higher in twins than singletons)
   b. Gestational diabetes (2 times higher in twins than singletons)
   c. Hospital admission
   d. Preterm labor and delivery (most significant cause of morbidity in multiple gestations)
      i. Twins: 35–36 weeks
      ii. Triplets: 32–33 weeks
      iii. Quadruplets: 28–29 weeks
   e. Anemia
   f. Preeclampsia (3 times higher in twins)
   g. Pulmonary edema (complication of preeclampsia, tocolytics)
   h. Cesarean delivery

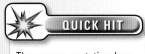

QUICK HIT

The average gestational age of delivery decreases by 4 weeks with each additional fetus.

2. Postpartum complications
   a. Hemorrhage
   b. Endometritis
B. Fetal
   1. Spontaneous abortion (2 times higher in twins)
      a. No antenatal monitoring protocol shown to predict twin losses
      b. If loss occurs remote from term, expectant management of remaining fetus(es) is likely appropriate
   2. Morbidity and mortality (~5 times higher in twins) related to premature birth (dependent on gestational age at delivery) including hyperbilirubinemia, respiratory distress syndrome, intraventricular hemorrhage, patent ductus arteriosus, necrotizing enterocolitis, sepsis, bronchopulmonary dysplasia, death
   3. Intrauterine growth restriction (IUGR)
   4. Congenital anomalies (2 times higher in twins)
   5. Placental abruption
   6. Cord accidents/cord prolapse
   7. Pathology related to monochorionic twins
      a. Twin–twin transfusion syndrome (TTTS)
         i. Results from imbalance of vascular anastomoses of placental vessels between fetuses leading to "loss" of volume/blood from 1 twin (donor) to other (recipient)
            (a) Donor twin characteristics: often smaller with lower amniotic fluid volume (AFV) (**oligohydramnios**); may develop heart failure due to anemia and hypovolemia
            (b) Recipient twin characteristics: often larger with higher AFV (polyhydramnios); may develop heart failure due to polycythemia and volume overload
         ii. Staging (Table 19.2)
         iii. Treatment
            (a) Serial amnioreduction
            (b) In utero laser ablation of intertwin vascular anastomoses
      b. Monoamniotic twins
         i. 40%–70% mortality (2%–5% risk every week after 15 weeks)
         ii. Elective delivery at 32–34 weeks recommended
      c. Acardiac twin (twin reversed arterial perfusion [TRAP])
         i. <1% of monochorionic twin pregnancies
         ii. Results from arterial-to-arterial placental anastomosis
            (a) Arterial blood from "pump" twin flows directly into placental artery of "acardiac" twin (in reverse direction)

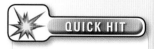

QUICK HIT

In monochorionic gestation, death of a twin can lead to death or permanent neurologic injury of the surviving fetus (due to acute blood loss into the dead fetus); even immediate delivery is unlikely to prevent injury.

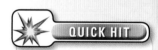

QUICK HIT

TTTS occurs in 10%–15% of monochorionic twins.

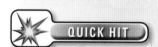

QUICK HIT

Lack of a dividing membrane places the pregnancy at risk of cord entanglement and fetal death due to cord accident.

Stage	Polyhydramnios/Oligohydramnios[a]	Absent Bladder in Donor	Critically Abnormal Doppler Studies[b]	Hydrops	Demise
I	+	−	−	−	−
II	+	+	−	−	−
III	+	+	+	−	−
IV	+	+	+	+	−
V	+	+	+	+	+

TABLE **19.2** **Twin–Twin Transfusion Syndrome Quintero Staging System**

[a]Polyhydramnios = maximum vertical pocket >8 cm; oligohydramnios = maximum vertical pocket <2 cm.
[b]Critically abnormal Doppler studies = umbilical artery: absent end-diastolic flow or reversed end-diastolic flow; ductus venosus: reversed end-diastolic flow, pulsatile umbilical venous flow.

(b) Leads to severe malformation (i.e., often no development of structures cephalad of abdomen)

   iii. May lead to high output cardiac failure in pump twin

   iv. Size of acardiac twin in relation to pump twin determines prognosis (high risk if acardiac twin is >70% size of pump twin)

   v. Treatment options

     (a) Expectant management (if low risk and no cardiac failure in pump twin)

     (b) Radio frequency ablation of circulatory loop in acardiac twin

     (c) Cord ligation of acardiac twin (if umbilical cord present)

  d. Conjoined twins

   i. 1/70,000 deliveries

   ii. Named for point of union of twins

     (a) Thoracopagus (40%): anterior union of upper trunk

     (b) Omphalopagus (33%): anterior union of middle of trunk

     (c) Pygopagus (19%): joining of posterior rumps

     (d) Ischiopagus (6%): anterior union of lower 1/2 of body

     (e) Craniopagus (2%): joining of heads

     (f) Cephalopagus (rare): anterior union of upper 1/2 of body with conjoined head (may result in 2 faces on opposite sides—Janiceps twins)

     (g) Parapagus (rare): lateral union of lower 1/2 of body extending variable distance upwards (in extreme cases 2 faces side by side on 1 head)

   iii. Survival

     (a) 40%–60% stillborn

     (b) 35% die within 24 hours of birth

IV. Diagnosis and Management

  A. Diagnosis (by ultrasound)

   1. Suspect if uterine size > dates

   2. Determination of chorionicity is critical for management

    a. Separate gestational sacs = dichorionic

    b. Single gestational sac with separate amniotic sacs = monochorionic

    c. 2nd/3rd-trimester findings (Table 19.3)

   3. Dating of pregnancy crucial because treatment of complications (e.g., preterm labor) depends on gestational age

  B. Antenatal care

   1. Nutrition

    a. Balanced diet with additional 300 kcal daily

    b. Weight gain 35–45 lb (if normal weight prior to conception)

    c. Multivitamins, folic acid, calcium, iron

   2. Anemia

    a. Increased blood volume with twins (= 3 L or more) as compared to singleton (= 2 L)

    b. Increased blood loss at delivery anticipated

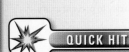

QUICK HIT

The survival of conjoined twins depends on the severity of malformations both at the site of union and distant from the site of union.

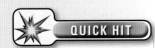

QUICK HIT

It is easiest to determine chorionicity in the first trimester.

TABLE **19.3**	**Determination of Chorionicity by Second/Third Trimester Ultrasound**	
Finding	**Dichorionic**	**Monochorionic**
Separate placentas	Often (but may approximate one another, thus appearing to be one placenta)	Never
Dividing membrane	Thick with "lambda" or "twin peak sign"	Thin with "T sign"
Discordant fetal sex	Sometimes (~1/3)	Never (extremely rare, case reports due to postzygotic genetic events)

3. Fetal growth
   a. Serial ultrasounds every 3–4 weeks
      i. Fundal heights not accurate in predicting fetal growth
      ii. IUGR more common in multiple gestations
   b. Assessment of fetal discordance
      i. (Weight of larger fetus – weight of smaller fetus)/weight of larger fetus = up to 20% discordance is normal
      ii. If >20% discordance, more frequent ultrasounds
4. Surveillance for preterm labor
   a. Educate patient regarding symptoms (cramping, back pain, vaginal discharge, bleeding)
   b. Cervical examinations (digital or sonographic)
   c. Fetal fibronectin testing may be useful
5. Surveillance for preeclampsia: blood pressure assessment and urine protein assessment at each visit
6. Surveillance for complications of monochorionic twinning (TTTS)
   a. Serial ultrasounds every 2 weeks to assess AFVs
   b. Umbilical cord Dopplers
C. Intrapartum management
   1. Each fetal heart rate should be monitored separately during labor
   2. Cesarean delivery (electively) is option for *all* twins
      a. Maneuvers necessary for delivery of 2nd nonvertex fetus dependent on operator experience
      b. Possibly emergent Cesarean delivery may be necessary for delivery of 2nd fetus even after vaginal delivery of 1st fetus
      c. Generally route of choice for higher order multiple deliveries
   3. Assessment of fetal presentations and sizes
      a. If 1st fetus is nonvertex (20% of twin pregnancies) → Cesarean delivery recommended
      b. If 1st fetus vertex presentation
         i. 2nd fetus is vertex (40% of twin pregnancies)
            (a) May deliver vaginally
            (b) If 2nd fetus were to convert to nonvertex with delivery of 1st fetus, breech extraction should only be attempted if 2nd fetus is not significantly larger than 1st
         ii. 2nd fetus is nonvertex (40% of twin pregnancies)
            (a) Concordant with or smaller than 1st fetus → may deliver vaginally (delivery of 2nd fetus by breech extraction)
            (b) Discordant with and larger than 1st fetus → Cesarean delivery

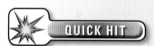

Monoamniotic twins should all be delivered by Cesarean delivery.

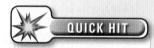

There is an increased risk for postpartum hemorrhage from atony due to uterine overdistension regardless of route of delivery with multiple gestation.

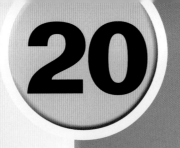

20 Fetal Growth Abnormalities: Fetal Growth Restriction and Macrosomia

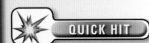
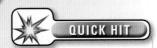
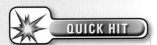
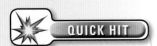
I. Fetal Growth Restriction

A. Definitions
1. **Fetal growth restriction (FGR):** estimated weight is <10th percentile of specific population at given gestational age (Table 20.1)
2. **Small for gestational age (SGA):** birth weight <10th percentile for gestational age (see Table 20.1)

B. Significance
1. Recognizing FGR can identify infants at risk for increased short-term and long-term morbidity and mortality
2. Limitations in use of gestational age percentiles
   a. By definition, prevalence of FGR will be 10%, but not all small neonates are growth restricted; over 2/3 of smaller neonates are constitutionally small
   b. Does not take into account growth *rate*, which may be more important
   c. FGR at earlier gestational age = greater effects on morbidity and mortality

C. Etiology
1. Early-onset growth restriction
   a. More commonly associated with heritable factors, immunologic abnormalities, chronic maternal disease, fetal infection, and multiple pregnancies
   b. Early in pregnancy, fetal growth occurs primarily through cellular hyperplasia or cell division; FGR leads to irreversible diminution of organ size and function
   c. More associated with symmetric growth restriction
2. Late-onset FGR
   a. More commonly associated with uteroplacental insufficiency
   b. Later in pregnancy, fetal growth occurs through cellular hypertrophy; delayed-onset FGR caused by decreased cell size; adequate nutrition can restore fetal size
   c. More associated with asymmetric growth restriction due to shunting of blood and nutrients to fetal head
   d. Typically has better prognosis than earlier growth restriction

TABLE 20.1 Fetal Growth Descriptors	
Term	**Definition**
Fetal growth restriction	Estimated fetal weight <10th percentile for gestational age
Small for gestational age	Infant birth weight <2,500 g at term or <10th percentile for gestational age
Macrosomia	Estimated fetal weight >4,000–4,500 g
Large for gestational age	Infant birth weight >90th percentile for gestational age

TABLE 20.2	**Risk Factors Associated With Intrauterine Growth Restriction**	
Maternal Factors	**Fetal Factors**	**Placental Factors**

• Medical conditions
  • Hypertension
  • Renal disease
  • Restrictive lung disease
  • Long-standing diabetes
  • Cyanotic heart disease
• Viral infections
• Drug/alcohol abuse
• Cigarette smoking
• Malnutrition
• Teratogen exposure
	• Genetic disorders
	• Multiple gestation
	• Constitutional
		• Primary placental disease
		• Uterine anomalies affecting placental implantation
		• Uteroplacental insufficiency/microinfarctions

D. Risk factors (Table 20.2)
1. Maternal factors
   a. Viral infections: rubella, varicella, cytomegalovirus, parvovirus B19; early infections can have associated structural anomalies (see Chapter 17)
   b. Substance abuse: alcohol, illicit drugs
   c. Cigarette smoking
   d. Prescription medications: anticonvulsants, warfarin, folic acid antagonists
   e. Maternal medical conditions: hypertension, cyanotic heart disease, long-standing diabetes, collagen vascular disease
   f. Extremes in maternal age (<16 years or >35 years)
   g. Nutritional deficiencies and inadequate weight gain
2. Fetal factors
   a. Chromosomal abnormalities (e.g., trisomies 13 and 18, Turner syndrome)
   b. Multifetal pregnancies
   c. Genetic/constitutional
   d. Female gender
3. Placental factors
   a. Placental abnormalities: chronic abruption, placental mosaicism
   b. Uterine anomalies: uterine septum or fibroids that can affect placental implantation
   c. Uteroplacental insufficiency: usually caused by microinfarctions
E. Diagnosis: if FGR suspected, ultrasonography done to assess fetal size and growth
1. Physical exam
   a. Fundal height: useful screening test for abnormal height but with high rates of false-negative and false-positive predictive values
   b. Maternal weight: low maternal weight associated with poor weight gain can be associated with FGR
   c. Ultrasound
      i. Biometry: fetal biometry measurements, including biparietal diameter, head circumference, abdominal circumference, and femur length used to calculate estimated fetal weight and possible FGR
      ii. Determine growth rate: serial fetal biometric parameters provide estimated growth rate, which can assess progression and severity of growth restriction
      iii. Amniotic fluid volume (AFV): like FGR, oligohydramnios (decreased amniotic fluid) can be caused by uteroplacental insufficiency
   d. Doppler velocimetry (Figure 20.1)
      i. Umbilical artery systolic/diastolic (S/D) ratio: indirectly measures resistance within placental vessels; FGR fetuses with absent or reverse end-diastolic flow have progressively worse perinatal outcomes

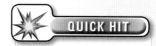

QUICK HIT

A small fetus with normal AFV and a normal growth rate is likely to be a normal, constitutionally small neonate. "Customized" growth curves have been generated for different populations to account for ethnic and geographic differences.

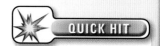

QUICK HIT

Early-onset FGR is caused by fetal factors (e.g., chromosomal abnormalities, congenital anomalies, early fetal infections), has a worse prognosis, and is less responsive to intervention.

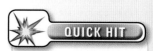

QUICK HIT

The etiology of FGR cannot be found in 50% of cases.

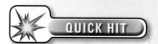

QUICK HIT

Less than 5% of FGR is related to early viral infections.

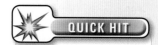

QUICK HIT

Drug abuse (e.g., narcotics, heroin, methadone, cocaine) causes FGR in 30%–50% of cases. Smoking increases growth restriction three- to fourfold.

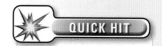

QUICK HIT

Fetal karyotyping is advised if structural anomalies are present or early/severe growth restriction is identified.

Fetal Growth Abnormalities

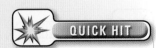

QUICK HIT

Accurate early assessment of gestational age is crucial in diagnosing FGR. Dating is increasingly imprecise at later gestational ages.

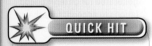

QUICK HIT

Between 20 and 36 weeks of gestation, fundal height in centimeters should approximate gestational age in weeks. Any discrepancy >2 cm warrants ultrasound examination.

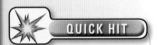

QUICK HIT

Normal abdominal circumference measurement excludes growth restriction, with a false-negative rate <10%.

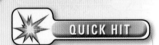

QUICK HIT

Ultrasound evaluation should include detailed anatomic survey to rule out structural abnormalities. About 10% of FGR cases have associated congenital anomalies.

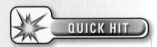

QUICK HIT

FGR associated with oligohydramnios is generally more severe with increased neonatal morbidity.

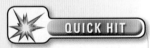

QUICK HIT

As placental resistance increases, diastolic flow decreases and the S/D ratio increases. Normal S/D ratio at term is 1.8–2.0. As the S/D ratio increases and worsens, it can progress to absent end-diastolic flow or even reverse end-diastolic flow. Fetuses with reverse end-diastolic flow are at increased risk of fetal death.

FIGURE 20.1 Doppler velocimetry.

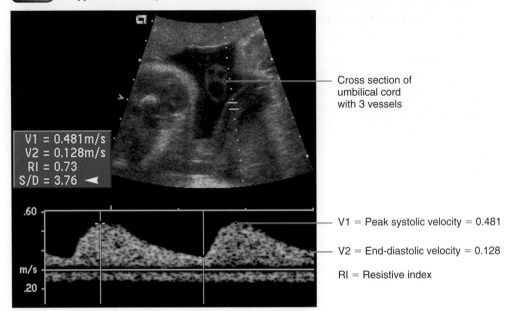

V1 = 0.481m/s
V2 = 0.128m/s
RI = 0.73
S/D = 3.76

Cross section of umbilical cord with 3 vessels

V1 = Peak systolic velocity = 0.481

V2 = End-diastolic velocity = 0.128

RI = Resistive index

Umbilical artery Doppler of a 35-week fetus demonstrates an elevated S/D ratio of 3.76.

 ii. Fetal middle cerebral artery (MCA): decreased placental perfusion generally spares fetal brain; shunting to brain causes increase of diastolic and mean blood flow velocity in MCA

 iii. Ductus venosus: fetus with highly abnormal ductus flow at risk of impending acidemia and death

F. Management

 1. Antepartum fetal management

  a. Fetal surveillance

   i. Fetal movement counts, nonstress tests, biophysical profiles, Doppler velocimetry studies

   ii. Frequency of fetal monitoring based on degree of growth restriction and severity of fetal testing findings: range from daily to weekly

  b. Serial biometry ultrasound: every 3–4 weeks to assess fetal growth curve and follow extent of growth restriction

  c. Antenatal steroid administration if preterm delivery before 34 weeks likely

  d. Timing of delivery based on gestational age and fetal condition

   i. Deliver when risk of fetal morbidity/mortality exceeds that of neonatal morbidity/mortality

   ii. Mode of delivery: if antenatal testing reassuring, attempt labor and vaginal delivery; increased risk for fetal intolerance of labor

 2. Neonatal management: depends on severity of growth restriction and gestational age

  a. Preparation for neonatal respiratory compromise

  b. Management of possible hypoglycemia, hypothermia, polycythemia

  c. Assessment for possible structural anomalies

G. Potential outcomes

 1. Antepartum outcomes: intrauterine fetal death, asphyxia, acidemia, intolerance to labor

 2. Neonatal outcomes: low Apgar scores, polycythemia, hypoglycemia, hypothermia, respiratory distress, seizures, sepsis, meconium aspiration, intravascular hemorrhage, neonatal death

 3. Long-term outcomes

  a. Cognitive impairment

  b. Sequelae from prematurity or congenital/structural anomalies

  c. Fetal origins of adult disease (**Barker hypothesis**): weight abnormalities, hypertension, dyslipidemia, insulin resistance, cardiovascular disease

II. Macrosomia

A. Definitions
1. **Macrosomia** = estimated fetal weight >4,000–4,500 g (see Table 20.1)
2. **Large for gestational age (LGA)** = estimated weight >90th percentile of specific population at given gestational age (see Table 20.1)

B. Significance
1. Recognizing macrosomia allows providers to diagnose and manage cause (e.g., gestational diabetes, maternal obesity)
2. Allows providers to prepare for possible delivery complications
3. Limitations
   a. Most macrosomic neonates not pathologically large but constitutionally large
   b. Birth weights have increased over time, making older birth weight percentiles less accurate
   c. Birth weight depends on race/ethnicity and gender

C. Risk factors (Table 20.3)
1. Maternal factors
   a. Prior history of macrosomia
   b. Maternal prepregnancy obesity
   c. Multiparity
   d. Ethnicity
   e. Glucose intolerance/gestational diabetes
   f. Dyslipidemia
2. Fetal factors
   a. Genetic/constitutional
   b. Genetic syndromes including **Beckwith-Wiedemann syndrome** (large bodies, large tongues, midline abdominal wall defect, neonatal hypoglycemia)
   c. Male gender
   d. Gestational age >40 weeks

D. Diagnosis
1. Physical exam
   a. Fundal height: useful screening test for abnormal fetal growth but poor predictor of macrosomia
   b. Leopold maneuvers (see Figure 10.2)
2. Ultrasound
   a. Biometry: fetal biometry measurements, including biparietal diameter, head circumference, abdominal circumference, and femur length, used to calculate estimated fetal weight and possible macrosomia
   b. AFV: gestational diabetes can be associated with polyhydramnios

E. Management
1. Rule out maternal diabetes; if diabetes diagnosed, optimal diabetic management of pregnancy necessary
2. Early induction or early delivery *not* indicated for suspected macrosomia
   a. Early induction of labor does not decrease maternal or neonatal morbidity
   b. Early induction does increase rate of Cesarean delivery

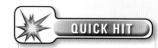

QUICK HIT

No therapies are proven beneficial in FGR. The goal of antepartum management is to determine the optimal time for delivery.

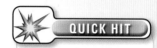

QUICK HIT

At <34 weeks, timing of delivery is based on gestational age and fetal testing. At 34–37 weeks, deliver if risk factors for adverse outcomes are present (e.g., worsening maternal condition, poor/absent fetal growth, poor Doppler velocimetry studies). At >37 weeks, the fetus should be delivered.

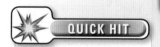

QUICK HIT

Most growth-restricted fetuses are constitutionally small and have good outcomes.

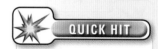

QUICK HIT

Macrosomia is associated with increased risk for Cesarean delivery, postpartum hemorrhage, vaginal lacerations, uterine rupture, shoulder dystocia, and lower Apgar scores.

QUICK HIT

Neonatal risks depend on the etiology of the macrosomia. Constitutionally large neonates generally have good outcomes. With maternal diabetes, there are increased neonatal risks, including hypoglycemia, hypothermia, prematurity, and fetal death.

TABLE 20.3 Risk Factors for Macrosomia	
Maternal Factors	**Fetal Factors**
• Previous pregnancy with macrosomia	• Constitutional/genetic potential
• Diabetes/glucose intolerance	• Genetic disorder
• Maternal obesity	• Male gender
• Parity	• >40 weeks' gestation

Fetal Growth Abnormalities

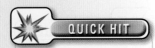

The differential diagnosis of increased fundal height includes wrong due date, macrosomia, polyhydramnios, multiple gestation, large placenta, uterine fibroids, and error due to maternal habitus/obesity.

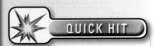

Ultrasound estimates of macrosomic fetal weights are associated with significant errors. Although no specific biometric parameter is highly sensitive and specific, **abdominal circumference** is the *most reliable* measurement to assess for macrosomia.

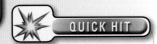

For pregnancies without diabetes, no interventions have been shown to lessen fetal growth when macrosomia is suspected.

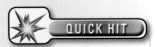

Currently, no evidence supports early induction or early delivery for suspected macrosomia.

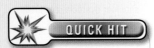

Macrosomia leads to potential risks in adulthood, such as impaired glucose tolerance, obesity, metabolic syndrome, and cardiovascular disease.

3. Cesarean delivery
   a. Mother without diabetes: Cesarean delivery should be offered when estimated fetal weight >5,000 g
   b. Mother with diabetes: Cesarean delivery should be offered when estimated fetal weight >4,500 g
4. Neonatal management depends on gestational age of neonate and underlying etiology of macrosomia

Fetal Growth Abnormalities

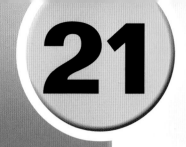

Isoimmunization

I. Natural History

A. Can be caused by any blood group antigen system

B. Most common cause: Rh system (composed of 5 different antigens)
1. C, c, E, e antigens
2. D antigen most frequently associated with isoimmunization
   a. Rh positive (Rh+): patient has D antigen on red blood cells (RBCs)
   b. Rh negative (Rh−): patient lacks D antigen on RBC (gene deletion)
   c. Weak D antigen: variant of D antigen; manage as Rh+

C. <0.1 mL Rh+ blood needed to cause isoimmunization

D. Events in which isoimmunization can occur
1. Delivery of baby and placenta: *most common*
2. Threatened, spontaneous, elective, or therapeutic abortion
3. Ectopic pregnancy
4. Bleeding associated with placenta previa or abruption
5. Invasive fetal procedure (e.g., amniocentesis/chorionic villus sampling)
6. Abdominal trauma
7. External cephalic version

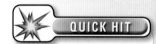

> **QUICK HIT**
>
> Isoimmunization occurs when an Rh− pregnant woman carrying an Rh+ fetus (paternally inherited) is exposed to fetal RBCs.

II. Effects of Antibody Development on Fetus and Newborn

A. Generally, 2 exposures needed to cause significant immune response

B. 1st "at-risk" pregnancy (when fetus Rh+)
1. Low risk for significant anemia
2. Spontaneous pregnancy loss and elective termination

C. Subsequent "at-risk" pregnancy
1. Reexposure to Rh+ fetal blood produces anamnestic response
2. More robust and rapid than initial response

D. IgM: 1st immunoglobulin (Ig) produced (does not cross placenta)

E. IgG: secondary antibody response
1. Crosses placenta into fetal circulation
2. Binds to D-antigen site on fetal RBCs
3. Fetal RBCs bound by antibody are hemolyzed
   a. Fetal reticuloendothelial system
   b. Complement mediated pathways
4. Resultant fetal hyperbilirubinemia
   a. Bilirubin may deposit in basal ganglia leading to kernicterus
   b. Postnatal treatment
      i. Ultraviolet light
      ii. Exchange transfusion
5. Anemia may result in hydrops fetalis
   a. **Hydrops fetalis**: fluid accumulation in 2 or more extravascular compartments
      i. Pericardial effusion
      ii. Pleural effusion

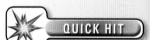

> **QUICK HIT**
>
> Spontaneous pregnancy loss and elective termination can be sources of maternal exposure to fetal RBCs.

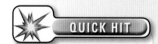

> **QUICK HIT**
>
> Subsequent pregnancies with an Rh+ fetus put an Rh− mother at risk for more significant hemolysis and anemia.

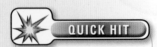

When the mother is Rh−, paternal antigen status determines the likelihood of the fetus carrying D antigen.

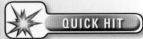

If a fetus does not carry paternal antigen, regardless of the quantity of maternal antibody, the fetus will not be at risk for hemolysis.

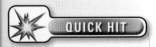

All pregnant women should be tested at their first prenatal visit for ABO blood group and their Rh−D type as well as screened for RBC antibodies.

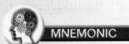

To distinguish antibodies, remember that Lewis is IgM and does not cross the placenta: Kell kills, Duffy dies, Lewis lives.

    iii. Ascites
    iv. Subcutaneous edema
  b. Pathophysiology of hydrops fetalis
    i. Decreased oncotic pressure due to fetal anemia
    ii. Extramedullary hematopoiesis in liver
      (a) Decreased protein production in liver
      (b) Increased intravascular resistance to flow due to islands of hematopoietic cells
    iii. Cardiac failure
      (a) High output failure secondary to anemia
      (b) Decreased oxygen delivery to myocardium

III. Significance of Paternal Antigen Status (When Mother is Rh−)

A. Essential in assessing if fetus is at risk for developing anemia
B. Paternal antigen status
  1. Homozygous D: 100% chance fetus carries paternal antigen
  2. Heterozygous D: 50% chance fetus carries paternal antigen
  3. Lacks D (Rh−): 0% chance fetus carries paternal antigen
C. Determination of antigen status
  1. For antigen other than D, antigen testing performed
  2. For D antigen, genotyping necessary to determine zygosity
  3. If paternal D heterozygote, amniocentesis can be performed to determine fetal RBC antigen status by genotyping of fetal cells in amniotic fluid

IV. Diagnosis

A. Initial antibody screen at 1st prenatal visit
B. Repeat antibody screening
  1. At 28 weeks before administration of anti-D Ig
  2. Postpartum
  3. Time of any event in pregnancy (see "Natural History" section)
C. Identified antibodies that can cause fetal hemolysis should be quantified and reported in titer format (e.g., 1:4, 1:8, 1:16); higher titer indicates more significant antibody response
D. Some antibodies identified are *not* associated with fetal hemolytic disease, and no further evaluation is warranted (e.g., anti-Lewis, anti-I)

V. Assessment of Abnormal Antibody Screen

A. Maternal antibody identification and titer
  1. Titers quantify amount of antibody
  2. Titers do *not* provide information about fetal status
B. Paternal antigen testing, possible fetal DNA testing
C. History of affected fetus/neonate obtained
  1. Prior affected fetus/neonate
    a. Titers not predictive of severity of disease
    b. Fetal assessment initiated irrespective of titer
  2. No prior affected fetus/neonate
    a. Serial antibody titers
    b. Critical titer associated with significant risk; severe fetal hemolytic disease usually >1:8 (specific level varies from center to center)
    c. Titers of 1:8 or less should be followed every 2–4 weeks
D. Assessment of risk for fetal anemia if critical titer reached, or if prior affected fetus/neonate
  1. **Serial middle cerebral artery (MCA) Doppler assessment**
    a. Most commonly used assessment tool
    b. Measure peak systolic velocity in MCA
    c. If anemic
      i. Blood less viscous (fewer cells)
      ii. Velocity of flow increases

iii. High peak systolic velocity = moderate to severe anemia

iv. Degree of velocity elevation above median for gestational age correlates inversely with fetal hematocrit (Hct)

v. Useful to detect moderate to severe anemia only

2. Amniotic fluid bilirubin assessment
   a. Performed through serial amniocentesis
   b. Bilirubin normally deceases in 2nd 1/2 of pregnancy
   c. Fetal hemolysis increases amniotic fluid bilirubin levels
   d. Replaced by MCA assessment in many centers

3. Serial ultrasonography
   a. Monitor fetal growth and well-being, even if MCA normal
   b. Useful to detect hydrops fetalis: indicates severe anemia

4. Percutaneous umbilical blood sampling (PUBS) under ultrasound guidance performed if previously mentioned assessment testing abnormal
   a. Needle advanced into umbilical vein
   b. Hct of sampled fetal blood measured
   c. Intrauterine transfusion if fetus anemic

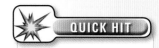

QUICK HIT

If hydrops fetalis is seen on ultrasound, expect Hct to be <15%.

VI. Management (*Figure 21.1*)

A. Historically, blood transfused into fetal peritoneal cavity (RBCs absorbed into fetal circulation via lymphatic channels)

B. Currently, blood transfusion into umbilical vein is preferred technique
   1. Antigen-negative blood (depending on blood group involved)
   2. Transfusion when PUBS confirms fetal anemia
   3. 1%–3% procedure complication rate (e.g., fetal death, preterm delivery)
   4. Determinants of volume of transfusion
      a. Gestational age
      b. Estimated fetal weight
      c. Hct of donor blood
      d. Fetal Hct
   5. Determinants of timing of subsequent transfusions
      a. Severity of disease
      b. Serial MCA Doppler assessment
   6. After 2–3 transfusions, most blood in fetal circulation will be transfused antigen-negative blood, resulting in less frequent need for further transfusion

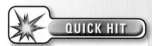

QUICK HIT

Administer 300 µg of anti-D Ig in any circumstance in which fetomaternal hemorrhage can occur.

VII. Prevention

A. Awareness that maternal exposure and sensitization to fetal RBC antigens *most often* happens during delivery but can occur at any time in pregnancy

B. Administration of anti-D Ig during pregnancy
   1. At 28 weeks' gestation: further reduces risk of sensitization to 0.2%
   2. If delivery has not occurred within 12 weeks of anti-D Ig injection at 28 weeks, administering 2nd dose should be considered
   3. Each dose provides protection for up to 30 mL fetal blood or 15 mL fetal RBCs
   4. **Kleihauer-Betke (KB) test**
      a. KB test: number of fetal cells as proportion of total cells (maternal + fetal) used to calculate dose of anti-D Ig needed
      b. **Indirect Coombs test** useful postadministration
         i. If positive, sufficient unbound antibody present, indicating adequate anti-D Ig dose given
         ii. Direct Coombs test, by contrast, detects antibodies adhered to RBCs

C. Administration of anti-D Ig within 72 hours of delivery to prevent Rh− D isoimmunization in most cases
   1. Reduces sensitization from 16% to 2%
   2. Residual 2% risk is likely from sensitization during pregnancy

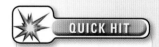

QUICK HIT

The KB test can quantify fetal RBCs in the maternal circulation.

Isoimmunization

FIGURE 21.1   Algorithm for management of the red cell alloimmunized pregnancy.

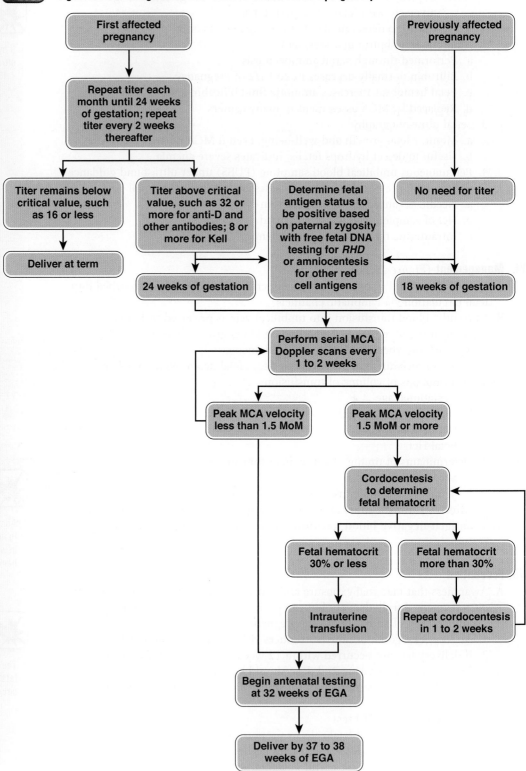

EGA, estimated gestational age; MCA, middle cerebral artery; MoM, multiples of the median.
(Reproduced with permission from Moise KJ Jr, Argoti PS. Management and prevention of red cell alloimmunization in pregnancy: a systematic review. *Obstet Gynecol.* 2012;120:1132. Copyright © 2012 Lippincott Williams & Wilkins.)

VIII. Management of Isoimmunization to Other RBC Antigens

A. Anti-D Ig effective only for preventing sensitization to D antigen (i.e., not effective in preventing sensitization to other red cell antigens)

B. Anti-D Ig has reduced D isoimmunization, but *isoimmunization to other groups has proportionally increased*

C. Factors determining likelihood of antibodies causing fetal hemolysis

1. Size of fetomaternal hemorrhage
2. Potency of antigen
3. Isoform of antibody response (IgG *versus* IgM)

D. Most important cause of hemolytic disease of fetus not associated with D antigen is isoimmunization to **Kell antigen**

1. Most often due to prior blood transfusion, not pregnancy related
2. If anti-Kell detected in antibody screen
   a. Paternal blood typing for Kell antigen indicated: if heterozygous, amniocentesis indicated to determine fetal Kell status by genotyping
   b. Anemia for Kell isoimmunization unique
      i. Not primarily due to hemolysis
      ii. Primarily destruction and suppression of bone marrow hematopoietic precursor cells
      iii. Monitoring amniotic fluid bilirubin not useful
      iv. Poor correlation between titer and fetal risk
      v. Lower critical titer (1:8 or less) often used to initiate monitoring

E. ABO incompatibility may cause hemolytic disease

1. Usually mild fetal anemia
2. Mild due to fewer A and B antigens on fetal RBCs and majority of antibody IgM
3. Associated with newborn hyperbilirubinemia

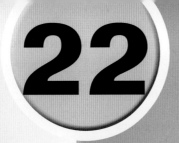

22 Preterm Labor

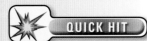

QUICK HIT

About 12% of babies in the United States are born prematurely.

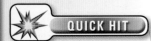

QUICK HIT

Usually, no cause or risk factor for preterm labor is identified.

I. Background

A. Definitions
   1. **Preterm birth:** delivery prior to 37 weeks
   2. **Preterm labor:** preterm gestation with regular contractions and cervical changes (dilation and effacement)
B. Fetal complications associated with prematurity
   1. Respiratory distress syndrome
   2. Intraventricular hemorrhage
   3. Necrotizing enterocolitis
   4. Sepsis
   5. Neurologic impairment/seizures

II. Causes and Risk Factors

A. Causes
   1. Premature activation of maternal or fetal hypothalamic–pituitary–adrenal axis
      a. Maternal stress
      b. Fetal stress
   2. Infection
   3. Decidual hemorrhage
   4. Pathologic uterine distention
B. Risk factors
   1. Prior history of preterm delivery
   2. Premature rupture of membranes (PROM)
   3. Infection
      a. Intra-amniotic
      b. Urinary
      c. Bacterial vaginosis
         i. Symptomatic patients should be treated
         ii. Asymptomatic screening has not shown to be effective
      d. Sexually transmitted infections
      e. Periodontal disease
   4. Excessive uterine enlargement
      a. Multiple gestation
      b. Polyhydramnios
   5. Uterine distortion
      a. Leiomyomas
      b. Septate uterus or other anomaly
   6. Fetal
      a. Congenital anomaly
      b. Growth restriction (fetal stress)
   7. Placental abnormalities
      a. Placental abruption
      b. Placenta previa

8. Miscellaneous
   a. Smoking or substance abuse
   b. African American
   c. Age <18 or >40 years

III. Evaluation

A. Monitor contractions with tocometer
B. Evaluate for cervical change with speculum or digital exam
C. Look for signs of infection
   1. Urinalysis
   2. Complete blood count
   3. Consider gonorrhea and chlamydia cultures
   4. Evaluate for bacterial vaginosis
   5. Evaluate for chorioamnionitis
      a. Clinical diagnosis (2 or more)
         i. Maternal tachycardia
         ii. Fetal tachycardia
         iii. Fever
         iv. Uterine tenderness
      b. Amniocentesis may be performed
         i. Presence of bacteria
         ii. Presence of white blood cells
         iii. Elevated lactate dehydrogenase
         iv. Decreased glucose
D. Consider fetal fibronectin (fFN) at 24–34 weeks' gestation
   1. fFN: glycoprotein that functions to bind chorionic–decidual interface
   2. Increased concentration of fFN in cervicovaginal secretions is found with preterm labor

IV. Management

A. Assess fetal well-being
   1. Fetal heart rate monitoring
   2. Ultrasound
      a. Fetal presentation
      b. Estimated fetal weight
B. Tocolysis (Table 22.1)
   1. Tocolytics do not prolong pregnancy beyond 2–7 days
   2. Contraindications
      a. Advanced labor
      b. Mature fetus (tocolysis rarely used after 34 weeks or after corticosteroids completed)

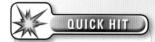

When a cervical fFN test is negative, the risk of delivering in the next 7–14 days is low.

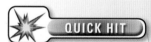

fFN must be collected during the speculum exam, prior to the digital exam.

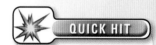

The fFN test has good negative predictive value but poor positive predictive value.

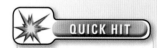

The main goal of tocolytic therapy is to prolong pregnancy for 48 hours to allow for administration of corticosteroids.

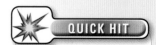

About 50% of patients with preterm contractions have spontaneous resolution of contractions.

TABLE 22.1	Tocolytic Agents Used in Management of Preterm Labor		
Tocolytic	**Mechanism of Action**	**Route Given**	**Potential Side Effects**
Magnesium sulfate	Antagonizes effects of free intracellular calcium	IV	Hypotonia, respiratory depression or cardiac arrest at high levels
Calcium channel blocker (nifedipine)	Block calcium channels	PO	Hypotension, headaches
β-Mimetic (terbutaline)	Decreases free intracellular calcium	SQ, IV, PO	Tachycardia, arrhythmias, tremor, hypokalemia, hyperglycemia
Prostaglandin synthetase inhibitors (indomethacin)	Decreases prostaglandin production	PO, PR	GI distress, premature closure of ductus arteriosus, oligohydramnios

GI, gastrointestinal; IV, intravenous; PO, by mouth; PR, rectally; SQ, subcutaneously.

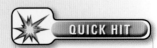

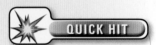

    c. Intrauterine infection
    d. Significant vaginal bleeding
    e. Severe preeclampsia
C. Administer corticosteroids
    1. 2 doses of betamethasone or 4 doses of dexamethasone (48 hours to complete dosing)
    2. Decreases incidence of respiratory distress syndrome
    3. Decreases incidence of intraventricular hemorrhage
D. Group B *Streptococcus* (GBS) prophylaxis
    1. GBS culture usually obtained in clinic at 36–37 weeks
    2. If GBS status unknown
        a. Perform culture on admission
        b. Start antibiotics for prophylaxis if positive culture or unknown status

V. Prevention

A. 17-α-hydroxyprogesterone caproate
    1. Weekly injections starting at 16–20 weeks' gestation
    2. Reduces rate of recurrent preterm delivery
B. Vaginal progesterone supplementation

Preterm Labor

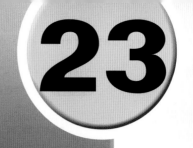

Third-Trimester Bleeding

I. Evaluation of Third-Trimester Bleeding

A. History
1. Quantify bleeding (# of pads)
2. Associated symptoms (e.g., contractions or abdominal pain)
3. Personal or family history of bleeding disorders
4. Other possible sources for bleeding
5. Recent intercourse or pelvic exam

B. Physical exam
1. Vital signs
2. Fetal heart rate
3. General exam
   a. Abdominal exam: Is there tenderness or a palpable contraction?
   b. Bruising or petechiae may be indicative of bleeding disorder
4. Speculum exam: after placenta located

C. Differential diagnosis
1. Vulva
   a. Varicose veins
   b. Tears or lacerations
2. Vagina: lacerations
3. Cervix
   a. Polyp
   b. Cervicitis
   c. Carcinoma
   d. Ectropion
      i. Eversion of endocervix secondary to progesterone in pregnancy
      ii. Glandular cells exposed to vaginal acidity
      iii. Reddened and raw appearance
4. Intrauterine
   a. Placenta previa
   b. Placental abruption
   c. Vasa previa
   d. Uterine rupture

D. Management
1. 2 large-bore IVs for crystalloid fluid
2. Labs
   a. Complete blood count
   b. Coagulation studies
   c. Type and cross
3. Determine need for delivery
   a. Bleeding significant
      i. Move toward delivery
      ii. Likely emergent Cesarean delivery

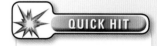

QUICK HIT

Third-trimester bleeding occurs in 4%–5% of all pregnancies.

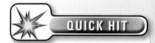

QUICK HIT

The pelvic exam should not be performed until placental location is confirmed (usually with ultrasound).

FIGURE
23.1 Placenta accreta, increta, and percreta.

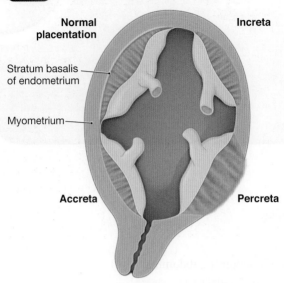

Normal placentation

Increta

Stratum basalis of endometrium

Myometrium

Accreta

Percreta

(From Beckmann CRB, Ling FW, et al. *Obstetrics and Gynecology*, 7th ed. Baltimore: Lippincott Williams & Wilkins; 2014.)

b. Bleeding insufficient to warrant emergency delivery
  i. Admit patient
  ii. Close observation of mother and fetus
4. Determine blood type for Rh status
  a. Rh– patients may need immunoglobulin (Ig) to protect against Rh D antigen
  b. **Kleihauer-Betke test** can be done to determine amount of fetal blood in maternal circulation and, therefore, how much Ig needed (see Chapter 21)

II. **Placenta Previa**
  A. Definitions (Figure 23.1)
    1. **Complete previa:** placenta completely covers cervical os
    2. **Partial previa:** placenta overlies part but not all of cervical os
    3. **Low-lying placenta:** placental edge in lower uterine segment but does not reach internal os
  B. Incidence and etiology
    1. 1/200 pregnancies
    2. 75% of patients with previa will have 1 or more episodes of bleeding (1st episode usually 29–30 weeks' gestation)
    3. Unknown etiology but may be associated with abnormal vascularization
  C. Risk factors
    1. Previa in prior pregnancy
    2. Prior uterine surgery including Cesarean delivery
    3. Multiparity
    4. Advanced maternal age
    5. Tobacco or cocaine use
  D. Presentation (Table 23.1)
  E. Management
    1. 1st or 2nd episode of bleeding often managed with close observation (each subsequent bleed is usually heavier than prior)
    2. 3rd bleed often leads to delivery
    3. Delivery via Cesarean delivery
  F. Complications
    1. **Placenta accreta:** placental tissue extends into superficial layer of myometrium
    2. **Placenta increta:** placental tissue extends further into myometrium
    3. **Placenta percreta:** placental tissue extends through myometrium into serosa and may involve adjacent organs such as bladder

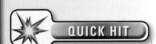
QUICK HIT

Placenta previa occurs when the placenta is located close to or over the cervical os.

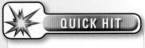
QUICK HIT

The classic presentation of placenta previa is *painless* vaginal bleeding.

TABLE 23.1	**Characteristics of Placenta Previa and Placental Abruption**	
Characteristic	**Placenta Previa**	**Placental Abruption**
Magnitude of blood loss	Variable	Variable
Duration	Often ceases within 1–2 hours	Usually continuous
Abdominal discomfort	None	Can be severe
Fetal heart rate pattern on electronic monitoring	Normal	Tachycardia, then bradycardia; loss of variability; decelerations frequently present; intrauterine demise not rare
Coagulation defects	Rare	Associated, but infrequent; DIC often severe when present
Associated history	None	Cocaine use, abdominal trauma, maternal hypotension, multiple gestation, polyhydramnios

DIC, disseminated intravascular coagulation.
(From Beckmann CRB, Ling FW, et al. *Obstetrics and Gynecology*, 7th ed. Baltimore: Lippincott Williams & Wilkins; 2014.)

III. Placental Abruption

A. Definitions (Figure 23.2)
   1. **Complete** abruption: entire placenta separates from uterine wall
   2. **Partial** abruption: part of placenta separates from uterine wall
   3. **Marginal** abruption: separation limited to edge of placenta
B. Incidence and etiology
   1. Significant enough to warrant delivery; occurs in 1% pregnancies
   2. Etiology: premature separation of *normally* implanted placenta
C. Risk factors
   1. *Chronic hypertension or preeclampsia*
   2. Multiple gestation
   3. Advanced maternal age
   4. *Tobacco or cocaine use*
   5. Premature rupture of membranes
   6. Chorioamnionitis
   7. *Trauma*
   8. Abruption in prior pregnancy
   9. Increased α-fetoprotein in 2nd-trimester screen
D. Presentation (see Table 23.1)

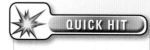

QUICK HIT

Maternal hypertension and history of trauma or tobacco or cocaine use are significant risk factors for placental abruption.

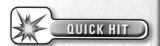

QUICK HIT

The classic presentation of placental abruption is abdominal pain and vaginal bleeding.

Third-Trimester Bleeding

FIGURE 23.2 Types of placental abruption.

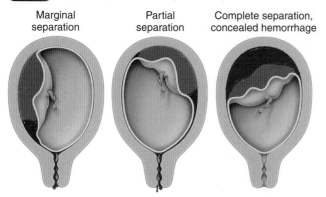

Marginal separation | Partial separation | Complete separation, concealed hemorrhage

Note that vaginal bleeding is absent when the hemorrhage is concealed. (From Beckmann CRB, Ling FW, et al. *Obstetrics and Gynecology*, 7th ed. Baltimore: Lippincott Williams & Wilkins; 2014.)

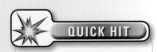

Placental abruption is the most common cause of coagulopathy in pregnancy.

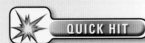

Vasa previa occurs with passage of fetal blood vessels over the cervical os and below the presenting fetal part.

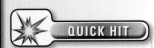

Uterine rupture can be life threatening for both mother and fetus.

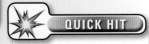

Most cases of uterine rupture occur at the site of a prior Cesarean delivery scar.

E. Management
   1. Severe hemorrhage and/or fetal distress: delivery (likely Cesarean)
   2. Minimal bleeding and reassuring fetal tracing: expectant management may be appropriate
F. Complications
   1. **Couvelaire uterus:** blood penetrates uterus; uterine serosa becomes blue-purple in coloration
   2. **Disseminated intravascular coagulation:** rare but should be ruled out
   3. Fetal demise

IV. Vasa Previa
A. Incidence and etiology: 1/2,500 pregnancies
B. Risk factors
   1. **Velamentous cord insertion:** fetal blood vessels insert into membranes rather than into placenta
   2. **Succenturiate lobe:** extra lobe of placenta separate from main placenta with fetal vessels passing between
C. Presentation
   1. Vaginal bleeding (*fetal blood*) immediately after rupture of membranes
   2. Fetal distress at onset of vaginal bleeding/rupture of membranes
   3. Sometimes detected by ultrasound in prenatal period
D. Management
   1. Emergent Cesarean delivery
   2. **Apt test** can be performed to distinguish fetal blood from maternal blood
      a. Blood mixed in water for hemolysis
      b. Sodium hydroxide (NaOH) applied
         i. Fetal blood remains pink
         ii. Maternal blood turns brown
E. Complications
   1. Rupture of fetal vessels can quickly result in fetal death given small fetal blood volume
   2. Fetal mortality = 60%

V. Uterine Rupture
A. Incidence and etiology
   1. Overall incidence 0.003%
   2. Spontaneous
   3. Associated with trauma
   4. Associated with prior uterine scar
      a. Most ruptures occur during labor
      b. Incidence of rupture ranges from 0.5% to 3.7% and depends on number of prior Cesarean deliveries and events surrounding labor (i.e., use of augmentation or induction agents)
      c. Trial of labor after prior *classical* (vertical uterine incision through upper, contractile portion of uterus) Cesarean delivery is *not* recommended
B. Presentation
   1. Vaginal bleeding
   2. Abdominal pain
   3. Loss of station of presenting fetal part
   4. May have fetal distress/demise
C. Management: emergent Cesarean delivery
D. Complications
   1. Fetal mortality = 50%–75%
   2. Maternal mortality = ~1%

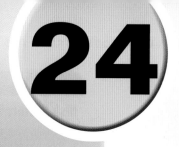

Premature Rupture of Membranes

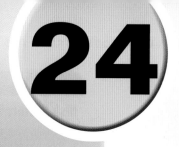

24

I. Background
A. Amniotic fluid
1. Primarily composed of fetal urine after 16 weeks
2. Small contribution from other sources
a. Passage of fluid across fetal membranes, skin, and umbilical cord
b. Fetal saliva
c. Fetal pulmonary effluent
3. Protects fetus from infection, trauma, and umbilical cord compression
4. Allows for fetal movement and breathing
a. Musculoskeletal development facilitated
b. Lung development promoted
B. **Premature rupture of membranes (PROM)**: rupture of chorioamniotic membrane before onset of labor
1. Associated with 12% of all pregnancies
2. Occurs in 8% of term pregnancies
C. Preterm PROM: PROM before 37 weeks' gestation
1. Among leading causes of neonatal morbidity and mortality
2. Associated with 30% of preterm deliveries
D. Consequences of PROM: depends on gestational age at time of occurrence and amniotic fluid level after occurrence
1. Intrauterine infection (major complication of PROM): risk increased with lower genital tract infections
a. *Neisseria gonorrhoeae*
b. Group B *Streptococcus* (GBS)
c. Bacterial vaginosis
2. Umbilical cord prolapse
3. Abruptio placentae
4. PROM after amniocentesis: likely to reseal with reaccumulation of fluid
5. If persistent oligohydramnios <22 weeks
a. Incomplete alveolar development
b. High risk of pulmonary hypoplasia (infants cannot be adequately ventilated)
6. Survival likely at 24–26 weeks' gestation, but morbidity rates high due to extreme prematurity

II. Etiology
A. Cause not clearly understood
B. Risk factors (Box 24.1)
C. Factors determining latency (time from PROM to delivery)
1. Older gestational age associated with shorter latency
2. Less amniotic fluid after PROM associated with greater risk of infection and shorter latency

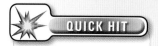

QUICK HIT

Amniotic fluid after 16 weeks' gestation consists primarily of fetal urine.

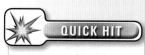

QUICK HIT

PROM is a leading cause of neonatal morbidity/mortality.

BOX 24.1

Risk Factors for Premature Rupture of Membranes (PROM)

- Sexually transmissible disease
- Other lower genital tract infections (e.g., bacterial vaginosis)
- Cigarette smoking during pregnancy
- Prior PROM
- Short cervical length
- Prior preterm delivery
- Hydramnios
- Multifetal gestation
- Bleeding in early pregnancy

> **QUICK HIT**
>
> Treatment of chorioamnionitis is IV antibiotics and prompt delivery no matter what gestational age.

> **QUICK HIT**
>
> Fluid passing though the vagina must be presumed to be amniotic fluid until proven otherwise.

D. **Chorioamnionitis:** infection of fetal membranes and amniotic fluid
  1. Increased risk of sepsis
     a. Fetal: associated with periventricular leukomalacia and cerebral palsy
     b. Maternal
  2. Clinical findings
     a. Fever
     b. Tachycardia (maternal and fetal)
     c. Uterine tenderness
     d. Purulent cervical discharge (late finding)
     e. Elevated white blood cell (WBC) count
     f. Labor (often dysfunctional)
  3. Treatment: *intravenous (IV) antibiotics and prompt delivery, irrespective of gestational age*

III. Diagnosis

A. Sterile vaginal speculum exam
  1. Pooling of amniotic fluid in vagina
  2. Visualization of amniotic fluid leaking per cervical os
B. Nitrazine test
  1. Uses pH to distinguish amniotic fluid
  2. Vaginal fluid placed on strip of nitrazine paper
     a. Paper turns dark blue: amniotic fluid (pH >7.1)
     b. Paper remains same color (yellow)
        i. Normal vaginal secretions (pH 4.5–6.0)
        ii. Urine (pH ≤6.0)
  3. Causes of false-positive and false-negative nitrazine tests (Table 24.1)
C. Fern test
  1. Pattern of arborization seen on microscopy when amniotic fluid placed on slide and dried in room air (Figure 24.1)

TABLE 24.1 Causes of False-Positive and False-Negative Nitrazine Tests

False Positives	False Negatives
Basic urine	Remote PROM with no residual fluid
Semen	Minimal amniotic fluid leakage
Cervical mucus	
Blood contamination	
Some antiseptic solutions	
Vaginitis (especially trichomonas)	
PROM, premature rupture of membranes.	

FIGURE
24.1 Ferning pattern from amniotic fluid.

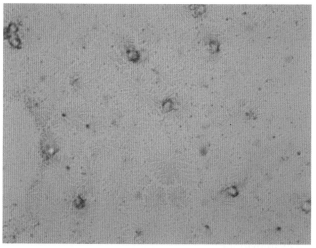

(From Beckmann CRB, Ling FW, et al. *Obstetrics and Gynecology*, 7th ed. Baltimore: Lippincott Williams & Wilkins; 2014.)

 2. Due to sodium chloride content of amniotic fluid
 3. Cervical mucus can also fern but often thicker pattern with less branching
 4. More specific than nitrazine test
 E. Ultrasonography
  1. Assessment of amniotic fluid index
  2. Ruptured membranes less likely if amniotic fluid volume normal
 F. Transabdominal injection of indigo carmine dye into uterine cavity
  1. Passage of blue fluid from vagina demonstrates ruptured membranes
  2. *Gold standard for diagnosis* (but involves invasive procedure)
  3. Useful when clinical history or physical exam unclear
 G. Differential diagnosis (Box 24.2)

IV. Evaluation and Management
 A. Key factors in evaluation
  1. Gestational age at PROM
  2. Assessment of fetal well-being
  3. Presence of uterine contractions
  4. Likelihood of chorioamnionitis
  5. Amount of remaining amniotic fluid
  6. Degree of fetal maturity
 B. Physical exam
  1. Palpation of uterus for tenderness
  2. Fundal height measurement (approximate gestational age and identify fetal lie)
  3. Sterile speculum exam
   a. Visualize presence of amniotic fluid
   b. Test for vaginal infection (including GBS)
   c. Test for cervical infection (*N. gonorrhoeae* and *Chlamydia trachomatis*)
   d. Visualize degree of cervical dilation
  4. Digital exam avoided (unless in labor) to reduce infection risk

BOX 24.2

Differential Diagnosis of Premature Rupture of Membranes

- Urinary incontinence
- Increased physiologic vaginal secretions during pregnancy
- Increased cervical discharge (e.g., infection)
- Exogenous fluids (e.g., semen, douche)
- Vesicovaginal fistula

Premature Rupture of Membranes

C. Ultrasound exam
  1. More accurate gestational age assessment
  2. Identification of fetal lie/presentation
  3. Measurement of amniotic fluid index
D. Amniocentesis (only if remaining fluid is adequate and accessible)
  1. Assessment of fetal lung maturity: can also be done on vaginal fluid
  2. Evidence of intra-amniotic infection
    a. Gram stain
    b. Elevated WBC count
    c. Low glucose level
    d. Positive culture
E. **Term PROM** (≥37 weeks' gestation)
  1. Spontaneous labor within 24 hours: 90%
  2. Awaiting spontaneous labor for 12–24 hours reasonable
  3. Induction of labor in presence of infection risk factors
    a. Previous or concurrent vaginal infections
    b. GBS colonization
    c. Multiple digital pelvic examinations
F. **Preterm premature rupture of membranes (PPROM)**
  1. Latency period: inversely related to gestational age
    a. 28–40 weeks
      i. 50%: spontaneous labor within 24 hours
      ii. 80%: spontaneous labor within 1 week
    b. 24–28 weeks (50%: spontaneous labor within 1 week)
  2. Delivery and IV broad-spectrum antibiotics indicated if intrauterine infection strongly suspected (regardless of gestational age)
  3. Use of tocolytics controversial
  4. Management: gestational-age dependent (Table 24.2)
  5. Additional considerations with PROM before 20–22 weeks
    a. Pulmonary hypoplasia
      i. Fetal breathing of amniotic fluid vital to lung development
      ii. Pulmonary development can be arrested at stage of development when rupture occurred
    b. Skeletal deformities (inability of fetus to move within amniotic sac)
    c. Antenatal steroids when age of viability reached

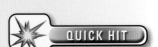

QUICK HIT

If the decision for delivery is made, GBS prophylaxis is indicated based on prior culture results or risk factors if cultures are not performed.

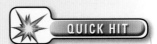

QUICK HIT

The latency period in cases of PROM is inversely related to gestational age.

TABLE **24.2**	**Management of Premature Rupture of Membranes**
Gestational Age at PROM	**Management**
≥34 weeks' gestation	• Proceed to delivery • GBS prophylaxis in labor as indicated
32–34 weeks' gestation	• Expectant management, unless evidence of fetal lung maturity or contraindication to expectant management • Antibiotics to prolong latency • GBS prophylaxis in labor as indicated • Corticosteroid administration; some experts recommend tocolysis to complete steroid course
24–32 weeks' gestation	• Expectant management, unless contraindicated • Antibiotics to prolong latency • Corticosteroid administration • No consensus for tocolytic therapy • GBS prophylaxis in labor as indicated
<24 weeks' gestation	• Patient counseling • Expectant management versus induction of labor • No data regarding antibiotics to prolong latency • GBS prophylaxis not indicated

GBS, group B *Streptococcus*; PROM, premature rupture of membranes.

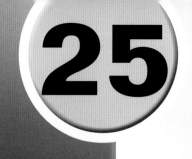

Postterm Pregnancy and Intrauterine Fetal Demise

I. Postterm Pregnancy

A. Definitions
1. **Term pregnancy**: >37 completed weeks' gestation
2. **Estimated date of delivery (EDD)** calculated as 40 weeks from 1st day of **last menstrual period (LMP)**
   a. Assumes regular menses, 28-day cycles
   b. Assumes no recent oral contraceptive pill (OCP) usage
3. **Postterm pregnancy**: pregnancy that continues >42 weeks

B. Etiology, causes, and risk factors
1. Inaccurate dating = most common "cause"
   a. Irregular menses (inconsistent ovulation)
   b. Recent discontinuation of OCPs
   c. Poor memory of LMP
   d. Late or no prenatal care
2. Anencephaly
3. Fetal adrenal hypoplasia
4. Extrauterine pregnancy
5. Maternal obesity
6. Nulliparity
7. Prior postterm delivery

C. Maternal risks
1. Labor dysfunction
2. Obstetric trauma (3rd- and 4th-degree perineal lacerations)
3. Increased rate of Cesarean delivery (with attendant risks)
   a. Infection
   b. Bleeding
   c. Thromboembolic disease (deep vein thrombosis/pulmonary embolism)
   d. Damage to surrounding structures

D. Fetal risks
1. Stillbirth (**intrauterine fetal demise [IUFD]**)
2. Macrosomia
   a. Abnormally large infant (>4,000–4,500 g)
   b. 2.5%–10% of postterm pregnancies
   c. Associated with shoulder dystocia/birth injury
3. Shoulder dystocia
   a. Increased ~20-fold if macrosomia
   b. Impaction of anterior shoulder behind pubic symphysis
   c. Brachial plexus injury
      i. **Erb-Duchenne palsy**: injury to upper roots of brachial plexus (C5, C6) (arm hangs to side, rotated medially; also known as "waiter's tip" position
      ii. **Klumpke paralysis**: injury to C8, T1 ("claw hand" where forearm supinated with hands/wrists flexed)

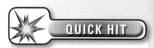

The terminology "post-dates" is misleading and should not be used.

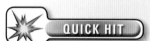

The majority of postterm pregnancies occur for unknown reasons.

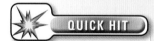

The risk of IUFD is approximately 1:300 at 42 weeks.

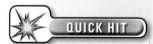

Shoulder dystocia is an obstetric emergency!

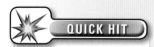

Among cases of brachial plexus injury from shoulder dystocia, 80%–90% resolve within 1 year.

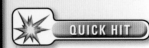

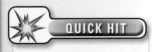

4. Meconium aspiration syndrome
   a. Respiratory distress due to small and large airway obstruction
   b. Chemical pneumonitis
5. Dysmaturity syndrome
6. Oligohydramnios (decreased amniotic fluid)
   a. Amniotic fluid index (AFI) <5 cm
   b. Poorer outcomes associated with cord compression, meconium aspiration, uteroplacental insufficiency
   c. Indication for delivery at term

E. Diagnosis
   1. Diagnosis rests on establishment of gestational age >42 weeks
   2. Dating criteria
      a. LMP alone often unreliable
      b. Early ultrasound (6–12 weeks) more accurate to establish EDD than later
      c. Early prenatal care useful in establishing accurate gestational age

F. Management
   1. Gestational age ≥41 weeks: induction/delivery versus continued antepartum care
      a. Induction/delivery appropriate in some circumstances
         i. Influenced by patient concerns
         ii. Fetal well-being: delivery indicated if testing abnormal
         iii. Status of cervix determined using Bishop score
      b. Antepartum surveillance continued only if fetal well-being established
         i. Nonstress test (NST)
         ii. Biophysical profile (BPP)/modified BPP
         iii. Oxytocin challenge test
         iv. Daily fetal movement counts
         v. **Umbilical** artery Dopplers *not* used
   2. Gestational age ≥42 weeks: induction of labor/delivery

II. Intrauterine Fetal Demise

A. Definitions
   1. Death of fetus in utero >20 weeks' gestation
   2. <20 weeks = miscarriage/spontaneous abortion
   3. Also known as *stillbirth, fetal demise, fetal death*

B. Diagnosis
   1. Confirmed by ultrasound: absence of fetal cardiac activity
   2. Signs/symptoms
      a. Absent fetal movement
      b. Decrease in pregnancy symptoms (e.g., nausea, breast tenderness)
      c. Vaginal bleeding
      d. Labor/contractions

C. Causes and risk factors
   1. Unexplained (most common reason); not readily attributed to any cause
      a. Closer to term IUFD, more likely to be "unexplained"
      b. Depends on how aggressively cause is investigated
   2. Intrauterine growth restriction/placental insufficiency
   3. Abruptio placenta/feto–maternal hemorrhage
   4. Infection: fetal death caused by direct infection or severe maternal illness
      a. More common cause in developing countries
      b. Acquired transplacentally or through ascending infection
      c. Specific infections
         i. Parvovirus
         ii. Cytomegalovirus
         iii. *Toxoplasma*
         iv. *Listeria, Escherichia coli*, group B *Streptococcus*, other bacteria
         v. Herpes simplex virus
         vi. Malaria (placental invasion and insufficiency)
         vii. Influenza, varicella (severe maternal illness)
         viii. Syphilis

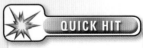

5. Congenital anomalies
6. Immune and nonimmune hydrops
7. Genetic abnormalities: more common with advanced maternal age
8. Umbilical cord accidents
   a. Nuchal cord
   b. True knot
   c. Cord abnormalities
   d. Often cited as reason for demise but should only do so after detailed evaluation for other causes
9. Uterine rupture
10. Maternal medical and pregnancy complications
    a. Hypertensive disorders/preeclampsia
    b. Diabetes
    c. Obesity
    d. Renal disease
    e. Systemic lupus erythematosus
    f. Thrombophilia/antiphospholipid antibody syndrome
    g. Cholestasis of pregnancy
    h. Thyroid disorders
    i. Cardiac disease
    j. Asthma/other pulmonary diseases
    k. Drug abuse/dependence
    l. Smoking
11. Trauma/abuse
12. African American
13. Low socioeconomic status
14. Advanced maternal age
15. Multiple gestation (e.g., twin–twin transfusion, cord entanglement)
16. Prior stillbirth
17. Postterm pregnancy

D. Management and treatment
1. Offer induction/delivery after diagnosis is made
   a. Method of induction depends on gestational age
      i. Mechanical ripening prior to induction may be used
      ii. Pitocin
      iii. Prostaglandins (may use for induction and ripening in appropriate cases)
   b. Dilation and evacuation may be required (<24 weeks)
   c. Risk of uterine rupture if prior Cesarean delivery
   d. Cesarean delivery may be required in some cases
2. If induction or immediate delivery declined, then may await spontaneous labor
   a. Immediate delivery usually not medically necessary
   b. Majority of patients will go into labor within 1–2 weeks
   c. At risk for developing consumptive coagulopathy (disseminated intravascular coagulation)
      i. Typically occurs 3–4 weeks after demise but can happen sooner
      ii. Monitor for coagulopathy: fibrinogen, platelet count, prothrombin time/partial thromboplastin time
      iii. May require transfusion of blood components, aggressive fluid resuscitation, critical care to deal with massive hemorrhage
      iv. Limits pain control options (e.g., epidural)
3. Provide emotional support, grief counseling, religious support if desired for patient and family
4. Investigation for cause
   a. Chromosome analysis (fetal karyotype)
      i. Amniocentesis prior to delivery: often yields best results
      ii. Biopsy of fetal tissue
      iii. Cord blood/placental tissue

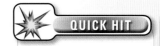

QUICK HIT

The most common genetic abnormality is aneuploidy, and the most common aneuploidies are trisomies 21, 18, and 13.

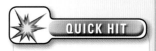

QUICK HIT

Many healthy babies are born with nuchal cords and umbilical knots.

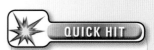

QUICK HIT

Coagulopathy is caused by the release of thromboplastin (tissue factor) from the placenta into the maternal circulation.

Postterm Pregnancy

      b. Evaluation of fetus, placenta, and umbilical cord
        i. Gross examination of fetus
        ii. Autopsy if desired
        iii. Maternal lab evaluation and investigation for underlying medical conditions

E. Prevention
  1. No good intervention in general population
  2. High-risk populations
    a. Control/optimize maternal medical condition (e.g., good glycemic control, blood pressure control)
    b. Antenatal testing when indicated: BPP, NST, fetal Dopplers
    c. Induction of labor at term or sooner when indicated

I. Informed Consent

A. Procedure explained in detail, including possible risks and complications, alternatives to procedure, as well as how patient will benefit from procedure

B. Should be obtained in writing (consent form)

C. Patient should be allowed to ask questions and have them answered to her satisfaction

D. Language patient can understand
1. Avoid medical jargon when possible
2. Use translator if needed

E. Patient should be competent to give consent

II. Ultrasound

A. Uses high-frequency sound waves to produce images of various structures and organs
1. Transvaginal
2. Transabdominal

B. Indications for obstetric ultrasound
1. Determination of location and viability of pregnancy
   a. Intrauterine *versus* ectopic pregnancy (Figure 26.1)
   b. Molar pregnancy

FIGURE 26.1 Sites at which an ectopic pregnancy may occur.

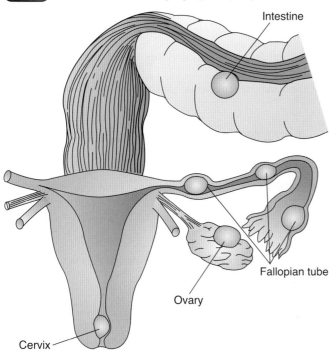

Intestine

Fallopian tube

Ovary

Cervix

(From Pillitteri A. *Maternal and Child Nursing*, 4th ed. Philadelphia: Lippincott, Williams & Wilkins; 2003.)

FIGURE 26.2 Fetal gestational age measurements.

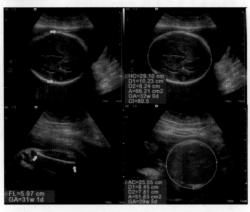

BPD: Biparietal diameter   HC: Head circumference
FL: Femur length   AC: Abdominal circumference

Ultrasound provides accurate distance measurements. Fetal age is often determined by biparietal diameter, circumference measurements *(top)*, femur length, and abdominal circumference measurements *(bottom)*. Based on known correlation methods, the gestational age (GA) can be calculated for each of the measurements. (From Jerrold T, Bushberg JT, Seibert JA, Leidholdt EM, Boone JM. *Essential Physics of Medical Imaging.* Baltimore: Lippincott Williams & Wilkins; 2011.)

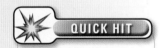

QUICK HIT

Placental lacunae are often predictive of placenta accreta.

2. Determining number of fetuses, chorionicity
3. Gestational age determination (Figure 26.2)
4. Fetal anatomy (evaluation for birth defects/anomalies)
5. Placental location and evaluation
   a. Normal location
   b. Placenta previa or low lying
   c. Accreta, increta, or percreta (see Figure 23.1)
   d. Vasa previa
6. Evaluation of fetal growth
7. Genetic screening
   a. 1st-trimester screening (nuchal translucency)
   b. Anomalies associated with genetic syndromes
   c. Used in tests to obtain chromosomes: amniocentesis, chorionic villus sampling (CVS)
8. Antenatal testing
   a. Biophysical profile
   b. Dopplers (middle cerebral artery [MCA] and umbilical artery)
9. Cervical length measurement
10. Evaluation of uterine abnormalities, maternal structures (leiomyoma, adnexal masses)
C. Risks and complications
   1. Generally accepted as safe with few risks but should only be used when medically necessary
   2. Possible maternal anxiety if abnormalities found
   3. Possibility of missing abnormalities

III. Chorionic Villus Sampling *(Figure 26.3)*

A. Performed in 1st trimester (usually 10–12 weeks)
   1. Sample placenta to obtain tissue (chorionic villi) for prenatal genetic diagnosis
   2. Ultrasound used for guidance
   3. Transabdominal approach uses spinal needle
   4. Transcervical approach transcervical catheter
   5. Indications: high risk for fetus with genetic diseases, abnormal 1st-trimester screening/ultrasound

FIGURE
26.3 Chorionic villus sampling.

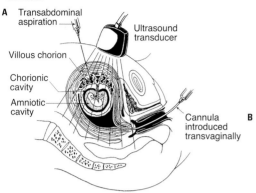

A Transabdominal aspiration

Ultrasound transducer

Villous chorion

Chorionic cavity

Amniotic cavity

Cannula introduced transvaginally

B

(**A**) Transabdominal approach. (**B**) Transvaginal approach. (From Beckmann CRB, Ling FW, et al. *Obstetrics and Gynecology*, 5th ed. Baltimore: Lippincott Williams & Wilkins; 2006.)

B. Performed earlier in pregnancy than genetic amniocentesis
  1. Decreases risks of pregnancy termination because able to terminate earlier in pregnancy
  2. Decreases potential maternal emotional distress if termination done earlier
C. Risks and complications
  1. Diagnostic error: maternal cell contamination, placental mosaicism
  2. Pregnancy loss (approximately 2.5%); depends on operator experience
  3. Bleeding or subchorionic hematoma
  4. Infection
  5. Rupture of membranes (rare in experienced centers)
  6. Limb reduction defects (LRDs) *not* thought to be increased when CVS performed after 10 weeks

IV. Amniocentesis
A. Needle (20- or 22-gauge) passed through maternal abdomen into amniotic sac to obtain amniotic fluid under ultrasound guidance
B. Indications for amniocentesis
  1. Genetic (usually performed at 15–20 weeks)
     a. Discard first 1–2 mL to avoid maternal cell contamination
     b. Fetal skin cells and cells from urinary, respiratory, and gastrointestinal tracts
     c. Cells placed in tissue culture
     d. Fluorescence in situ hybridization (FISH): quicker results for certain chromosomes (13, 18, 21, X, Y)
  2. Amnioreduction for polyhydramnios
  3. Amniotic fluid to assess fetal lung maturity (3rd-trimester test)
  4. Evaluation for intra-amniotic infection
     a. Preterm labor/preterm premature rupture of membranes
     b. "TORCH" infections
  5. Isoimmunization monitoring: measurement of bilirubin to assess fetal anemia
C. Risks and complications
  1. Pain or cramping: usually transient and not severe
  2. Chorioamnionitis
     a. Introduction of skin flora or bowel flora if bowel accidentally pierced
     b. Rare: approximately 0.1% of cases
     c. May lead to maternal sepsis, death
  3. Leakage of fluid (2%–3% of cases)
     a. Often resolves if puncture site "reseals"
     b. Successful pregnancy outcomes common despite leakage
     c. May lead to chorioamnionitis
  4. Vaginal bleeding
  5. Isoimmunization: give RhoGAM to minimize risk

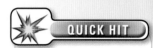

QUICK HIT

RhoGAM is given to all Rh-negative nonsensitized patients after CVS.

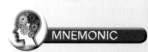

MNEMONIC

TORCH infections
Toxoplasmosis
Other
Rubella
Cytomegalovirus
Herpes simplex virus 2

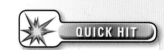

QUICK HIT

"Other infections" in the TORCH acronym include coxsackievirus, varicella-zoster virus (chickenpox), HIV, chlamydia, parvovirus B19, and syphilis.

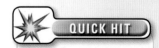

QUICK HIT

Amniocentesis for assessment of fetal anemia is being replaced by the use of MCA Doppler monitoring.

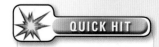

QUICK HIT

Chorioamnionitis should be treated aggressively if suspected.

Obstetric Procedures

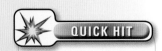

Amniocentesis <15 weeks' gestation is associated with more pregnancy losses and clubfoot deformities.

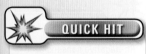

Shoulder dystocia occurs when the anterior shoulder is unable to be delivered with gentle traction and is an *obstetric emergency*!

6. Pregnancy loss (spontaneous abortion, stillbirth, neonatal death)
7. Fetal injury with needle
8. Early amniocentesis

V. Spontaneous Vaginal Delivery (SVD)

A. Fetus delivered with aid of maternal pushing
B. Procedure for "routine" delivery
   1. Patient usually in lithotomy position
   2. Vagina and perineum prepped and bladder drained if needed
   3. Fetal head gently flexed while crowning to minimize perineal trauma
   4. Head allowed to restitute (external rotation) and nuchal cord reduced if needed
   5. Anterior shoulder delivered with gentle downward traction
   6. Posterior shoulder delivered with upward traction, and remainder of body then delivered
   7. Cord clamped and cut, suction of mouth and nares
   8. Infant handed to waiting attendant or placed on maternal abdomen
   9. Placenta delivered (3rd stage of labor)
   10. Uterine massage and monitoring of bleeding
   11. Repair of laceration or episiotomy
C. **Shoulder dystocia**
D. Episiotomy and perineal lacerations
   1. Episiotomy sometimes required to expedite delivery, prevent uncontrolled laceration, or help in dealing with shoulder dystocia
      a. Midline episiotomy: vertical incision made with scissors from posterior fourchette toward anus/rectum
      b. Mediolateral episiotomy: incision made with scissors at 45° angle on perineum away from hymenal ring
   2. Perineal laceration
      a. 1st degree: superficial tear involving epithelial layer
      b. 2nd degree: involves perineal body but not into external anal sphincter
      c. 3rd degree: extends into anal sphincter but not into rectal mucosa
      d. 4th degree: extends into anal sphincter and rectal mucosa
E. Complications of SVD
   1. Maternal lacerations, hemorrhage, hematoma
   2. Shoulder dystocia
   3. Retained placenta or products of conception
   4. Metritis
   5. Pelvic organ prolapse, incontinence (long-term outcome)
   6. Thromboembolism

VI. Vaginal Birth After Cesarean Delivery (VBAC)

A. **Trial of labor after Cesarean (TOLAC)** possible in certain patients
   1. 1 previous low transverse uterine incision (2 prior low transverse incisions acceptable in certain cases)
   2. No other uterine scars (myomectomy, wedge resection for cornual ectopic)
   3. Adequate maternal pelvis
   4. Obstetrician and appropriate support staff immediately available for potentially emergent Cesarean delivery
B. TOLAC not advised and contraindicated in some cases
   1. Prior classical uterine incision or extension into active segment of uterus
   2. Prior uterine dehiscence or rupture
   3. Lack of resources to perform emergent Cesarean delivery
   4. Obstetric or maternal contraindications to vaginal delivery
   5. Macrosomia and twin gestation considered relative contraindications
C. Success rate approximately 60%–80%
   1. Successful VBAC more likely in those with prior vaginal delivery
   2. Factors associated with greater likelihood of VBAC success
      a. Original Cesarean delivery indication nonrecurring (e.g., malpresentation, nonreassuring fetal status)

b. Nonmacrosomic fetus

c. Patient admitted in labor

3. Factors associated with less likely VBAC success

a. Maternal obesity

b. Original Cesarean delivery for arrest of descent

D. Benefits of successful VBAC compared with repeat Cesarean delivery

1. Less risk of bleeding, damage to surrounding organs, infection, and future abnormal placentation due to repeat Cesarean deliveries

2. Less pain

3. Shorter hospital stay

4. Shorter convalescence

E. Risks and complications of TOLAC

1. Uterine rupture (~1% with low transverse uterine incision)

a. Risk greatly increased with incision involving active segment of uterus

b. Pitocin to be used with greater caution due to increased rupture risk

c. **Prostaglandins** avoided due to higher rupture risk

d. Neonatal encephalopathy or death in cases of uterine rupture

e. Possible need for hysterectomy

f. Transfusion

g. Maternal death

2. Risks associated with emergent Cesarean delivery

a. Febrile morbidity/infections

b. Damage to surrounding organs

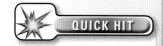

QUICK HIT

Reasons to suspect uterine rupture include severe abdominal pain, vaginal bleeding, fetal heart rate decelerations, and loss of fetal station.

VII. Operative Vaginal Delivery

A. Use of obstetric forceps or vacuum device to affect delivery

B. Prerequisites for operative delivery

1. Engaged fetal vertex

2. Ruptured membranes, fully dilated cervix, bladder drained

3. Adequate pain control

4. Adequate maternal pelvis

5. Certain knowledge of position of fetal head

6. Skilled operator

7. Appropriate support staff and immediate access to Cesarean delivery

8. Operative delivery contraindicated if previously mentioned prerequisites not met and/or suspected fetal coagulopathy

C. Indications for operative delivery

1. Prolonged 2nd stage of labor

2. Nonreassuring fetal heart tones or suspected fetal compromise

3. Need for shortened stage of labor: maternal cardiovascular disease, cerebrovascular disease, maternal exhaustion

D. Forceps

1. Types of forceps include classical, rotational, and those for delivery after coming head of breech

2. Outlet forceps

a. Scalp visible without separating labia

b. Fetal head on perineum

c. Rotation not >45°

d. Position: direct occiput anterior or posterior, left/right occiput anterior, left/right occiput posterior (Figure 26.4)

3. Low forceps: fetal skull at ≥+2 station

4. Mid-forceps: between 0 and +2 station

5. High forceps: higher than 0 station (no longer used in modern obstetrics)

6. Procedure

a. Forceps applied and proper placement confirmed; rotation performed if needed

b. Fetus delivered using gentle traction combined with maternal expulsive effort

Obstetric Procedures

FIGURE 26.4 Forceps delivery.

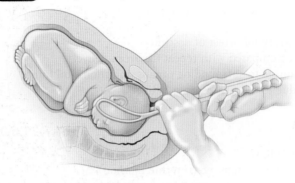

(From Beckmann CRB, Ling FW, et al. *Obstetrics and Gynecology*, 7th ed. Baltimore: Lippincott Williams & Wilkins; 2014.)

7. Risks and complications
   a. Vaginal and perineal lacerations; increased incidence or 3rd- and 4th-degree lacerations
   b. Bleeding
   c. Increased incidence of pelvic organ prolapse, fecal/urinary incontinence
   d. Fetal lacerations and bruising
   e. Intracranial hemorrhage, retinal hemorrhage
   f. Cephalohematoma
   g. Skull fracture
E. Vacuum extraction (indications for vacuum essentially same for forceps)
   1. Theoretical advantage compared to forceps
      a. Less maternal trauma and lacerations
      b. Less intracranial pressure during traction
      c. Requires less space compared to placing metal force blades in vagina
   2. Procedure (Figure 26.5)
      a. Vacuum cup applied ~3 cm anterior to posterior fontanelle and bisecting sagittal suture, suction applied, and correct placement verified
      b. Fetus delivered with gentle traction in concert with maternal pushing
   3. Risks and complications
      a. Scalp lacerations
      b. Cephalhematoma
      c. Intracranial hemorrhage
      d. Retinal hemorrhage
      e. Neonatal jaundice
      f. Shoulder dystocia
      g. Vaginal trauma, lacerations, prolapse/incontinence

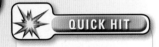

QUICK HIT

Avoid vacuum extraction in premature infants <34 weeks because of the risk of fetal intraventricular hemorrhage.

VIII. Breech Vaginal Delivery

A. Breech vaginal deliveries declining as fewer obstetricians trained in procedure
B. Types of breech presentations (see Figure 13.1)
   1. Complete breech: hips and knees flexed—**"cannonball"**
   2. Frank breech: hips flexed and knees extended
   3. Footling (incomplete) breech: 1 or both feet as presenting part
C. Requires skilled operator and often performed in operating room with ancillary and anesthesia support
D. **Head entrapment** may occur and requires immediate intervention
   1. Uterine relaxant
   2. May require **Dührssen** incision in cervix

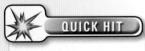

QUICK HIT

Cord prolapse is more likely with the footling breech presentation.

IX. Cesarean Delivery

A. Procedure in which infant delivered through incision in abdomen and uterus
B. Rate in United States: ~30%

FIGURE
26.5 Vacuum extraction.

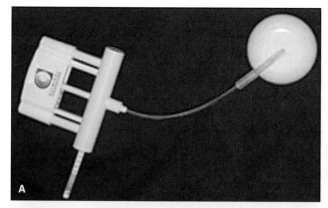
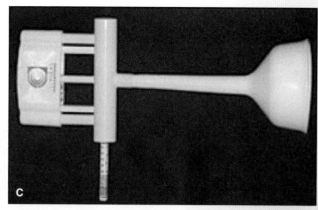
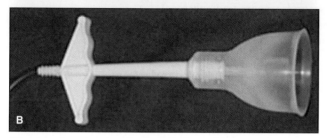

Different cup shapes have been developed. The flat cup (**A**) has been developed to allow for placement of the vacuum on a part of the fetal head not directly presenting. **B** and **C** represent two types of soft cups; **B** is designed to be used with a separate suction pump, **C** has a handheld pump attached. (From Hook CD, Damos JR. Vacuum-assisted vaginal delivery. *Am Fam Physician.* 2008;78[8]:953–960.)

C. Indications
1. Arrest disorders/labor abnormalities
2. Nonreassuring fetal testing
3. Malpresentation
4. Prior Cesarean delivery or uterine surgery
5. Some fetal anomalies
6. Maternal infections (active herpes, human immunodeficiency virus) and other medical disorders
7. High-order multiple gestation
8. Placenta previa
9. Macrosomia/cephalopelvic disproportion
10. Elective upon patient request (assuming full informed consent)

D. Procedure
1. Abdomen prepped and draped; adequate anesthesia confirmed
2. Skin incision made
   a. **Pfannenstiel incision** ("bikini cut"): transverse incision ~3 cm above pubic symphysis
   b. **Midline vertical incision**: often performed in emergent cases or when additional exposure may be needed
   c. **Maylard incision**: transverse incision similar to Pfannenstiel, but medial aspect of rectus abdominis muscle incised if additional exposure needed
3. Subcutaneous fat incision and rectus fascia exposed then incised
4. Fascial incision extended and dissected off underlying rectus muscles
5. Midline between rectus muscles identified and peritoneum entered
6. Bladder blade positioned, vesicouterine peritoneum incised and extended, bladder flap created, and bladder blade replaced
7. Hysterotomy made using scalpel
   a. Low transverse uterine incision (most common)
   b. Low vertical incision

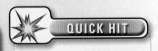

  c. Classical uterine incision (vertical hysterotomy in active segment)
   i. Transverse lie (back down)
   ii. Premature infant and poorly developed lower uterine segment
   iii. Fibroids obstructing lower uterine segment
   iv. Associated with higher rate of uterine rupture in following pregnancies
   v. Classical incision closed in multiple layers
  d. **J-incision** and **T-incision**: performed after attempted low transverse when additional room to deliver fetus is needed
 8. Infant delivered and placenta extracted along with membrane and other debris
 9. Hysterotomy closed using absorbable suture, and hemostasis assured
 10. Fascia and other incised layers closed
 11. Dressing applied and patient taken to recovery area
E. Risks and complications
 1. Bleeding, hematoma
 2. Damage to bowel, bladder, other surrounding structures
 3. Infection (metritis, wound, urinary tract, abscess)
 4. Need for future Cesarean delivery
 5. Uterine rupture in subsequent pregnancies
 6. Hysterectomy
 7. Abnormal placentation in future pregnancies (previa, accreta, etc.)
 8. Injury to fetus: scalpel lacerations
 9. Bowel obstruction, ileus (postoperative)
 10. Thromboembolism
 11. Death

X. Tubal Ligation

A. Method of **permanent sterilization** performed by ligating and excising portion of each fallopian tube
B. Performed after vaginal delivery (postpartum) or at time of Cesarean delivery
 1. Common techniques include Parkland, Pomeroy, and modified Pomeroy methods as well as others
 2. Postpartum tubal ligation performed through mini-laparotomy at level of uterine fundus: typically infra-umbilical and tube brought to incision site
  a. Advantage: single hospitalization and anesthesia for delivery and tubal
  b. Absorbable suture used so that tubal ends will separate after procedure
  c. **Fimbriated end** identified in order to confirm fallopian tube
  d. Complete transection of tubal lumen required
 3. Tubal ligation at time of Cesarean delivery
  a. Avoids need for separate procedure
  b. Tubes often easily identified but should still follow out to fimbriae
 4. Interval tubal ligation also possible via laparoscopy, laparotomy, or via hysteroscopy
C. Risks and complications
 1. Surgical risks: bleeding, infection, pain, damage to organs/surrounding structures, hernia
  a. Small incision makes it relatively "blind" procedure
  b. Deferring from postpartum to interval tubal ligation considered if potential distorted anatomy (pelvic/abdominal adhesions from past pelvic inflammatory disease, pelvic surgery)
  c. Procedure is elective; should not be performed if mother unstable
 2. Failure with subsequent pregnancy ($<$1%)
 3. Ectopic pregnancy
 4. **Regret**: patient must be absolutely sure and understand permanence
  a. Postpone if neonate doing poorly unless mother absolutely sure
  b. Counsel regarding all nonpermanent contraceptive options
 5. Anesthesia risks
 6. Posttubal ligation syndrome
  a. Menorrhagia and intermenstrual bleeding
  b. Controversial whether it actually exists

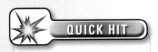

XI. Cervical Cerclage

A. Suture placed as reinforcement to prevent cervical dilation in patients with cervical insufficiency
1. Uses permanent suture (Mersilene tape, Prolene); typically removed prior to delivery or shortly thereafter (if Cesarean delivery performed)
2. May be placed vaginally or abdominally
3. Indications: poor obstetric history (cervical insufficiency), cervical changes on ultrasound, cervical changes on exam ("**rescue cerclage**")
4. Cerclage due to poor history typically placed at 12–14 weeks

B. Cerclage *avoided* in presence of
1. Labor
2. Cervical or intrauterine infection
3. Ruptured membranes
4. Chromosomal or major congenital anomalies
5. Vaginal bleeding of unknown etiology
6. Fetal demise

C. Types (Figure 26.6)
1. **McDonald cerclage** (see Figure 26.6A)
   a. Vaginal approach
   b. Cervix grasped anteriorly and posteriorly with ring forceps, and nonabsorbable suture placed as high as possible circumferentially in purse-string fashion
   c. Suture into cervical stroma but not into cervical canal
   d. Suture tied and end left long enough to allow future removal
2. **Shirodkar cerclage** (see Figure 26.6B)
   a. Vaginal approach
   b. Requires dissection of paracervical area anteriorly and posteriorly
   c. Nonabsorbable suture placed and also tied down after bladder and rectum dissected away from cervix
   d. Mucosa reapproximated with absorbable suture if needed
   e. Stitch sometimes left in place for use in future pregnancy if Cesarean performed
3. **Abdominal cerclage** (see Figure 26.6C)
   a. More invasive but stitch able to be placed higher at cervicoisthmic portion of uterus
   b. Used in patients with failed/poor outcome with prior vaginal cerclage
   c. May be performed laparoscopically or as open procedure

D. Risks and complications
1. Rupture of membranes (more likely if membranes prolapsing/bulging)
2. Pregnancy loss
3. Infection, chorioamnionitis, maternal sepsis
4. Bleeding
5. Damage to surrounding maternal structures (bladder, rectum)
6. Anesthesia risks
7. Fistula formation (rare)
8. Tearing through of stitch if in labor
9. "Cervical dystocia" in which cervix does not open during labor

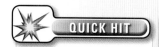

QUICK HIT

Cervical insufficiency is associated with recurrent painless cervical dilation and delivery in the second trimester.

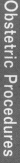

XII. External Cephalic Version

A. Procedure in which operator uses hands on maternal abdomen to convert malpresenting (breech/transverse) fetus to cephalic presentation (Figure 26.7)
B. 1 operator elevates breech and shifts it laterally while another manipulates fetus to perform forward or backward roll bringing head down to become presenting part
1. Ultrasound guidance used to monitor progress and intermittently monitor fetal heart rate
2. Mineral oil on maternal abdomen
3. Uterine relaxant (terbutaline, nitroglycerine) sometimes used
4. Epidural for pain control sometimes used: provides pain control, but must be cautious to avoid maternal injury/uterine rupture with excessive force

FIGURE
26.6 Incompetent cervix can be treated by three procedures.

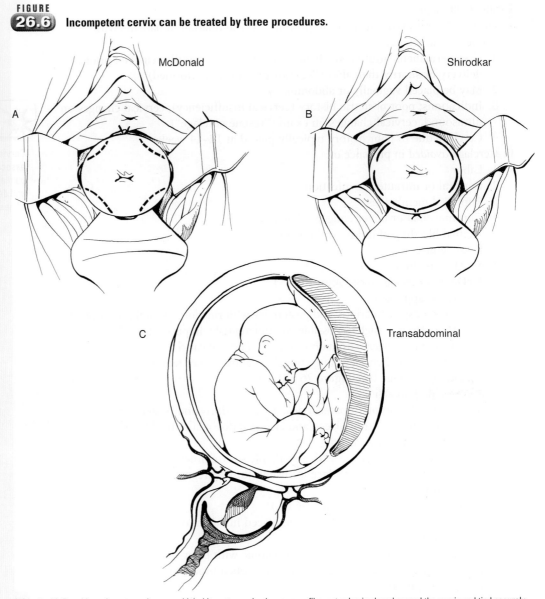

(A) In the McDonald cerclage procedure, a multiple-bite suture using large, monofilament nylon is placed around the cervix and tied securely to reduce the diameter of the cervical canal to a few millimeters. **(B)** In the Shirodkar procedure, Mersilene tape encircling the cervix is passed under the mucosa and anchored to the cervix anteriorly and posteriorly with interrupted sutures. **(C)** With transabdominal cervicoisthmic cerclage, a Mersilene band is placed in an avascular space medial to the uterine vessels at the level of the cervicouterine junction. (From Scott JR, Gibbs RS, Karlan BY, Haney AF. *Danforth's Obstetrics and Gynecology.* Baltimore: Lippincott Williams & Wilkins; 2008.)

5. Performed in hospital with immediate availability for emergency Cesarean delivery if needed
6. Performed ~36–37 weeks
7. Fetal heart rate monitored after successful procedure
8. Contraindications to version
   a. Placenta previa
   b. Nonreassuring fetal testing/uteroplacental insufficiency
   c. Prior uterine scar (relative)
   d. Uterine anomaly
   e. Multiple gestation
   f. Nuchal cord on ultrasound
   g. Oligohydramnios
   h. Obvious cephalopelvic disproportion
C. Factors associated with successful external cephalic version
   1. Multiparity
   2. Unengaged presenting part

FIGURE 26.7 External cephalic version.

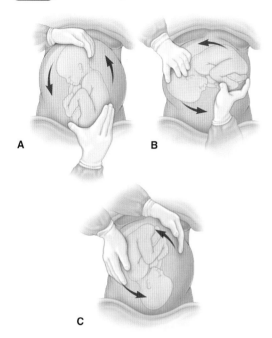

A

B

C

(A–C) In this maneuver, the fetus is converted from a breech to a vertex presentation. (From Beckmann CRB, Ling FW, et al. *Obstetrics and Gynecology*, 7th ed. Baltimore: Lippincott Williams & Wilkins; 2014.)

3. Normal amniotic fluid volume
4. Earlier gestation associated with higher success rate but also more conversion back to breech

D. Factors associated with failure
1. Well engaged breech in pelvis
2. Oligohydramnios
3. Maternal obesity
4. Anterior placenta
5. Fetus with spine either anterior or posterior
6. Large fetus
7. Advanced gestational age

E. Risks and complications
1. Placental abruption
2. Uterine rupture
3. Fetomaternal hemorrhage/isoimmunization: RhoGAM if Rh negative
4. Preterm labor
5. Fetal distress requiring emergent Cesarean delivery
6. Fetal injury
7. Amniotic fluid embolism

XIII. Surgical Management of Postpartum Hemorrhage (PPH)

A. PPH
1. Blood loss >500 mL after vaginal delivery or >1,000 mL after Cesarean delivery
2. Treatment dependent on treating underlying cause of bleeding
3. Requires maternal resuscitation as well as blood product replacement

B. Treatment of uterine atony (most common cause of PPH)
1. Uterotonics (oxytocin, methylergonovine, prostaglandins)
2. Bimanual uterine massage
   a. Operator's fist placed inside vagina
   b. Uterus compressed and massaged between fist and external hand placed at fundus

3. Uterine tamponade
   a. Gauze (Kerlix) packed into uterine cavity
   b. Balloon tamponade (Bakri, Cook)
      i. Balloon also inserted into uterine cavity
      ii. Inflated with saline to apply pressure to uterine lining
4. Selective artery embolization
   a. May be useful in cases of abnormal vasculature (arteriovenous malformation)
   b. Procedure performed by interventional radiologist
5. Arterial ligation
   a. Requires laparotomy if performed after vaginal delivery
   b. Works by decreasing perfusion to uterus
   c. Ascending uterine artery ligation (O'Leary)
      i. Relatively easy procedure and often 1st artery attempted when performing artery ligation
      ii. Can be performed bilaterally
      iii. Absorbable suture passed through myometrium of lower uterine segment, then tied down laterally around artery
   d. Utero-ovarian, infundibulopelvic ligaments: additional sites for ligation if needed
   e. Hypogastric artery ligation: technically difficult; requires experienced surgeon
6. Compression sutures
   a. B-Lynch: suture placed to fold uterus on itself in anterior/posterior plane to create "artificial" tone
   b. Additional technique described in which suture placed through and through and anterior and posterior uterus sewn together
7. Hysterectomy
   a. Procedure of last resort when other measures have failed
   b. Abnormal placentation (accreta, increta, percreta) most common indication
   c. Risk of damage to ureter and bladder and other surrounding structures
C. Genital tract lacerations (most common: perineal, vulvar, vaginal, periurethral, and cervical)
   1. Should be suspected if bleeding continues despite adequate uterine tone
   2. Diagnosis made by thorough inspection
   3. Pain control and visualization key to adequate repair; surgical assistance and operating room possibly required
   4. Laceration repaired with absorbable suture (Vicryl, Chromic gut) to obtain hemostasis
      a. Red rubber catheter in urethra if needed for lacerations close to urethra to avoid urethral occlusion
      b. 4th-degree perineal laceration: reapproximation of rectal mucosa and anal sphincter essential for good repair
D. Retained products of conception
   1. Uterine curettage or manual extraction to remove membranes/placental tissue
   2. Large sharp curette (banjo, bovine) advanced into uterine cavity, and gentle curettage performed to remove products
      a. Ultrasound guidance often useful to avoid perforation and verify removal of all products
      b. Uterotonic agents if needed

Gynecology

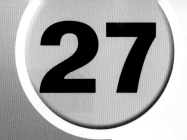

Contraception

I. General

A. Goal to prevent sperm and oocyte from uniting
1. Inhibiting development and release of egg
2. Imposing mechanical, chemical, or temporal barrier between sperm and egg
3. Altering ability of fertilized egg to implant and grow

B. Failure rates (Table 27.1)
1. **Method failure rate:** failure rate inherent in method if patient uses it correctly 100% of time
2. **Typical failure rate:** failure rate seen as method if actually used by patients

C. Factors affecting choice of contraceptive method (Figure 27.1)
1. Efficacy
2. Safety
   a. Health risks
   b. Side effects
3. Availability
4. Cost
5. Personal acceptability
6. Reversibility
7. Noncontraceptive advantages

II. Combination Hormonal Contraceptives

A. General
1. Used by 1/3 of sexually active women in United States
2. Combination of an estrogen + progestin (acts like progesterone)

B. Mechanism of action
1. Estrogen: ethinyl estradiol
   a. ↓ Follicle-stimulating hormone
   b. Prevents maturation of follicle
   c. Potentiates progestin effects
2. Progestin
   a. ↓ Luteinizing hormone (LH)
   b. Inhibits ovulation
   c. Thickens cervical mucus
   d. Alters peristalsis of fallopian tube
3. Daily opposition of estrogen by progestin results in endometrial atrophy (thinning)

C. Effectiveness
1. Typical use = 92%
2. Perfect use = 99.7%

D. Varieties of combination oral pills
1. **Dose of ethinyl estradiol**
   a. Low dose = 30–35 μg
      i. More complete suppression of ovulation
      ii. More estrogen-related side effects

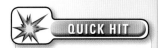

QUICK HIT

None of the currently available combination contraceptives contains a true progesterone (21-carbon steroid) but use a progestin—that is, a steroid hormone that acts on progesterone receptors.

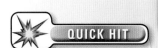

QUICK HIT

Because estrogen opposed by constant progestin causes atrophy, the purpose of the placebo week in oral contraceptives (OCPs) is to allow the ovary that has been suppressed during the active pills to spontaneously restart unopposed estrogen production to reprolifer-ate the endometrium to get ready for another 3 weeks of atrophy. At the same time that withdrawal bleeding is occurring, proliferation of the basal layer of the endo-metrium is occurring.

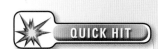

QUICK HIT

Method failure rates for oral, transdermal, and transvaginal combination contraceptives are in the range of ≤1%.

TABLE **27.1** Contraceptive Technique Pregnancy Rates in the First Year of Use in the United States		
	Percentage of Women Experiencing an Unintended Pregnancy Within the First Year of Use	
Method	**Typical Use**[a]	**Perfect Use**[b]
No method of contraception	85.0	85.0
Withdrawal	27.0	4.0
Hormonal contraceptives		
Combination pill	8.0	0.3
Progestin-only pill	8.0	0.3
Contraceptive patch	8.0	0.3
Contraceptive ring	8.0	0.3
DMPA	3.0	0.3
Implantable contraceptive rods	0.05	0.05
Barrier contraceptives		
Spermicides	29.0	18.0
Male condom (without spermicide)	15.0	2.0
Female condom	21.0	5.0
Diaphragm and spermicide	16.0	6.0
Sponge (parous)	32.0	20.0
Sponge (nulliparous)	16.0	9.0
Intrauterine devices (IUDs)		
Progesterone IUD	0.2	0.2
Copper T-380A	0.8	0.6
Natural family planning		
Calendar	5.0	
Ovulation method	3.0	
Symptothermal	2.0	
Postcoital contraception/emergency	25.0	
Permanent—sterilization		
Male	0.15	0.10
Female	0.5	0.5

DMPA, depot medroxyprogesterone acetate.

[a]Among typical couples who initiate use of a method (not necessarily for the first time); the percentage who experience an accidental pregnancy during the first year if they do not stop use for any other reason.

[b]Among couples who initiate use of a method (not necessarily for the first time) and who use it perfectly (both consistently and correctly); the percentage who experience an accidental pregnancy during the first year if they do not stop use for any other reason.

(Adapted from American College of Obstetricians and Gynecologists. *Guidelines for Women's Health Care*, 3rd ed. Washington, DC: American College of Obstetricians and Gynecologists; 2007:184–185.)

b. Ultra-low dose = 15–25 μg
   i. More breakthrough bleeding (BTB)
   ii. Require more adherence to every 24-hour dosing
c. High dose = 50 μg: used rarely to control persistent BTB
2. **Type of progestin**
   a. **1st generation:** norgestrel, norethindrone, ethynodiol diacetate
   b. **2nd generation:** levonorgestrel, norethindrone acetate
   c. **3rd generation:** desogestrel, noregestimate
   d. **Drosperinone** (not steroid hormone)
      i. Has antimineralocorticoid properties
      ii. Need to monitor potassium levels
3. **Sequencing of placebo interval**
   a. **Standard (21/7):** 3 weeks active pills, 1 week off (placebo)
      i. Excellent cycle control similar to normal ovulatory cycles
      ii. Disadvantage of monthly periods

FIGURE 27.1 Decision tree for choosing a contraceptive method.

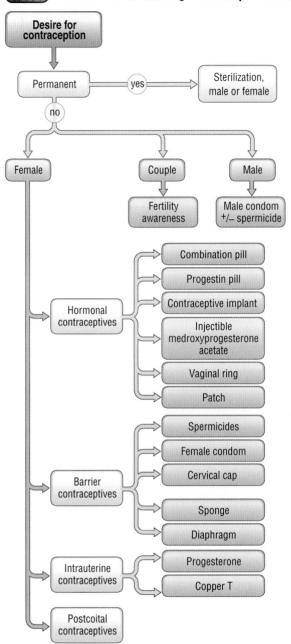

(From Beckmann CRB, Ling FW, et al. *Obstetrics and Gynecology*, 7th ed. Baltimore: Lippincott Williams & Wilkins; 2014.)

    b. **Extended duration (84/7):** 12 weeks active pills, 1 week off
        i. Spaces cycles to every 3 months
        ii. BTB can be common (secondary to more prolonged atrophy)
    c. **Continuous (365/0):** active pills
        i. No predictable cycles
        ii. BTB can happen anytime
  4. **Phasic formulations (biphasic and triphasic pills)**
    a. Increasing doses of progestin
        i. More BTB
        ii. Can only be used in standard 28-day regimen (no extended duration)
    b. Increasing doses of ethinyl estradiol: less BTB
    c. Ethinyl estradiol in placebo week: used to control vasomotor symptoms
       during placebo week in perimenopausal women on OCPs

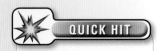

Contraception

E. Different delivery routes
   1. Combination contraceptive **pills**
   2. Combination contraceptive vaginal **ring**
   3. Combination contraceptive **patch**
F. Indications
   1. Contraception
      a. Nonpermanent
      b. Easily reversed: should be off for 2–3 cycles before attempting pregnancy because of endometrial atrophy
   2. Noncontraceptive uses
      a. ↓ Dysmenorrhea
      b. Control irregular menstrual cycles
      c. ↓ Menorrhagia
      d. Cycle control in patients with chronic anovulation
      e. Treatment of polycystic ovary syndrome
      f. ↓ Hirsutism (via ↑ sex hormone–binding globulin [SHBG])
      g. ↓ Acne
      h. ↓ Pelvic pain
      i. Suppression of endometriosis
      j. ↓ Ovarian cancer risk (via fewer lifetime ovulations)
      k. ↓ Endometrial cancer risk (via atrophy through progestin opposition)
      l. ↓ Premenstrual syndrome symptoms
      m. ↓ Mastalgia and benign breast disease
      n. ↓ Functional ovarian cyst formation
G. Contraindications (Box 27.1)

BOX 27.1

Absolute and Relative Contraindications to the Use of Combination Oral Contraceptives[a]

Absolute
- Thrombophlebitis, thromboembolic disease
- Undiagnosed abnormal vaginal bleeding
- Cerebral vascular disease
- Known or suspected pregnancy
- Coronary occlusion
- Smokers >35 years old
- Impaired liver function
- Congenital hyperlipidemia
- Known or suspected breast cancer
- Hepatic neoplasm

Relative
- Severe vascular headache (classic migraine, cluster)
- Severe hypertension (if <35–40 years of age and in good medical control, can elect OCP)
- Diabetes mellitus (prevention of pregnancy outweighs the risk of complicating vascular disease in diabetics younger than 35–40 years)
- Gallbladder disease (may exacerbate emergence of symptoms when gallstones are present)
- Hx of obstructive jaundice in pregnancy (some patients will develop jaundice)
- Epilepsy (do not exacerbate epilepsy, but antiepileptic drugs may decrease effectiveness of OCPs)
- Morbid obesity (must monitor glucose and lipoprotein profiles regularly)

Conditions No Longer Considered Contraindications
- Uterine leiomyoma (low-dose formulations not associated with growth; reduced bleeding may help in management)
- Sickle cell disease or sickle C disease
- Before elective surgery (theoretical association with thrombosis outweighed in most cases by avoiding pregnancy)

OCP, oral contraceptive.
[a]Risk primarily related to the estrogenic component.

H. Major complications
   1. Thromboembolic disease
      a. Deep venous thromboembolism
      b. Pulmonary embolism
   2. Stroke
   3. Myocardial infarction
   4. Cholestasis and gallbladder disease
   5. Hepatic adenoma (extremely rare)
I. Side effects
   1. BTB
      a. 10%–30% incidence in 1st 3 cycles
      b. Likely to occur if pill missed for 1 day
      c. Can occur if more than 4–6 hours late taking pill
   2. Bloating
   3. Weight gain: limited to 1–2 lb of cyclical water retention; no cumulative weight gain
   4. Breast tenderness
   5. Nausea
   6. Fatigue
   7. Headaches
J. Advantages
   1. Predictable menstrual periods
   2. ↓ Menstrual flow
   3. Shortens menstrual cycle
   4. ↓ Cramping
   5. ↓ Iron-deficiency anemia
   6. ↓ Cancer risk
      a. Endometrial
      b. Ovarian
   7. ↓ Ovarian cyst formation
   8. ↓ Pelvic infection
   9. Prevent intrauterine and ectopic pregnancies
   10. Amenorrhea rates
      a. 1st year: 1%
      b. 1st 5 years: 5%
K. Disadvantages
   1. Estrogens
      a. Affect lipid metabolism (↑ triglycerides)
      b. Potentiate Na^+ and H_2O retention
      c. ↑ Renin substrate
      d. Stimulate cytochrome P450 system
      e. Can reduce antithrombin III
      f. ↑ SHBG; can ↓ libido
   2. Progestins
      a. ↑ Sebum formation
      b. ↑ Cholestatic jaundice
      c. Induce smooth muscle relaxation
   3. Interaction with other medications
      a. ↓ Efficacy with concomitant use of
         i. Barbiturates
         ii. Benzodiazepines
         iii. Phenytoin
         iv. Carbamazepine
         v. Rifampin
         vi. Sulfonamides
      b. ↓ Biotransformation (↑ effect) with concomitant use of
         i. Anticoagulants
         ii. Methyldopa

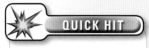

QUICK HIT

All complications of combination contraceptives are increased in smokers. Therefore, combination OCPs are contraindicated after age 35 years in smokers.

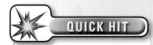

QUICK HIT

Combination contraceptives prevent pregnancies. IUDs only prevent intrauterine pregnancies.

Contraception

iii. Phenothiazines

iv. Reserpine

v. Tricyclic antidepressants

III. Progestin-only Contraceptives

A. General: good choice for women in whom estrogen-containing formulations are contraindicated

B. Mechanism of action

1. ↓ LH

2. Inhibits ovulation

3. Thickens cervical mucus

4. Alters peristalsis of fallopian tube

5. Decidualization (atrophy) of endometrium

C. Effectiveness: varies per method; see below

D. Indications: women for whom estrogen-containing preparations are contraindicated

1. Migraine headaches, especially those with focal neurologic signs or aura

2. Cigarette smoking age ≥35 years

3. History of thromboembolic disease

4. Hypertension in women with vascular disease or age ≥35 years

5. Systemic lupus erythematosus with vascular disease, nephritis, or antiphospholipid antibodies

6. Hypertriglyceridemia

7. Coronary artery disease

8. Congestive heart failure

9. Cerebrovascular disease

E. Contraindications

1. Breast malignancy

2. Liver dysfunction

F. Delivery routes

1. Progestin only oral pill

a. General

i. Norethindrone: only progestin pill marketed in United States

ii. Act primarily by ↑ cervical mucus thickness

iii. Ovulation continues in about 40% of patients

b. Advantages

i. Ideal for lactating women

ii. May be started immediately after delivery in breastfeeding mother

iii. Good choice for women age >40 years

iv. Little effect on coagulation factors, blood pressure, or lipid profile

c. Disadvantages

i. Must be taken at same time each day, starting on 1st day of menses

ii. If >3 hours late taking minipill, backup contraceptive method should be used for 48 hours

d. Side effects

i. BTB

ii. Ovarian follicular cysts

iii. Acne

e. Major complication: if pregnancy occurs, likelihood of ectopic pregnancy is higher

f. Effectiveness

i. Typical use = 92%

ii. Perfect use = 99.7%

2. Depot medroxyprogesterone acetate (DMPA)

a. General (Box 27.2)

i. Injectable progesterone given intramuscularly or subcutaneously every 3 months

ii. Maintains contraceptive level for at least 14 weeks

BOX 27.2

Indications and Contraindications for DMPA Contraception

Indications

Desire for >1 year of contraception has been one of the indications until the recent concerns about effect on bone density. Now, use beyond 2 years should be individualized and considered carefully.

Women for whom compliance with other methods has been problematic

Breastfeeding

Women for whom estrogen-containing preparations are contraindicated

Women with seizure disorders

Sickle cell anemia

Anemia secondary to menorrhagia

Contraindications

- High risk for osteoporosis
- Known or suspected pregnancy
- Undiagnosed vaginal bleeding
- Known or suspected malignancy of the breast
- Active thrombophlebitis, current or past history of thromboembolic disorders, or cerebral vascular disease
- Liver dysfunction or disease
- Known sensitivity to DMPA or any of its other ingredients

Discussion

Short- or long-term use of DMPA should not be considered as an indication for dual-energy X-ray absorptiometry or other tests that assess bone mineral density.

One injection every 3 months, 2-week "safety" interval (i.e., can be delayed up to 2 weeks without loss of efficacy)

No effect on quality of breast milk or on baby; increases quantity of breast milk; can be administered immediately postpartum

See below for absolute contraindications

Antiseizure medications unaffected, and sedative effects of progestins may aid in seizure control

Probable in vivo inhibition of suckling

Decreased menstrual flow

DMPA, depot medroxyprogesterone acetate.

---

   b. Advantages

     i. ↓ Risk of endometrial hyperplasia, endometrial cancer, and iron-deficiency anemia

     ii. Improves pain associated with endometriosis and dysmenorrhea

     iii. ↑ Quantity of breast milk; can be administered immediately postpartum

   c. Disadvantages

     i. After discontinuation, only 50% of patients resume normal menses within 6 months

     ii. 25% do not resume menses for >1 year; further workup might be indicated

   d. Side effects

     i. BTB

     ii. ↓ Bone mineral density (BMD) with long term use

     iii. Dual-energy X-ray absorptiometry (DEXA) or other tests to assess BMD not indicated

     iv. Can exacerbate mood disorders such as depression

     v. Can exacerbate headaches

   e. Major complications

     i. ↑ Body mass index (BMI)

     ii. ↓ BMD but does *not* ↑ risk of fractures

   f. Effectiveness

     i. Typical use = 97%

     ii. Perfect use = 99.7%

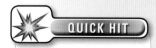

QUICK HIT

Short- or long-term use of DMPA should *not* be considered as an indication for DEXA or other tests to assess BMD.

Contraception

FIGURE 27.2 Subcutaneous contraceptive implant using etonogestrel.

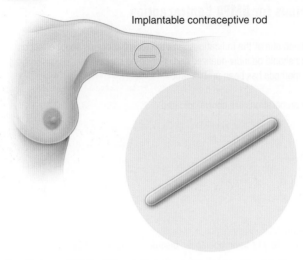

Implantable contraceptive rod

(From Beckmann CRB, Ling FW, et al. *Obstetrics and Gynecology*, 7th ed. Baltimore: Lippincott Williams & Wilkins; 2014.)

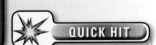

> **QUICK HIT**
>
> Injections, implants, and intrauterine contraception have effectiveness rates that equal or even surpass those of sterilization.

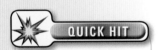

> **QUICK HIT**
>
> Injectable contraception, subcutaneous rods, and IUDs are often referred to as *LARCs*—long-active reversible contraception.

3. Implantable contraceptive rod (Figure 27.2)
   a. General
      i. Releases daily dose of progestin
      ii. Works primarily by thickening cervical mucus and inhibiting ovulation
   b. Advantages
      i. Unlike DMPA, it does not affect BMD
      ii. Effective contraception for 3 years
      iii. Possibly less weight gain than with injectable DMPA
   c. Disadvantages
      i. Insertion and removal are office procedures
      ii. Placement requires trained provider
   d. Side effects
      i. BTB
      ii. Local irritation
      iii. ↑ Pigmentation of skin overlying rod
   e. Major complications
      i. Nerve injury during placement
      ii. Difficult removal
   f. Effectiveness
      i. Typical use = 99.7%
      ii. Perfect use = 99.7%

IV. Intrauterine Devices (IUDs)

A. General (Figure 27.3)
   1. 3 types of IUDs available in United States
   2. All IUD insertion techniques share same basic rules
      a. Prophylactic antibiotics not indicated for insertion
      b. Sterile technique and vaginal prep should be used prior to insertion
      c. Bimanual examination before insertion to determine direction of insertion into endometrial cavity
      d. Proper inserter removal while leaving IUD in place
   3. Removed by simply pulling on strings
   4. If pregnancy does occur, risk for ectopic pregnancy will be higher, but IUDs do not increase overall risk of ectopic pregnancy because of contraception effect

B. Mechanism of action
   1. Copper T-380A
      a. Releases copper into uterus
      b. Creates unfavorable uterine environment

FIGURE
 27.3 Intrauterine devices using copper or levonorgestrel.

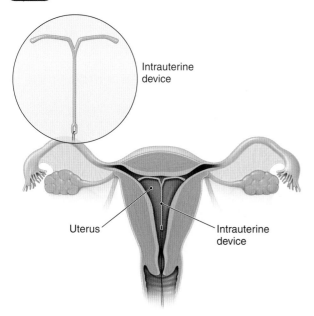

Intrauterine
device

Uterus

Intrauterine
device

(From Beckmann CRB, Ling FW, et al. *Obstetrics and Gynecology*, 7th ed. Baltimore: Lippincott Williams & Wilkins; 2014.)

Contraception

    c. Prevents sperm from going into uterus and fallopian tube, reducing sperm's
      ability to fertilize egg

  2. Levonorgestrel-releasing Intrauterine System

    a. Releases levonorgestrel into uterus

    b. Thickens cervical mucus

    c. Creates unfavorable uterine environment, preventing sperm and egg from
      meeting

C. Effectiveness: rates equal or even surpass those of sterilization

D. Indications (Box 27.3)

  1. Multiparous and nulliparous women at low risk for sexually transmitted
    diseases (STDs)

  2. Women who desire long-term reversible contraception

  3. Women with certain medical conditions such as

    a. Diabetes

    b. Thromboembolism

    c. Menorrhagia/dysmenorrhea

    d. Breastfeeding

    e. Breast cancer (copper only)

    f. Liver disease (copper only)

E. Contraindications

  1. Pregnancy

  2. Pelvic inflammatory disease (current or within past 3 months)

  3. STDs (current)

  4. Puerperal or postabortion sepsis (current or within past 3 months)

  5. Purulent cervicitis

  6. Undiagnosed abnormal uterine bleeding

  7. Malignancy of the genital tract

  8. Known uterine anomalies or fibroids distorting endometrial cavity

  9. Allergy to any component of IUD or Wilson disease (for copper-containing IUDs)

F. Types of IUDs

  1. Copper T-380A

    a. General

      i. Lifespan of 10 years

      ii. Risk of STDs is most important factor in patient selection, not age or parity

BOX 27.3

Indications and Contraindications for Intrauterine Device Use

Indications
- Multiparous and nulliparous women at low risk for sexually transmitted diseases
- Women who desire long-term reversible contraception
- Women with the following medical conditions, for which an intrauterine device may be an optimal method:
  - Diabetes
  - Thromboembolism
  - Menorrhagia/dysmenorrhea
  - Breastfeeding[§]
  - Breast cancer[‖]
  - Liver disease[¶]

Contraindications
- Pregnancy
- Pelvic inflammatory disease (current or within the past 3 months)
- Sexually transmitted diseases (current)
- Puerperal or postabortion sepsis (current or within the past 3 months)
- Purulent cervicitis
- Undiagnosed abnormal vaginal bleeding
- Malignancy of the genital tract
- Known uterine anomalies or fibroids distorting the cavity in a way incompatible with intrauterine device (IUD) insertion
- Allergy to any component of the IUD or Wilson disease (for copper-containing IUDs)

[§]Copper only until 4–6 weeks postpartum.
[‖]Copper only for current breast cancer.
[¶]The levonorgestrel intrauterine system is not recommended for current liver disease.
Data from The intra-uterine device: Canadian Consensus Conference on Contraception. *J SOGC.* 1998;20(7):769–773; IMAP statement on intrauterine devices. International Planned Parenthood Federation (IPPF). International Medical Advisory Panel (IMAP). *IPPF Med Bull.* 1995;29(6):1–4; and World Health Organization. Medical eligibility criteria for contraceptive use. 3rd ed. Geneva: WHO; 2004.
Adapted from American College of Obstetricians and Gynecologists. *Guidelines for Women's Health Care,* 3rd ed. Washington, DC: American College of Obstetricians and Gynecologists;2007:192–193.

  b. Advantages
    i. **Lack of hormone**
    ii. **Can be used as emergency contraception**
    iii. Can be placed in breastfeeding women
    iv. Does not require everyday effort
    v. Rapid return of fertility after removal
  c. Disadvantages
    i. Placement requires in-office procedure
    ii. Ovulation and menses continue
  d. Side effects
    i. Abnormal uterine bleeding
    ii. Dysmenorrhea
  e. Major complications
    i. Expulsion resulting in pregnancy
    ii. Can become embedded in uterine wall, requiring hysteroscopic removal
    iii. Can perforate uterus (at insertion, or can migrate), requires laparoscopic removal
  f. Effectiveness
    i. Typical use = 99.2%
    ii. Perfect use = 99.4%
 2. Levonorgestrel-releasing Intrauterine System
  a. Types
    i. Mirena® – good for 5 years
      52 mg LNG
      32 mm long x 32 mm wide

ii. Skyla® – good for 3 years
13.5 mg LNG
30 mm long x 28 mm wide

b. Advantages
i. Removal followed by rapid return to normal fertility
ii. ↓ Menstrual blood due to effect of progesterone on endometrium
iii. ↓ Dysmenorrhea

c. Noncontraceptive indications
i. Endometrial hyperplasia without atypia
ii. Menorrhagia
iii. Women on chronic anticoagulation

d. Disadvantages
i. Placement requires in-office procedure
ii. Ovulation continues

e. Side effects
i. Serum progesterone levels unaffected, but hormone-related effects such as headaches, nausea, breast tenderness, depression, and cyst formation have been reported
ii. Same as for copper

f. Effectiveness
i. Typical use = 99.8%
ii. Perfect use = 99.8%

V. Barrier Contraceptives

A. General: among oldest and most widely used contraceptive methods

B. Mechanism of action: provide barrier between sperm and egg

C. Effectiveness
1. Each method depends on proper use before or at time of intercourse
2. Higher failure rate than non–coitus-dependent methods

D. Indications
1. Contraception
2. Protection against transmission of STDs

E. Contraindications
1. Allergy to material
2. Unable to properly use them

F. Types
1. Spermicides
a. Contain active chemical that kills sperm (nonoxynol-9) + some type of carrier or base (gel, foam, cream, suppository, or tablet)
b. Foams and tablets should be inserted high into the vagina from 10–30 minutes before each act of intercourse
c. Duration of maximal spermicidal effectiveness no more than 1 hour
d. Douching should be avoided for at least 8 hours after use
e. No known association between spermicide use and congenital malformation
f. Effectiveness
i. Typical use = 71%
ii. Perfect use = 82%
g. Spermicides + condoms: have failure rates similar to hormonal methods
h. Spermicides may increase HIV transmission through disruption of genital epithelium

2. Male condom (without spermicide)
a. Only reliable, nonpermanent method of contraception available to men
b. May be made of latex, nonlatex, or animal membrane
c. Animal membrane ineffective against human immunodeficiency virus
d. Side effects: skin irritation or allergic reaction
e. Slippage and breakage rate in normal use ~5%–8% (couple should be counseled to seek medical care within 72 hours so that emergency contraception can be used)

Contraception

FIGURE 27.4 The female condom.

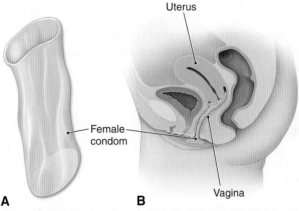

A **B**

(A) Preparation for insertion. (B) Condom in proper position. (From Beckmann CRB, Ling FW, et al. *Obstetrics and Gynecology*, 7th ed. Baltimore: Lippincott Williams & Wilkins; 2014.)

Contraception

    f. Effectiveness
      i. Typical use = 85%
      ii. Perfect use = 98%
3. Female condom (Figure 27.4A,B)
    a. Sheath or vaginal liner that fits into vagina before intercourse
    b. Slippage and breakage rate ~3%
    c. Can be placed before intercourse and can be removed any time after ejaculation
    d. Effectiveness
      i. Typical use = 79%
      ii. Perfect use = 95%
4. Diaphragm (Figure 27.5A–C)
    a. Small, latex-covered, dome-shaped device
    b. Proper use: apply contraceptive jelly or spermicide into center and along rim of device, which is then inserted into vagina, over cervix, and behind pubic symphysis covering anterior vaginal wall and cervix
    c. Can be inserted up to 6 hours before intercourse and must be left in place for 6–8 hours afterward but no more than 24 hours
    d. Can be removed, washed, and stored
    e. If additional intercourse is desired during 6–8-hour waiting time, additional spermicide should be applied without removing diaphragm, and waiting time should be restarted
    f. Several sizes of diaphragms available; must be fitted to individual patient
    g. ↑ Risk of urinary tract infections due to ↑ pressure against urethra and effect of spermicides
    h. Effectiveness
      i. Typical use = 84%
      ii. Perfect use = 94%
5. Cervical cap (Figure 27.6)
    a. Smaller version of diaphragm applied to cervix itself
    b. Associated with displacement, cervicitis, and toxic shock syndrome (TSS)
    c. Should be used with spermicide
    d. Must be left in place for 6 hours after intercourse but no longer than 48 hours
    e. Patient has to be able to correctly place it
6. Contraceptive sponge
    a. Small, pillow-shaped sponge containing spermicide
    b. Designed to fit over cervix and remain in place during intercourse

FIGURE 27.5 Diaphragm.

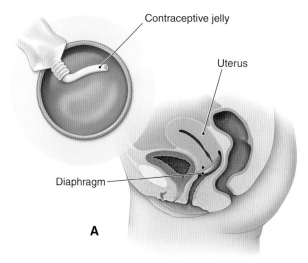

Contractive jelly

Uterus

Diaphragm

A

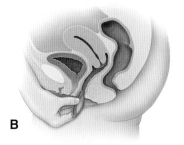

B

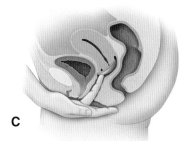

C

(**A**) Diaphragm in place. (**B**) Insertion of the diaphragm. (**C**) Checking to ensure the diaphragm covers the cervix. (From Beckmann CRB, Ling FW, et al. *Obstetrics and Gynecology*, 7th ed. Baltimore: Lippincott Williams & Wilkins; 2014.)

Contraception

    c. Only 1 size available

    d. Should be moistened prior to insertion and can be used for repeated acts of intercourse in 24-hour period

    e. Should be left in place for at least 6 hours after intercourse but no longer than 24 hours due to risk of TSS

VI. Natural Family Planning

  A. General

    1. Methods are safe and inexpensive

    2. Provide acceptable contraception in highly motivated couples and in women with regular menstrual cycle

    3. Several methods in use; all based on estimation of woman's fertile period

  B. Mechanism of action: prevent pregnancy by either avoiding intercourse around time of ovulation or using knowledge of time of ovulation to augment other methods, such as barriers or spermicides

FIGURE 27.6 Cervical cap.

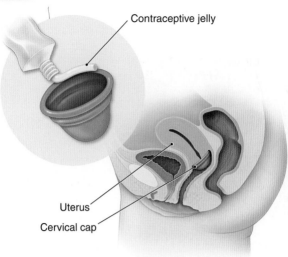

Contraceptive jelly

Uterus

Cervical cap

(From Beckmann CRB, Ling FW, et al. *Obstetrics and Gynecology*, 7th ed. Baltimore: Lippincott Williams & Wilkins; 2014.)

C. Effectiveness: failure rate with typical use is high
D. Indications: women able to identify their fertile days and have concerns about side effects and complications related to other methods
E. Contraindications
    1. Inability to predict ovulation time
        a. Recent delivery
        b. Breastfeeding
        c. Irregular cycles
    2. Unable to learn methodology
F. Types
    1. Calendar
        a. For woman with regular 28-day cycle, fertile period would last from days 10 through 17
        b. Additional days added to fertile period based on time of shortest and longest menstrual interval
    2. Basal body temperature: rise in basal body temperature of 0.5°–1°F indicates ovulation
    3. Cervical mucus: presence of thin, "stretchy," clear cervical mucus indicates ovulation
    4. Symptothermal: combines assessment of cervical mucus and basal body temperatures methods
    5. Lactation
        a. May temporarily suppress ovulation for up to 6 months in exclusively breastfeeding women
        b. Woman may begin ovulation before she resumes menstruation

VII. Emergency Contraception
A. General: employed after coitus has occurred
    1. If woman is already pregnant, these medications have no ill effect on fetus
    2. Amount of hormone not associated with alterations in clotting factors or teratogenic risk
B. Mechanism of action: prevents ovulation and fertilization and will not terminate existing pregnancy

Contraception

C. Effectiveness
1. Only effective before implantation has taken place
2. ↓ Effectiveness
a. Multiple unprotected coital events
b. Timing
i. Most effective if used within 72 hours of unprotected coitus
ii. Effectiveness ↓ >72 to <120 hours after unprotected intercourse
D. Indications: pregnancy prevention after unprotected or inadequately protected sex
E. Contraindications: known established pregnancy
F. Types
1. Yuzpe method
a. Combined oral contraceptive regimen
b. 100-mcg ethinyl estradiol + 0.5-mg levonorgestrel every 12 hours × 2 doses
c. Should be taken within 72 hours of unprotected intercourse
d. Side effects
i. Nausea
ii. Vomiting
iii. Irregular vaginal bleeding
e. Efficacy: 75%–80%
2. Plan B
a. Progestin-only regimen, approved for over-the-counter dispensing without prescription
b. 0.75-mg levonorgestrel every 12 hours × 2 doses
c. 1.5-mg levonorgestrel once (not Food and Drug Administration approved)
d. Lower incidence of nausea and vomiting than Yuzpe method and greater effectiveness
e. Efficacy: 89%
3. Copper-containing IUD
a. Can be inserted up to 5 days after unprotected intercourse
b. Contraindicated in patients with Wilson disease
c. Efficacy: >90%

VIII. Ineffective Methods
A. Postcoital douching
B. Coitus interruptus (withdrawal before ejaculation)
C. Makeshift barriers (such as food wrap)
D. Various coital positions

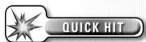

QUICK HIT

Before using a copper-containing IUD for emergency contraception, a pregnancy test is required because of the risk to an implanted pregnancy.

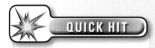

QUICK HIT

Among all of the emergency contraceptive methods, the copper T IUD is the most effective method when inserted up to 5 days after unprotected intercourse.

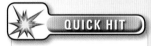

QUICK HIT

The levonorgestrel-releasing intrauterine system is not effective as an emergency contraceptive.

Contraception

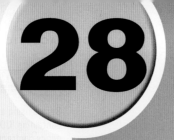

28 Sterilization

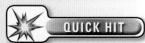

QUICK HIT

Sterilization should be considered permanent and irreversible.

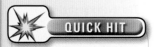

QUICK HIT

One third of surgical sterilization procedures are on men.

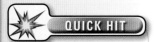

QUICK HIT

Because vasectomy is performed outside the abdominal cavity, the procedure has fewer risks than female sterilization.

I. General

A. *Most frequent method of birth control* used in United States
   1. ~1 in 3 couples rely on sterilization
   2. More common in women who are married, divorced, age >30 years, or African American
   3. Should be considered permanent and irreversible
   4. Prevents union of sperm and egg
      a. Vasectomy: prevents passage of sperm into ejaculate
      b. Tubal ligation or hysteroscopic sterilization permanently occlude fallopian tube

II. Male Sterilization: Vasectomy

A. Ligation of vas deferens via small incision in scrotum (Figure 28.1)
   1. Performed with local anesthesia
      a. Bleeding and hematoma formation
      b. Local skin infection
      c. Granuloma formation
B. Efficacy
   1. *Not immediately effective*
      a. Multiple ejaculations required to empty proximal collecting system
      b. Couples must use another form of contraception until azoospermia is confirmed by semen analysis (50% at 8 weeks and 100% at 10 weeks)
   2. Pregnancy occurs after vasectomy in about 1% of cases

FIGURE 28.1 **Vasectomy.**

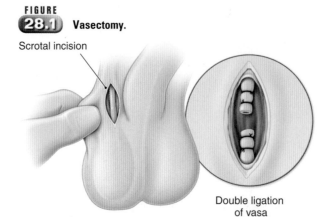

Scrotal incision

Double ligation of vasa

(From Beckmann CRB, Ling FW, et al. *Obstetrics and Gynecology*, 7th ed. Baltimore: Lippincott Williams & Wilkins; 2014.)

III. **Female Sterilization**

    A. Timing

        1. "Interval procedure" (not associated with a pregnancy)

        2. After spontaneous or elective abortion

        3. Postpartum procedure: after vaginal delivery, or at time of Cesarean delivery

    B. Methods of tubal occlusion

        1. **Laparoscopy**

            a. Electrocautery (unipolar or bipolar) (Figure 28.2A–C)

                i. Must completely coagulate 3-cm section of isthmic portion of tube

                ii. Unipolar has lower failure rate, but bipolar is safer

                iii. Risk of electrical damage to adjacent structures

            b. Falope ring (Figure 28.3A)

                i. Must be able to draw a sufficient "knuckle" of tube into Falope ring applicator

                ii. Bleeding is potential complication if too much pressure is placed on mesosalpinx during ring application

                iii. Higher incidence of postoperative pain

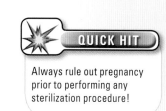

QUICK HIT

Always rule out pregnancy prior to performing any sterilization procedure!

FIGURE 28.2 Electrocautery.

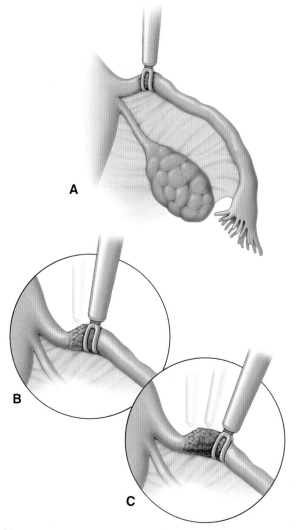

A

B

C

(A) Placement of electrocautery forceps. **(B)** Cauterization of the fallopian tube. **(C)** Tube coagulated to >3 cm in length. (From Beckmann CRB, Ling FW, et al. *Obstetrics and Gynecology*, 7th ed. Baltimore: Lippincott Williams & Wilkins; 2014.)

Sterilization

FIGURE
28.3 **Falope ring and Filshie clip.**

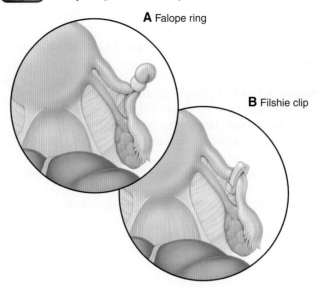

A Falope ring

B Filshie clip

(A) Falope ring. **(B)** Filshie clip. (From Beckmann CRB, Ling FW, et al. *Obstetrics and Gynecology*, 7th ed. Baltimore: Lippincott Williams & Wilkins; 2014.)

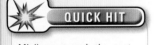

Minilaparotomy is the most common surgical approach for tubal ligation worldwide.

   c. Filshie or Hulka clip (Figure 28.3B)
      i. Clip placed around isthmic portion of tube
      ii. Least damage to tube but associated with higher rates of failure
  2. **Minilaparotomy**
      i. Performed by making small infraumbilical incision in postpartum period or small lower abdominal suprapubic incision as interval procedure
      ii. Most commonly, occlusion is accomplished by excision of all or part of fallopian tube, but use of clips, rings, or cautery can be done
      iii. Parkland (Figure 28.4) or Pomeroy method (Figure 28.5A–D)
         (a) Segment of tube is excised
         (b) With healing, there remains a 1–2-cm gap between the closed tubal segments
         (c) Important to distinguish fallopian tube from round ligament (always send tubal segments to pathology for histologic confirmation)

FIGURE
28.4 **The Parkland (modified Pomeroy) method.**

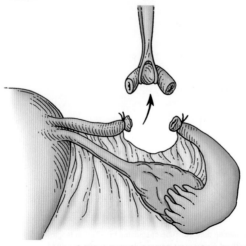

A 2- to 3-cm segment of the tube is doubly ligated, and the intervening segment is removed. (From Rock J, Jones H. *TeLinde's Operative Gynecology*, 10th ed. Philadelphia: Lippincott Williams & Wilkins; 2008.)

FIGURE 28.5 The Pomeroy method.

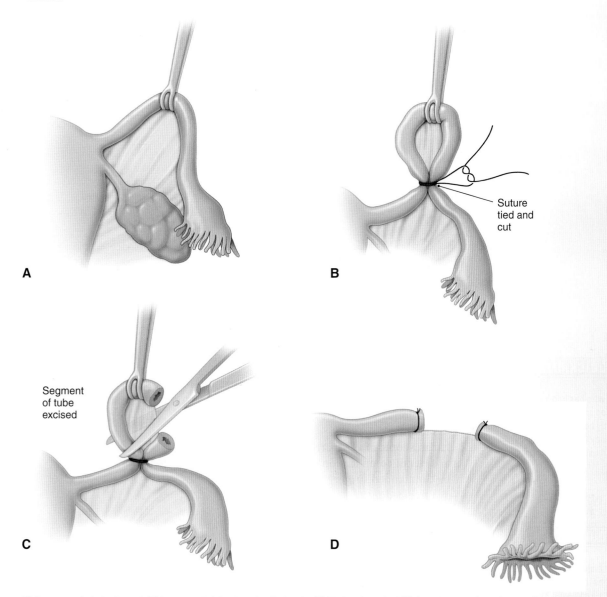

A

B

Suture tied and cut

Segment of tube excised

C

D

(A) A segment of tube is elevated. (B) A suture is tied, forming a loop in the tube. (C) The loop is excised. (D) A 1- to 2-cm gap forms between the ends of the cut tube when healing is complete. (From Beckmann CRB, Ling FW, et al. *Obstetrics and Gynecology*, 7th ed. Baltimore: Lippincott Williams & Wilkins; 2014.)

3. Sterilization at time of Cesarean delivery: same methods as used with minilaparotomy
4. **Hysteroscopy:** transcervical approach to gain access to fallopian tube ostia from within endometrial cavity—only Essure™ is available in United States
   a. Microinsertion system with a titanium-Dacron spring device
   b. Rod within the device causes tubal inflammation, resulting in tissue ingrowth, and tubal occlusion over time (at least 3 months)
   c. Patients must use another form of contraception until tubal occlusion is confirmed with hysterosalpingogram (HSG) at 3 months postprocedure
5. Transvaginal approach: rarely performed now
   a. Entry into peritoneal cavity via vagina into posterior cul-de-sac
   b. Requires adequate vaginal surgical training to avoid/minimize potential complications
C. Failure rates (Table 28.1)
   1. Overall failure rate for all methods is 18.5 per 1,000 procedures at year 10

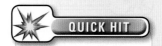

QUICK HIT

Tubal ligation has been found to decrease the risk of ovarian cancer and may offer some protection against pelvic inflammatory disease.

Sterilization

TABLE **28.1**	**Sterilization Failure Rates**	
Tubal Ligation Method	**10-Year Failure Rates per 1,000 Procedures**	**Complications**
Bipolar coagulation	24.8	
Unipolar coagulation	7.5	
Falope ring	17.7	
Interval partial salpingectomy	20.5	
Postpartum partial salpingectomy	7.5	
All methods	18.5	Injury to bowel or bladder, anesthesia-related complications, bleeding, infection, failure, ectopic pregnancy
Microinsert (by hysteroscopy)	Not yet available	Uterine or tubal perforation, bleeding, infection, inability to place the microinserts, nonocclusion over time
Filshie clip	9.7 at 2 years	

Sterilization

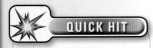

QUICK HIT

If a patient who has had a sterilization procedure subsequently has a positive pregnancy test, ectopic pregnancy must be ruled out.

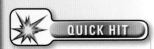

QUICK HIT

The risk for major complications is higher with an intra-abdominal procedure than with either vasectomy or transcervical approaches.

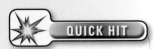

QUICK HIT

Although the risks for major complications are higher for an intra-abdominal procedure than a transcervical procedure, the transcervical approach is not successful in ~5% of patients.

2. Although pregnancy is rare after female sterilization, risk for ectopic pregnancy higher if failure does occur
   a. Ectopic risk varies by method: cauterization methods have highest risk
   b. Overall, 10-year cumulative probability for ectopic pregnancy after tubal ligation is 7.3 per 1,000 procedures
D. Complications
   1. Laparoscopic or postpartum sterilization
      a. Overall complication rate = 1.6%
      b. Unintended surgery = 0.9%
         i. Bleeding
         ii. Bowel injury
         iii. Bladder injury
      c. Rehospitalization = 0.6%
      d. Febrile morbidity = 0.1%
      e. Transfusion = <0.1%
      f. Mortality risk = 1–4 per 100,000 procedures
   2. Hysteroscopic approach
      a. Perforation of uterus: 1%
      b. Inability to place coils into tubes: 3%–5%
      c. Lack of tubal occlusion: 5% at 3 months and 1% at 6 months
      d. Perforation of fallopian tube: 1%–3%
   3. Independent risk factors for complications include
      a. Use of general anesthesia
      b. Obesity
      c. Diabetes
      d. Previous abdominal/pelvic surgery
   4. Risk for regret
      a. Important to discuss potential for regret during counseling
      b. Overall *risk for regret after sterilization is 12.7%*; 20% if age <30 years; and 5.9% if age >30 years at time of sterilization
      c. Factors associated with increased risk for regret
         i. Age <25 years at time of sterilization
         ii. Less access to, information about, or support for other types of nonpermanent contraceptives

      iii. Incomplete or inadequate information about procedure

      iv. Decision made under pressure from partner/spouse or because of medical indications

E. Reversal of tubal ligation

  1. Only 1% of women who undergo tubal ligation will request reversal

  2. Success rates for tubal patency range from 25% to 75%

  3. Many specialists recommend in vitro fertilization rather than attempt tubal reversal

  4. Most successful after sterilization procedure when minimal damage was done to smallest length of fallopian tube (i.e., clips or Falope rings)

IV. Counseling for Sterilization

A. Patients should be fully informed about procedure and its risks, effectiveness, long-term implications, and alternatives

B. Components of counseling

  1. Permanent nature of procedure

  2. Review reasons for choosing sterilization

  3. Screen for risk factors for regret

  4. Details of procedure, including risk for complications

  5. Possibility of failure, including risk for ectopic pregnancy

  6. Need for condom use to protect against sexually transmitted infections

  7. Alternative nonpermanent, contraceptive methods such as intrauterine devices (IUD) and implants are safe, long-acting options that are as effective as permanent sterilization but are reversible

  8. Completion of informed surgical consent

  9. State and federal regulations regarding timing of procedure after consent

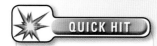

QUICK HIT

When a patient who has had tubal reversal becomes pregnant, she is presumed to have an ectopic pregnancy until intrauterine pregnancy is confirmed.

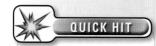

QUICK HIT

Counseling for sterilization should always include the options of *male and female* sterilization as well as long-acting contraceptive methods, like the IUDs and the subcutaneous implant.

Sterilization

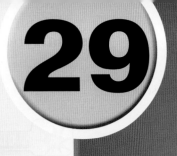

Reproductive Tract Congenital Anomalies

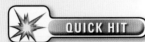

QUICK HIT

Incomplete or anomalous fusion of the paramesonephric ducts is the most common reproductive tract congenital anomaly (e.g., bicornuate uterus).

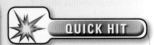

QUICK HIT

Because the paramesonephric and mesonephric (renal) systems develop alongside each other, an anomaly in one system frequently coexists with the other (e.g., renal and Müllerian agenesis).

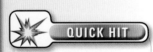

QUICK HIT

DES, which was used to prevent preterm labor from 1940 to 1971, was found to increase likelihood of vaginal adenosis, vaginal adenocarcinoma, and uterine malformations such as a "T-shaped" uterus and cervical hood.

I. Embryology

A. Upper vagina, cervix, uterus, and fallopian tubes formed by fusion of paramesonephric (Müllerian) ducts (Figure 29.1A–C)

1. Paramesonephric ducts 1st arise at 6 weeks' gestation lateral to cranial pole of mesonephric duct and expand caudally

2. By 9–10 weeks, they fuse in midline at urogenital septum to form uterovaginal primordium

3. Dissolution of septum between fused paramesonephric ducts leads to development of single uterus and cervix

B. Ovaries arise from genital ridge

C. Lower 1/3 of vagina arises from urogenital diaphragm

II. Epidemiology

A. Incidence: ~0.02% of female population

B. Fetuses exposed to maternal diethylstilbestrol (DES) from 1940 to 1971 had increased likelihood of abnormalities

1. Small, T-shaped endometrial cavity

2. Cervical hood

3. Fallopian tube abnormality

4. Vaginal adenosis

FIGURE 29.1 Formation of the uterus and vagina.

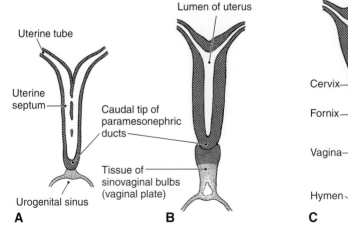

(A) 9 weeks. Note the disappearance of the uterine septum. **(B)** At the end of the third month. Note the tissue of the sinovaginal bulbs. **(C)** Newborn. The fornices and the upper portion of the vagina are formed by vacuolization of the paramesonephric tissue, and the lower portion of the vagina is formed by vacuolization of the sinovaginal bulbs. (From Sadler T. *Langman's Medical Embryology*, 9th ed. Baltimore: Lippincott Williams & Wilkins; 2003)

III. Clinical Manifestations

A. Some asymptomatic

B. Others discovered at expected onset of menarche or attempts to conceive
  1. If outlet obstruction: menstrual or pain-related symptoms
    a. Blood collects behind obstructed outlet for vagina (**hematocolpos**) or uterine cavity (**hematometra**)
    b. **Dysmenorrhea**
    c. **Dyspareunia**
  2. Pregnancy-related complications
    a. 1st- or 2nd-trimester loss
    b. Preterm labor
    c. Malpresentation of fetus

IV. Diagnostic Evaluation

A. Physical exam
  1. Evaluate secondary sexual characteristics
  2. Pelvic exam
    a. External genitalia
    b. Presence and/or patency of vagina
    c. Presence of uterus or duplication
    d. Presence of adnexa or mass
  3. Labs
    a. If presenting with primary amenorrhea: human chorionic gonadotropin, thyroid-stimulating hormone, prolactin, and follicle-stimulating hormone (see Chapter 40)
    b. Karyotype may be needed if Müllerian ducts absent and/or concern for XY chromosomes (see Chapter 40)

B. Imaging
  1. Pelvic ultrasound: lower cost evaluation of uterus and adnexa but unable to evaluate for intracavitary anomaly
  2. Computed tomography of abdomen and pelvis: lower cost than MRI but limited evaluation of uterine/adnexal structures
  3. Magnetic resonance imaging (MRI) of pelvis: more costly but better delineation of anatomy and/or anomalies
  4. Sonohystogram (saline infusion sonohysterography): better delineation of intracavitary anomaly
  5. Hysterosalpingogram: able to evaluate both intracavitary anomaly and tubal patency
  6. Hysteroscopy: both diagnostic and treatment of intracavitary anomalies such as uterine septum
  7. Laparoscopy: useful to inspect ovaries/gonads, fallopian tubes, and uterus to include rudimentary or 2nd horn
  8. Evaluation for urinary tract abnormalities is recommended if reproductive tract anomaly found

V. Treatment

A. May not require treatment if asymptomatic

B. Counseling if sexual dysfunction, genital ambiguity, infertility, or other chronic manifestations

C. Vaginal dilation if absent vagina

D. Surgical interventions
  1. **Imperforate hymen:** hymenotomy
  2. **Transverse vaginal septum:** colpotomy (incising vagina to treat hematocolpos)
  3. **Uterine** and/or **vaginal septum:** excision
  4. **Bicornuate uterus** or **uterine didelphys:** reunification procedure (Strassman procedure); recommended only in cases of unexplained repetitive pregnancy losses
  5. **Vaginal agenesis/hypoplasia:** creation of neovagina
    a. McIndoe procedure – surgical construction
    b. Frank Method – progressive pressure dilation

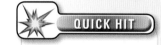

QUICK HIT

In young girls or adolescents, a rectal exam can allow palpation of uterus and preclude the need for a vaginal exam.

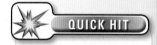

QUICK HIT

MRI is now regarded as the gold standard for diagnosing congenital anomalies of the reproductive tract because of its ability to visualize the adnexa, uterus, endometrium, cervix, and vagina as well as the genitourinary tract.

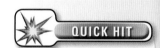

QUICK HIT

At the time of hysteroscopy, a bicornuate and a septate uterus can be impossible to differentiate, so laparoscopy is usually performed simultaneously to be able to look for a separate uterine horn as opposed to an arcuate single fundus, respectively.

Reproductive Tract Congenital Anomalies

FIGURE 29.2 Müllerian duct anomalies, hypoplasia/agenesis.

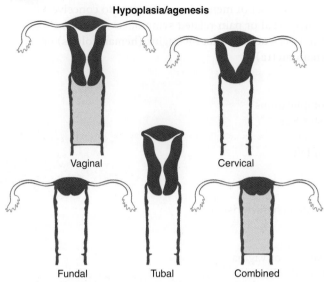

Schematic representation of developmental anomaly of the Müllerian duct involving hypoplasia or agenesis. (LifeART image copyright © 2015 Lippincott Williams & Wilkins. All rights reserved.)

VI. Müllerian Anomaly Classification

A. Class I: **Müllerian agenesis** or hypoplasia (Figure 29.2)
   1. Complete Müllerian agenesis: due to complete lack of development of paramesonephric structures
   2. Segmented Müllerian agenesis or hypoplasia
      a. Due to failure of formation
      b. Types
         i. Vaginal
         ii. Cervical
         iii. Fundal
         iv. Tubal
         v. Combined
B. Class II: **unicornuate uterus** (Figure 29.3)
   1. Due to unilateral failure of complete formation
   2. Types
      a. With rudimentary horn
      b. With communicating endometrial cavity

FIGURE 29.3 Müllerian duct anomaly, unicornuate.

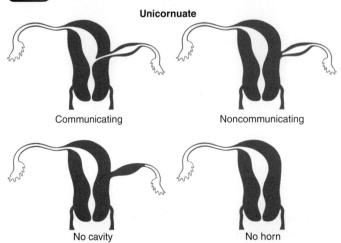

Schematic representation of developmental anomaly of the Müllerian duct involving one horn of the uterus. (LifeART image copyright © 2015 Lippincott Williams & Wilkins. All rights reserved.)

FIGURE 29.4 Müllerian duct anomaly, didelphys.

Didelphys

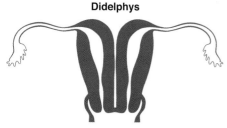

Schematic representation of developmental anomaly of the Müllerian duct involving a didelphic uterus. (LifeART image copyright © 2015 Lippincott Williams & Wilkins. All rights reserved.)

    c. With noncommunicating endometrial cavity

    d. Without cavity

    e. Without rudimentary horn

C. Class III: **uterine didelphys** (Figure 29.4)

    1. Due to failure of fusion of paramesonephric ducts

    2. 2 separate uterine bodies each with separate cervix, fallopian tube, and vagina

D. Class IV: **bicornuate uterus** (Figure 29.5)

    1. Due to failure of complete fusion

    2. Types

        a. **Complete bifurcation (bicollis):** cervix with each uterine horn

        b. **Partial bifurcation (unicollis):** single cervix with 2 uterine horns

E. Class V: **septate uterus** (Figure 29.6)

    1. Due to failure of dissolution of midline septum during fusion of paramesonephric ducts

    2. Types

        a. Complete septation

        b. Partial septation

F. Class VI: **arcuate uterus** (Figure 29.7)

G. Class VII: **DES-related anomalies** (Figure 29.8)

VII. Congenital Anomalies of Vulva and Vagina

A. Labial fusion

    1. May result in malpositioned vaginal orifice

    2. Most common etiology: excess androgens

        a. Exogenous androgens

        b. Endogenous androgen production

            i. **Congenital adrenal hyperplasia (CAH):** from enzyme deficiencies in steroid metabolic pathways

            ii. Androgen-producing tumors

    3. Often treated with reconstructive surgery

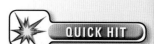

QUICK HIT

21-Hydroxylase deficiency is the most common form of CAH and leads to androgen overproduction and salt wasting due to mineralocorticoid deficiency (see Figure 41.2).

FIGURE 29.5 Müllerian duct anomaly, bicornuate.

Bicornuate

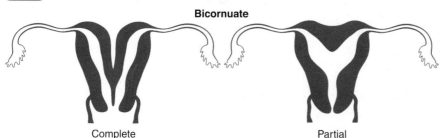

Complete   Partial

Schematic representation of developmental anomaly of the Müllerian duct involving a bicornuate uterus. (LifeART image copyright © 2015 Lippincott Williams & Wilkins. All rights reserved.)

FIGURE 29.6 Müllerian duct anomaly, septate.

Septate

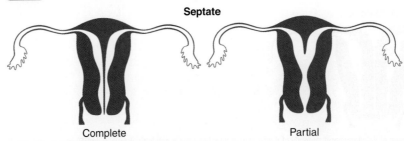

Complete   Partial

Schematic representation of developmental anomaly of the Müllerian duct involving a septate uterus. (LifeART image copyright © 2015 Lippincott Williams & Wilkins. All rights reserved.)

    B. Clitoromegaly
      1. Most common presentation of ambiguous genitalia
      2. Androgen excess: exogenous and endogenous
    C. Bifid clitoris

VIII. Congenital Anomalies of Hymen
    A. **Hymen:** junction between sinovaginal bulbs and urogenital sinus
    B. Anomalies occur when Müllerian tubercle is not canalized
    C. **Imperforate hymen:** opening does not develop in hymen
      1. Results in obstruction to outflow
      2. May present with menstrual symptoms: primary amenorrhea, dysmenorrhea, and abdominal/pelvic pain
      3. Before menarche: **hydrocolpos** or **mucocolpos** may occur (buildup of secretion behind hymen)
      4. After menarche: **hematocolpos/hematometra** may occur (buildup of blood behind hymen)
    D. Microperforations in hymen: do not present with hematometra but may require incision to open
    E. Septations in hymen: do not present with hematometra but may require excision

IX. Congenital Anomalies of Upper Vagina
    A. Vagina forms as paramesonephric system joins sinovaginal bulb at Müllerian tubercle
    B. Anomalies occur when Müllerian tubercle is not canalized
      1. Vaginal septum (transverse or longitudinal)
        a. Transverse: septal tissue occurs at junction between lower 2/3 and upper 1/3 of vagina
        b. Longitudinal
          i. May be present at various levels in upper and middle vagina
          ii. Variations include double vagina, blind pouch, or partial septum

FIGURE 29.7 Müllerian duct anomaly, arcuate.

Arcuate

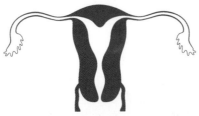

Schematic representation of developmental anomaly of the Müllerian duct involving an arcuate uterus. (LifeART image copyright © 2015 Lippincott Williams & Wilkins. All rights reserved.)

Reproductive Tract Congenital Anomalies

FIGURE 29.8 Müllerian duct anomaly, DES related.

DES related

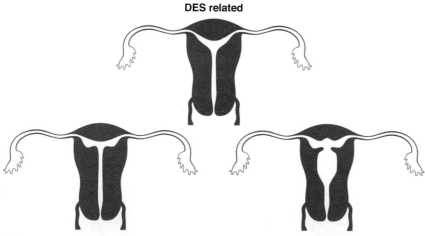

Schematic representation of developmental anomaly of the Müllerian duct related to DES. (LifeART image copyright © 2015 Lippincott Williams & Wilkins. All rights reserved.)

2. May occur with duplication of cervix or uterus (although not necessarily)
3. Similar symptoms as imperforate hymen: primary amenorrhea and dysmenorrhea
4. Treatment: surgical excision of septum

X. Congenital Anomalies of Lower Vagina

A. **Vaginal atresia**: occurs when urogenital sinus fails to contribute lower portion of vagina
   1. Absent lower vagina is replaced by fibrous tissue
   2. Similar symptoms as imperforate hymen: primary amenorrhea and dysmenorrhea
   3. Correction requires neovagina construction (see h. Treatment)

B. **Vaginal agenesis**
   1. **Mayer-Rokitansky-Küster-Hauser (MRKH) syndrome**
      a. Characterized by absence or hypoplasia of proximal vagina, cervix, uterus, fallopian tubes
      b. Clinically, patients have normal external genitalia with ridge of tissue representing hymen
      c. Rudimentary pouch of vagina may be present
      d. 10% have normal uterus with functioning endometrium
      e. Female karyotype: 46,XX
      f. Normal ovaries and ovarian function
      g. Normal secondary sexual characteristics
      h. Treatment
         i. Serial vaginal dilators used on perineum or blind vaginal pouch: may be used with or without surgery
         ii. McIndoe procedure: surgical creation of neovagina with placement of silicone mold lined by split-thickness skin graft
   2. **Androgen insensitivity syndrome (AIS)/testicular feminization**
      a. Nonfunctioning intracellular androgen receptors resulting in insensitivity to testosterone
      b. Male karyotype: 46,XY
      c. Normal male testosterone levels
      d. Lack of Wolffian (mesonephros) system development because of lack of androgen effect (Figure 29.9)
      e. However, due to Müllerian-inhibiting factor present in 46,XY lack of Müllerian system development also
      f. Phenotypically female: normal breast development, scant axillary and pubic hair

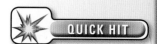

MRKH syndrome is also referred to as *Müllerian agenesis* and occurs because the paramesonephric system fails to form in an otherwise normal 46,XX woman.

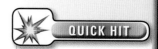

Patients with AIS appear as normal phenotypic females with breast development (estrogens) but no pubic hair (lack of androgen effects).

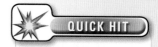

The most common tumors to develop in undescended male gonads are gonadoblastomas and malignant dysgerminomas.

FIGURE
29.9 Androgen insensitivity syndrome.

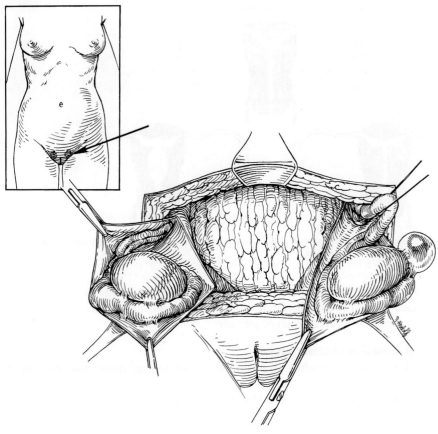

Operative findings in a patient with androgen insensitivity syndrome. (LifeART image copyright © 2015 Lippincott Williams & Wilkins. All rights reserved.)

    g. Rudimentary vaginal pouch

    h. Undescended male gonads

    i. Treatment

       i. Creation of vagina similar to MRKH patient

      ii. Surgical removal of undescended testes due to increased likelihood of malignancy

  C. **Vaginal adenosis**

    1. Vaginal wall consists of islands of columnar epithelium in normal squamous epithelium

    2. Most often located in upper 1/3 of vagina

    3. In utero DES exposure was risk factor

    4. Colposcopy and cytology surveillance indicated because of risk of developing adenocarcinoma

  D. **Dysontogenetic cysts** of vagina

    1. Soft cysts resulting from embryonic remnants

    2. **Gartner duct cyst:** most common, arising from remnants of Wolffian duct

      a. Varying sizes on anterolateral walls in upper 1/2 of vagina

      b. Most are asymptomatic and require no intervention

XI. Congenital Anomalies of Ovaries and Fallopian Tubes

  A. Abnormal embryologic development of ovaries is rare

    1. Congenital duplication or absence of ovarian tissue may occur

    2. Ectopic ovarian tissue and supernumerary ovaries: extremely rare

    3. Dual development of ovotestis: extremely rare

B. Genetic or chromosomal disorders may result in abnormal ovarian development
   1. **Turner syndrome (45,XO):** associated with rudimentary streaked ovaries, short stature, and early menopause
   2. **AIS/testicular feminization (46,XY):** results in undescended testes, which should be removed
C. Abnormal embryologic development of fallopian tubes is rare
   1. Aplasia or atresia usually of distal ampullary segment may occur and is usually unilateral
   2. Bilateral aplasia is usually accompanied by uterine and vaginal agenesis
   3. Complete duplication is rare; distal duplication and accessory ostia are more common
   4. In utero DES exposure often resulted in tubes that were shortened, distorted, or clubbed

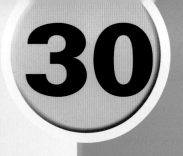

30 Reproductive Tract Benign Conditions

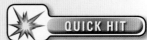

QUICK HIT

The clinical adage is: If it looks abnormal, then do a punch biopsy! Histologic examination is best to differentiate benign conditions, VIN, and cancers.

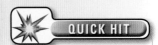

QUICK HIT

In general, ointments are more effective than creams in vulvar diseases because they are more occlusive as well as less irritating to sensitive skin.

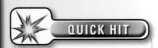

QUICK HIT

Because of the risk of progression to SCC, patients with lichen sclerosis need frequent surveillance, at least every 6 months even if symptoms are well controlled with steroid ointment.

I. Vulva (*Figure 30.1*)

A. Dermatoses (Table 30.1)

1. **Lichen sclerosis** (previously called Lichen Sclerosis et Atrophicus)
   a. Chronic skin condition mostly in genital and anal region
      i. Predominantly seen in postmenopausal women
      ii. Occasionally seen in adolescents and premenarchal girls
   b. Pruritus, burning, dyspareunia
   c. More common with autoimmune diseases and menopause; may be familial
   d. Bilaterally symmetric, thin, pale, crinkled skin similar to cigarette paper, onion skin, or parchment paper
   e. Also hyperkeratotic variety that is thick white (termed **leukoplakia**)
   f. Can extend from mons pubis to anus
   g. Eventually *destroys architecture*: loss of labial folds (particularly absence of labia minora), obliterates clitoris, and can lead to severe vaginal/introital stenosis
   h. Histology shows **loss of rete pegs**, chronic inflammation, and a very thin epithelial layer with or without overlying hyperkeratosis
   i. Can progress to **vulvar intraepithelial neoplasia (VIN)**; 5%–15% risk of **squamous cell carcinoma (SCC)** in postmenopausal women
   j. Therapy: potent topical steroids (0.05% clobetasol) often intermittently and indefinitely (Figure 30.2A–C)

 FIGURE 30.1 Biopsy of vulvar lesion.

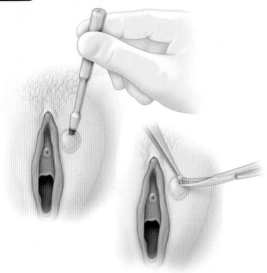

The punch is rotated in place to incise tissue. (From Beckmann CRB, Ling FW, et al. *Obstetrics and Gynecology*, 7th ed. Baltimore: Lippincott Williams & Wilkins; 2014.)

TABLE 30.1 Benign Epithelial Disorders of Vulva and Vagina

	Physical Findings	Symptoms	Treatment
Lichen sclerosis	Symmetric white, thinned skin on labia, perineum, and perianal region Shrinkage and agglutination of labia minora	Usually asymptomatic Occasional pruritus or dyspareunia	High-potency topical steroids (clobetasol or halobetasol 0.05%) 1–2×/day for 6–12 weeks
Squamous cell hyperplasia	Localized thickening of vulvar skin from edema Raised white lesions usually on labia majora and clitoris	Chronic pruritus and thickened skin	Medium-potency topical steroids 2×/day for 4–6 weeks
Lichen planus	Multiple shiny, flat, purple papules usually on inner aspects of labia minora, vagina, and vestibule Often erosive May have vaginal adhesions resulting in vaginal stenosis	Pruritus with mild inflammation to severe erosion	Vaginal hydrocortisone suppositories Surgical excision or vaginal dilators for vaginal adhesions Vaginal estrogen for vaginal atrophy
Lichen simplex chronicus	Thickened white epithelium, slight scaling usually unilateral and circumscribed	Vulvar pruritus	Medium-potency topical steroids 2×/day for 4–6 weeks
Vulvar psoriasis	Red, moist lesions, sometimes scaly May also be found on scalp, axilla, groin, and trunk	Asymptomatic or occasional pruritus	Ultraviolet light or topical steroids
Vaginal adenosis	Palpable red glandular spots and patches in upper 1/3 of vagina on anterior wall	None	Follow with serial exams

(From Callahan T, Caughey AB. *Blueprints: Obstetrics & Gynecology*, 5th ed. Baltimore: Lippincott Williams & Wilkins; 2009.)

2. **Lichen simplex chronicus** (also called *squamous cell hyperplasia*)
   a. Chronic skin thickening and edema arising from repetitive irritation
   b. Progressive pruritus and burning from prolonged irritation, leading to itch–scratch cycle
   c. Unilateral or symmetrically thickened, leathery white or reddish lesion(s) with excoriations

FIGURE 30.2 The three "lichens."

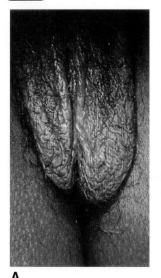 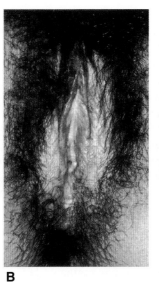 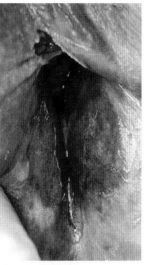

A   **B**   **C**

(A) Lichen simplex chronicus. **(B)** Lichen sclerosis. **(C)** Lichen planus. (From Beckmann CRB, Ling FW, et al. *Obstetrics and Gynecology*, 7th ed. Baltimore: Lippincott Williams & Wilkins; 2014.)

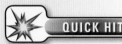

6 Ps of Lichen Planus
Purple
Polygonal
Pruritic
Planar
Papules
Plaques

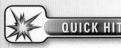

Skin excoriations and fissures can become infected; hygiene includes plain warm water soaks, loose cotton underwear, and avoidance of irritants (e.g., douches, "feminine" products).

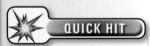

Patients presenting with vulvar ulcers should be screened for STDs (see Chapter 31).

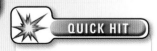

As part of the current and past medical history, ask about other general dermatologic conditions, oral symptoms, and allergies. These can be clues to vulvar disease.

QUICK HIT

Lack of estrogen in premenarchal, lactating, amenorrheic, and postmenopausal females plays a large role in vulvar/vaginal complaints.

d. Histology shows hyperkeratosis and **elongated rete pegs**

e. Therapy: topical steroids (from 1% hydrocortisone to 0.1% triamcinolone), antipruritic agents (antihistamines), and removing offending irritating agents

3. **Lichen planus**

a. Inflammatory, desquamative condition of vulva (may also involve vagina and/or gingival region of oral cavity)

b. Severe insertional dyspareunia, burning, and vaginal discharge

c. Ages 30–60 years

d. Drug induced and spontaneous forms

e. Inner labia with shiny, flat-topped, purplish/reddish papules +/− erosion → adhesions, vaginal stenosis

f. Can have white lacy bands (**Wickham striae**) near ulcerated lesions

g. Therapy: potent topical steroids (0.05% clobetasol) and occasionally systemic corticosteroids such as prednisone for 4–6 weeks, vaginal estrogen, surgery

4. Others: any dermatologic disorder can manifest on vulva

a. **Psoriasis**: autosomal-dominant disorder with velvety lesions
   i. May lack classic scaly patches due to vulva's moisture
   ii. Therapy: corticosteroids (betamethasone valerate 0.1%)

b. **Eczema** (atopic dermatitis): erythematous lesions

c. **Pemphigus**/bullous pemphigoid: autoimmune blisters

d. **Contact dermatitis**
   i. From soaps, lotions, deodorants, condoms, self-treatments
   ii. Therapy: remove offending agent; topical corticosteroids

e. **Seborrheic** dermatitis: pale red/yellow-pink lesions with oily, scaly yellow crust; seen also on scalp, chest, back, face

5. Ulcers

a. **Crohn disease**: vulvar ulcers may precede gastrointestinal (GI) symptoms; prominent edema, rectal abscesses, and fistulas may develop

b. **Aphthous ulcers** (*canker sores*): benign with unknown etiology; typically also in mouth

c. **Decubitus ulcers**: likely seen in chronically ill, those with limited mobility

d. **Behçet syndrome**: vulvar, oral, and ocular ulcerations (etiology and treatment unknown)

6. Atrophy

a. Postmenopausal women/others with estrogen deficiency (lactating women) → dyspareunia, dryness (see Chapter 42)

b. Therapy: topical estrogen

B. Structural

1. Agglutination

a. Premenarchal girls

b. Therapy: topical estrogen cream

2. **Urethral caruncle**: prolapsed urethral epithelium

a. Red, fleshy exophytic tissue at urethral meatus likely due to urogenital atrophy from estrogen deficiency

b. Children and elderly postmenopausal women

c. Therapy: topical estrogen

3. Cysts: generally no treatment required if asymptomatic; if infected/abscessed, antibiotics with incision/drainage (I&D) or excision

a. **Epidermal inclusion cysts**: solitary, mobile, nontender, pilosebaceous duct/ hair follicle
   i. Can be related to lacerations from birth trauma
   ii. Filled with keratinaceous material

b. **Sebaceous cysts**: multiple, nontender, usually appear yellow
   i. May be found on vulva or vagina
   ii. Caseous material (sebum)

c. Bartholin cyst/abscess
  i. Mucous glands at 4 and 8 o'clock, duct opens just external to hymenal ring
  ii. Small, minimal symptoms: warm soaks
  iii. Abscessed: simple I&D rarely successful
    (a) Need drainage via **Word catheter** for 4–6 weeks to create an epithelialized track
    (b) **Marsupialization:** cyst is opened and cyst walls sewn to skin on both sides to externalize cyst
  iv. Add antibiotics if cellulitis or sexually transmitted disease (STD)
  v. Bartholin gland cancer rare risk for woman age >40 years; biopsy cyst wall (Figure 30.3)
d. **Galactoceles:** milk line extends to vulva; milk-filled cyst can form postpartum
e. Varicosities: enlargement during pregnancy common
f. **Fox-Fordyce disease:** pruritic, inflamed, keratin-plugged apocrine sweat glands of axilla, mons, and/or labia (abscess = hidradenitis suppurativa)
g. **Hydrocele** or cyst of canal of Nuck: round ligament inserts into labium majus; can be site of peritoneal fluid collection

4. Masses
  a. Nevi (moles) and lentigo (freckles) found on labia: distinguish from melanoma (may require biopsy)
  b. **Fibroma:** slow-growing connective tissue tumor
  c. **Lipoma:** slow-growing adipose tumor; remove if symptomatic
  d. **Hemangioma**
    i. Soft, red, rapidly growing tumors in infants that bleed/ulcerate
    ii. Spontaneously involute, so should be left alone
  e. Others
    i. Hidradenoma papilliferum (apocrine gland tumor)
    ii. Neurofibroma (von Recklinghausen disease)
    iii. Granular cell tumor (previously called *myoblastoma* and *neural sheath Schwann cell tumor*)
    iv. Syringoma (eccrine gland tumor)
5. Clitoromegaly
  a. Excessive androgens (virilization); check testosterone levels
    i. Congenital adrenal hyperplasia
    ii. Androgen-producing ovarian or adrenal tumors
    iii. Cushing disease
  b. Normal size of clitoris 0.5 × <1.5 cm

FIGURE 30.3 Incision, drainage, and marsupialization of a Bartholin abscess.

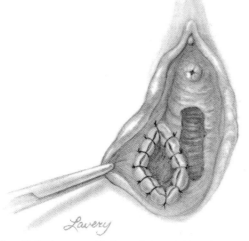

Reproductive Tract Benign Conditions

6. Trauma
   a. Assault, falls, motor vehicle accident → lacerations, hematomas: may require surgical evacuation and packing
   b. Female genital **mutilation**/female circumcision types I–IV (World Health Organization)
      i. Removal of clitoris and/or excising or appositioning labia to narrow vaginal orifice
      ii. Impacts infection risk, vaginal delivery, and sexual function
   c. Piercings: infections, scarring

C. Pain syndromes
   1. **Vulvodynia:** localized (provoked) or generalized (unprovoked) burning vulvar pain around introitus (if localized to vestibule = **vestibulitis**)
      a. Severe insertional dyspareunia: cotton-swab test identifies location and severity of pain
      b. Therapy: topical estrogen, topical lidocaine, lubricants, hydrocortisone, tricyclic antidepressants, gabapentin, physical therapy, surgical removal of vestibular glands
   2. **Vaginismus:** involuntary contraction of muscles surrounding vaginal orifice and pelvic floor
      a. Dyspareunia
      b. Treat infections or dermatitis, physical therapy, dilators, sexual therapist

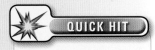

QUICK HIT

History of abuse is common in women with chronic pain conditions.

II. Vagina

A. Masses/lesions
   1. **Urethral diverticula**
      a. Obstructed periurethral glands (Skene glands) → "sacs" in anterior vagina; can drain into urethra, creating a suburethral diverticulum
      b. Symptoms: **chronic urinary tract infections (UTIs)**, dysuria, post-void dribbling
      c. Therapy: urethral dilation, diverticula excision
   2. **Gartner duct cyst**
      a. **Wolffian duct** (mesonephros) remnants form soft 1–5-cm cysts anteriorly in upper vagina and laterally in mid-vagina
      b. Mostly asymptomatic; excision may be indicated if symptomatic (e.g., dyspareunia)
   3. **Vaginal adenosis**
      a. Red glandular patches: upper 1/3 anterior vagina
      b. Associated with **diethylstilbestrol (DES)** exposure in utero
      c. Multiple cell types within lesions: biopsy mass or if bleeding to exclude adenocarcinoma
   4. **Endometriosis** (see Chapter 33): implants of endometrial tissue present in upper 1/3 vagina

B. Pelvic support defects (see Chapter 32)
   a. **Anterior vaginal prolapse (cystocele):** bladder bulges into vagina
   b. **Posterior vaginal prolapse (rectocele):** rectum bulges into vagina
   c. **Enterocele** (peritoneal sac containing bowel): bulges into vagina

C. Obstetric/surgical trauma
   1. **Fistula**
      a. Ureterovaginal, vesicovaginal, rectovaginal communications can form due to obstetric injury, surgery, radiation, and cancer; fistula tract often difficult to locate
      b. Symptoms: chronic discharge, irritation, and infection
      c. Treatment: surgical excision of tract and closure
   2. Inclusion cyst: infolding of vaginal epithelium in lower 1/3 posterior vagina resulting from imperfect approximation of lacerations or episiotomy
   3. Other traumas: prolonged pessary, diaphragm, or tampon use; foreign objects; sexual assault → ulceration, infection, laceration, hematoma

III. Cervix

A. Normal anatomy (Figure 30.4A–C)

1. **Squamocolumnar junction (SCJ):** outer squamous epithelium meets inner mucinous columnar epithelium of endocervix

   a. With menarche, columnar cells begin to undergo squamous metaplasia

   b. **Transformation zone (TZ):** represents area of change

2. Young women and women on estrogen (birth control pills, pregnancy) often have cervical **ectropion** (also called **eversion**)

   a. Visible reddish ring of mucinous columnar epithelium of endocervix appearing around cervical os

   b. As more cells undergo squamous metaplasia, TZ moves up endocervical canal

3. Columnar cells produce mucus

   a. Women with ectropion have more vaginal discharge

   b. Cells are very susceptible to trauma (postcoital spotting) and infection (e.g., human papillomavirus [HPV], chlamydia)

B. Cysts

1. **Nabothian cysts:** blocked mucinous endocervical glands, normal variant, no treatment needed

2. Mesonephric cysts: Wolffian duct remnants, no treatment needed

3. **Endometriosis:** can implant on cervix (see Chapter 33)

C. **Polyps** (see Chapter 40)

1. Benign pedunculated or broad-based (sessile) growth from either endocervix or endometrium

2. Potential for intermenstrual/postcoital bleeding; rarely obstructs canal (very rarely [<1%] can contain SCC or adenocarcinoma)

3. Twist off with ring forceps in office or sessile polyp can require dilation and curettage (D&C) +/− hysteroscopy

D. **Fibroids** (see Chapters 34 and 40)

1. **Leiomyomas** (**myomas**; **fibroids**): benign smooth muscle tumors of uterus (can also occur in cervix)

2. Irregular bleeding, dyspareunia, bladder/rectal pressure, pregnancy problems with dilation and malpresentation

3. Removal if symptomatic: hysterectomy *versus* myomectomy depends on size/location and desire to preserve reproductive capability

E. Stenosis

1. Etiology

   a. Congenital

   b. Scarring: surgery, cryosurgery, radiation

   c. Atrophy: secondary to lack of estrogen

   d. Obstruction: neoplasm, polyp, fibroid

2. Significant stenosis can prohibit normal menstrual flow (oligomenorrhea, amenorrhea, dysmenorrhea, hematometra)

3. Dilate if symptomatic to facilitate menstrual flow, uterine evaluation, vaginal delivery

F. Trauma: cervical laceration can occur with vaginal delivery, Cesarean delivery, gynecologic surgery, sexual assault

IV. Uterus

A. **Fibroids** (also called *leiomyomas* or *myomas*): benign monoclonal smooth muscle cell tumors of myometrium, pseudocapsule of compressed muscle fibers (see Chapters 34 and 40)

1. Abnormal **bleeding**, **pain (dysmenorrhea)**, **pressure** (in/on bowel, bladder, pelvis), pregnancy/fertility complications (spontaneous abortions, intrauterine growth restriction, fetal malpresentation), palpable **mass**

   a. Most common reason for hysterectomy

   b. Most asymptomatic: 45% women have fibroids by 5th decade

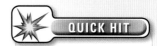

QUICK HIT

The transformation zone is the area most susceptible to HPV infection and neoplastic transformation.

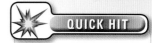

QUICK HIT

Fibroids are the most common reason for undergoing hysterectomy.

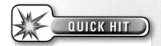

QUICK HIT

Distinguishing benign cervical lesions/masses from cervical cancer may require colposcopy, biopsy, and/or imaging (pelvic ultrasound, computed tomography [CT], magnetic resonance imaging [MRI]).

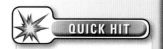

QUICK HIT

Cervical stenosis due to atrophy can prevent office endometrial biopsy during evaluation of postmenopausal bleeding and requires dilation in the operating room.

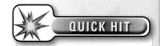

QUICK HIT

Large fibroids can be a source of hydronephrosis, urinary retention, and constipation. Fibroids can impair conception, implantation, fetal growth, and delivery but are the primary cause of infertility in <10% cases.

Reproductive Tract Benign Conditions

FIGURE 30.4 **Anatomy of the cervix.**

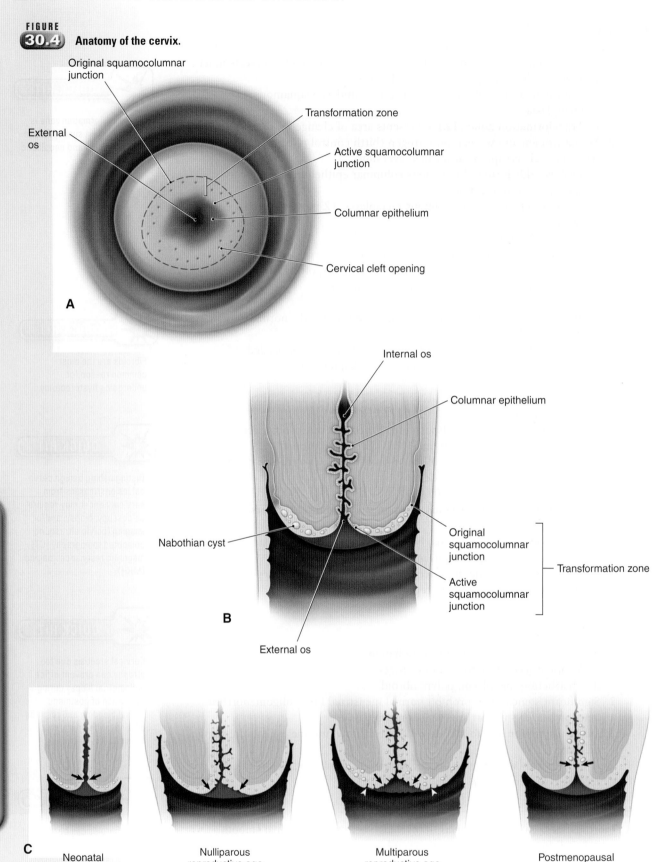

(A) The cervix and the transformation zone. (B) Anterior view of the cervix and exocervix. (C) Different locations of the transformation zone and the squamocolumnar junction during a woman's lifetime. (From Beckmann CRB, Ling FW, et al. *Obstetrics and Gynecology*, 7th ed. Baltimore: Lippincott Williams & Wilkins; 2014.)

2. Growth promoted by ovarian sex steroids (grow in pregnancy, stop growing postmenopause)
   a. Estrogen stimulates smooth muscle proliferation; progesterone interferes with apoptosis
   b. Sarcomas (malignancy) are rare <1/1,000 and probably are de novo neoplasms and not arising in benign fibroid
3. Risk factors
   a. Age, nulliparity, family history, race (African Americans 2–3 times higher than Caucasian women), obesity
   b. Oral contraceptive pills (OCPs), depot medroxyprogesterone acetate (DMPA), and smoking may decrease risk
4. Spherical, firm, white, well circumscribed (pseudocapsule)
5. Can outgrow blood supply and **degenerate** → hyalinization → cystic degeneration → calcification
   a. Fatty degeneration can occur but rare
   b. Carneous (red) degeneration occurs in 5%–10% pregnant women with fibroids = hemorrhage into fibroid
6. Locations
   a. **Intramural** (most common): alter shape and size of uterus
   b. **Subserosal**: project from uterine surface
   c. **Submucosal**: alter shape of endometrial cavity (heavy bleeding), pedunculated
   d. **Pedunculated**
      i. Subserosal: have stalk that attaches to uterus
      ii. Submucosal: have stalk that attaches to endometrium (Figure 30.5)
   e. Parasitic (attach to omental/mesenteric blood supply)
   f. Intraligamentous (in broad, round, or uterosacral ligaments)
   g. Intravenous (invade vena cava)
7. Diagnosis
   a. Fibroid uterus may be enlarged or irregularly shaped on exam
   b. Masses may be noted or further evaluated on imaging studies
      i. Transvaginal and abdominal ultrasound
      ii. Saline infusion sonohysterography: to evaluate endometrial cavity
      iii. Computed tomography (CT)
      iv. Magnetic resonance imaging (MRI)

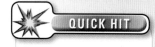

QUICK HIT

Degeneration of fibroids can be painful because it is a form of tissue infarction.

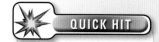

QUICK HIT

Pedunculated submucosal fibroids can prolapse through the cervix and "deliver"—*painfully!*

 FIGURE 30.5 **Common types of leiomyomata.**

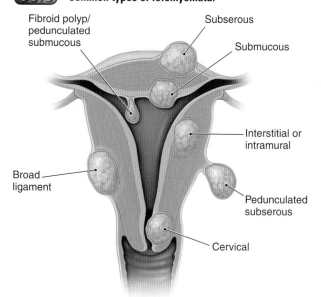

Fibroid polyp/pedunculated submucous

Subserous

Submucous

Interstitial or intramural

Broad ligament

Pedunculated subserous

Cervical

(From Beckmann CRB, Ling FW, et al. *Obstetrics and Gynecology*, 7th ed. Baltimore: Lippincott Williams & Wilkins; 2014.)

Reproductive Tract Benign Conditions

v. Hysterosalpingogram (HSG)

vi. Hysteroscopy

8. Differential diagnosis

   a. Uterine sarcoma

   b. Adenomyosis

   c. Endometrial polyp

   d. Ovarian mass/neoplasm

   e. Tubo-ovarian abscess (TOA)

   f. Bowel mass (diverticular disease, neoplasm)

   g. Pelvic kidney

9. Treatment: directed by patient symptoms; without symptoms, no therapy needed

   a. Medical management

     i. Hormonal management of heavy bleeding: hormonal contraceptives, oral/injected DMPA, levonorgestrel intrauterine device (IUD)

     ii. Gonadotropin-releasing hormone (GnRH) agonists: inhibit ovarian steroidogenesis

       (a) Significant vasomotor symptoms and adverse effect on bone mineral density (BMD)

       (b) Limited duration of use (6 months) and essentially 100% rebound to original size after discontinuation

       (c) Can be used to decrease fibroid size prior to surgery (i.e., 3-month course)

     iii. Mifepristone (RU 486): selective progesterone receptor antagonist (SPRM) may reduce fibroid volume without GnRH agonist side effects; use for this indication is experimental at this time

   b. Surgical management

     i. **Hysterectomy:** definitive therapy; abdominal, vaginal, laparoscopic, robotic modalities possible

     ii. **Myomectomy:** removal of fibroid(s), preservation of fertility (may/may not improve fertility)

       (a) Open, laparoscopic, robotic, hysteroscopic approach depends on size/location

       (b) >25% will need additional surgery for recurrent fibroids in future

     iii. **Endometrial ablation:** destruction of endometrial lining with heat, cold, radio frequency (see Chapter 36)

       (a) Decrease in uterine bleeding variable depending on fibroid size/location

       (b) Pregnancy after ablation not recommended

     iv. **Uterine artery embolization (UAE):** transcutaneous femoral placement of microspheres or coils into artery feeding fibroid → fibroid necrosis and shrinkage; pregnancy after UAE not recommended

     v. **MRI-focused ultrasound:** targeted ultrasound energy to create coagulative necrosis in fibroid; new modality

B. **Adenomyosis:** endometrial tissue grows into myometrial wall of uterus (see Chapters 33 and 34)

   1. Most often seen in multiparous women; heavy, painful menses and slightly enlarged and "**boggy**" uterus

   2. Can appear similar to uterine fibroids but lack pseudocapsule

C. **Endometrial polyps:** friable protrusions of endometrial tissue into cavity

   1. Irregular bleeding/postmenopausal bleeding

   2. Focal endometrial thickening on ultrasound

     a. Saline infusion sonography allows better visualization of endometrial cavity than simple transvaginal ultrasound

     b. Directly visualize with hysteroscopy

   3. Endometrial biopsy often misses polyps because polyps do not fit biopsy catheter opening

   4. *Hysteroscopy or D&C needed to remove*

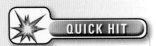

QUICK HIT

Fibroid growth is generally slow. Any rapidly enlarging pelvic mass needs careful follow-up and likely tissue diagnosis even if the patient is asymptomatic.

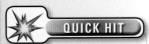

QUICK HIT

In patients on long-acting GnRH-agonist therapy, "add-back" therapy with norethindrone acetate can ameliorate the hot flashes and decrease the detrimental BMD effects, allowing a longer duration of use.

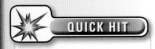

QUICK HIT

Intraoperative conversion to hysterectomy is always a risk in myomectomy cases. If the endometrial cavity is entered during myomectomy, the patient will need Cesarean delivery for any subsequent pregnancies.

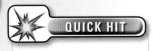

QUICK HIT

Diagnosis of adenomyosis can only be confirmed if a hysterectomy is performed.

QUICK HIT

Removal of endometrial polyps is indicated because of rare but possible endometrial hyperplasia, carcinoma, or carcinosarcoma.

D. **Endometrial hyperplasia**: abnormal proliferation of endometrium that can progress to endometrial carcinoma (see Chapter 49)
1. Risk factors: unopposed estrogen (in the absence of progesterone) drives endometrial proliferation and development of hyperplasia
   a. Chronic anovulation
   b. Polycystic ovarian syndrome (PCOS)
   c. Obesity
   d. Exogenous estrogen (estrogen-only hormone replacement therapy)
   e. Tamoxifen
   f. Granulosa-theca cell tumors
   g. Nulliparity
   h. Late menopause
   i. Diabetes mellitus
   j. Hypertension
2. Histologic types (Table 30.2)
   a. Simple and complex
   b. With and without cytologic atypia (complex atypical hyperplasia confers up to 30% malignant potential if untreated)
3. Intermenstrual or unexplained heavy/prolonged bleeding in women with risk factors, family history of colon/gynecologic cancer, or age >35 years should prompt **endometrial sampling**
   a. Sampling can be done with endometrial biopsy, D&C, or hysteroscopy with directed biopsy
   b. Ultrasound can be used to evaluate endometrial thickness but does not obviate need for a tissue diagnosis
   c. Women with postmenopausal bleeding need endometrial biopsy; endometrial stripe of <4 mm on ultrasound in postmenopausal woman is reassuring
   d. Women with Pap smears with atypical glandular cells need endometrial sampling
4. Treatment (endometrial hyperplasia *without* atypia)
   a. Medical
      i. Continuous progestins thin endometrial lining: inhibit/reverse hyperplasia
         (a) Oral (Provera, Megace, norethindrone)
         (b) Injectable (DMPA)
         (c) Levonorgestrel-releasing IUD
         (d) Repeat sampling to document normalization after 3–6 months of therapy
      ii. Cyclical progestins for 10–14 days each month: mimics ovulation and allows endometrium to completely slough each month
      iii. Combination OCPs can be used to treat simple hyperplasia that is due to anovulation: continuous opposition of estrogen by progestin leads to atrophy

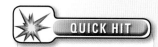

QUICK HIT

A long history of chronic anovulation should trigger endometrial biopsy prior to beginning hormonal therapy.

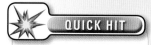

QUICK HIT

Women age <35 years who have abnormal uterine bleeding that does not respond to therapy (i.e., adequate OCP trial) should be considered for endometrial biopsy even if "low risk."

TABLE **30.2**	**Classification of Endometrial Hyperplasia and Progression to Endometrial Cancer**	
Architectural Type	**Cytologic Atypia**	**Progression to Endometrial Cancer**
Simple hyperplasia	Absent	1%
Complex hyperplasia	Absent	3%
Atypical simple hyperplasia	Present	8%
Atypical complex hyperplasia	Present	29%

(From Callahan T, Caughey AB. *Blueprints: Obstetrics & Gynecology*, 5th ed. Baltimore: Lippincott Williams & Wilkins; 2009.)

Reproductive Tract Benign Conditions

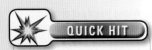

> **QUICK HIT**
>
> Endometrial ablation should not be performed in cases of hyperplasia or if the endometrium has not been sampled because these patients are still at risk for endometrial carcinoma.

b. Surgical

    i. D&C: may be used to obtain sample (in case of cervical stenosis), treat (simple hyperplasia), or more completely sample/evaluate cases of complex hyperplasia without atypia to exclude atypical hyperplasia or focus of carcinoma

5. Treatment (*atypical* hyperplasia)

    a. Surgical: hysterectomy is preferred treatment because of risk of progression to carcinoma or an undiagnosed coexisting carcinoma

    b. Medical: high-dose continuous progestins

        i. In patients who want to preserve reproductive capability

        ii. In patients who have severe medical comorbidities and are not good surgical candidates

        iii. Repeat sampling is imperative to document resolution

E. **Asherman syndrome**: intrauterine scarring in denuded endometrium (see Chapter 40)

    1. Irregular bleeding, amenorrhea, dysmenorrhea

    2. Can follow D&C, especially if infection present, endometrial ablation, or postpartum hemorrhage requiring D&C

    3. Treatment: hysteroscopy with resection of adhesions, estrogen

V. Fallopian Tubes and Ovaries (*see Chapter 50*)

A. **Hydrosalpinx/pyosalpinx**: infection/inflammation of fallopian tube, dilated, and filled with fluid or purulent material

    1. Often associated with pain and/or persistent cystic pelvic mass on ultrasound leading to surgical removal via laparoscopy or laparotomy

    2. If ovary also involved = TOA; active/acute TOA/infections require intravenous antibiotics prior to (or in place of) surgery

B. Tubal cysts: generally small incidental findings

    1. **Hydatid cysts of Morgagni** (paratubal cysts): can form near fimbriated ends of tube

    2. **Paraovarian cysts**: can form in mesosalpinx from vestigial remnants of Wolffian duct, tubal epithelium, and peritoneal inclusions

C. Ovarian cysts: 75% of ovarian masses are functional cysts; more common in reproductive-age women and smokers

    1. Generally asymptomatic; may be found incidentally on exam (palpable mass in thin patient) or pelvic imaging

    2. Can be source of pelvic/abdominal pain if hemorrhagic, ruptured, or torsed

    3. Can alter menstrual cycle length if associated with anovulation or progesterone production

        a. **Follicular cysts**: functional ovarian cysts form when maturing ovarian follicle does not rupture; 3–8-cm size (can be larger), "simple" unilocular (fluid-filled without internal septations)

        b. **Corpus luteum cysts**: functional ovarian cysts of enlarged/hemorrhagic corpus luteum that fails to regress after 14 days

            i. Menstruation can be delayed

            ii. Can be more firm that follicular cysts

            iii. When hemorrhagic (**corpus hemorrhagicum**), bleeding can be significant enough to cause hypovolemia, requiring surgery

        c. **Theca lutein cysts**: least common functional cysts; large (e.g., 30 cm) bilateral fluid-filled ovarian cysts

            i. Result from excessive β-human chorionic gonadotropin (β-hCG) levels (e.g., molar pregnancy, choriocarcinoma, ovulation induction, multiple gestations)

            ii. **Luteoma of pregnancy** (also called *hyperthecosis*): hyperplasic theca cells due to prolonged β-hCG exposure in pregnancy

                (a) Produces enlarged ovary that regresses postpartum

                (b) Can cause maternal virilization or ambiguous genitalia in female fetus

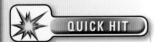

> **QUICK HIT**
>
> The ovaries should not be palpable in a postmenopausal woman.

d. **PCOS** (see Chapters 40 and 41)
    i. Endocrine disorder with chronic anovulation
    ii. Ovaries mildly enlarged with multiple small simple follicles throughout outer rim of ovarian cortex: "**ring of pearls**"
e. **Endometrioma:** "cyst" containing implants of endometriosis and blood generally associated with ovary, adnexa, and/or cul-de-sac; often associated with pain (see Chapter 33)

4. Differential
  a. Ectopic pregnancy
  b. Pelvic inflammatory disease/TOA
  c. Torsed adnexa
  d. Endometriosis
  e. Fibroids
  f. Ovarian neoplasm: benign or malignant
  g. Appendicitis
  h. Diverticular disease
  i. Other GI mass/process
  j. Dilations/stones/abnormalities of urinary tract (e.g., pelvic kidney)

5. Evaluation: pelvic ultrasound(s) to characterize and/or follow cyst
  a. Most functional cysts resolve in 60–90 days (2–3 menstrual cycles)
  b. **CA-125** can be drawn, depending on ovarian cancer risk factors, but is *never* screening test
  c. Pregnancy test will exclude ectopic from differential

6. Treatment (Table 30.3): depends on patient age, symptoms experienced, and cyst characteristics
  a. Expectant management with serial ultrasounds: appropriate for simple cysts without significant pain
    i. Reproductive-age women: cysts up to 8 cm (some say 10 cm) may be followed expectantly
    ii. Postmenopausal women: surgical removal more often recommended unless cyst very small
    iii. OCPs can suppress additional cyst formation in reproductive-age women
  b. Surgical evaluation/removal with laparoscopy/laparotomy: in postmenopausal women, persistent (>90 days), large or complex cysts (solid components, multiple septations), and cysts associated with ascites or significant bleeding
    i. Reproductive-age women: cystectomy
    ii. Postmenopausal women: oophorectomy

D. Benign ovarian tumors: slow-growing, generally asymptomatic unless ruptured, torsed, or endocrine-producing; rupture causes pain due to peritoneal irritation

1. Benign **germ cell** neoplasms
  a. Benign cystic teratoma (**dermoid**): most common benign ovarian tumor
    i. May contain various well-differentiated adult tissue types: most commonly, **ectodermal tissue** (sweat/sebaceous glands, hair follicles, teeth), brain, bronchus, thyroid, cartilage, intestine, bone

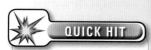

QUICK HIT

Ovarian masses are more likely to be benign than malignant in all age groups, but risk of malignancy increases with increasing age.

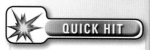

QUICK HIT

There are three categories of ovarian tumors: (1) Germ cell tumors arise from the actual germ cells (oocytes); (2) epithelial tumors originate from the surface (coelomic or mesothelial) lining the ovary; and (3) sex cord stromal tumors originate from the granulosa, theca, or mesenchymal cells of the ovarian cortex.

Reproductive Tract Benign Conditions

TABLE **30.3** **Management of Cystic Adnexal Mass**		
Age	**Size of Cyst**	**Management**
Premenarchal	>2 cm	Exploratory laparotomy
Reproductive	<6 cm	Observe for 8–12 weeks, then repeat ultrasound
	6–8 cm	Observe if unilocular; explore if multilocular or solid on ultrasound
	>8 cm	Exploratory laparoscopy/laparotomy for ovarian cystectomy
Postmenopausal	Palpable	Exploratory laparoscopy/laparotomy for ovarian oophorectomy

(From Callahan T, Caughey AB. *Blueprints: Obstetrics & Gynecology*, 5th ed. Baltimore: Lippincott Williams & Wilkins; 2009.)

ii. Mean age of occurrence = 30 years; 10%–15% bilateral, 15% will have torsion

iii. Frequently asymptomatic

iv. Treatment: surgical removal due to possibility of torsion and rupture

2. **Epithelial** ovarian neoplasms

a. Derived from mesothelial cells (line ovary and peritoneum)

b. Each epithelial type has benign, low malignant potential and frankly malignant varieties

   i. **Serous tumors: serous cystadenomas** most common

     (a) 70% benign, 5%–10% borderline, and 20%–25% malignant; 10% bilateral

     (b) May contain **psammoma bodies** (calcific concentric concretions)

   ii. **Mucinous tumors:** 85% benign, <10% bilateral

     (a) Can be large; associated with mucocele of appendix (perform appendectomy)

     (b) Rarely, pseudomyxoma peritonei develops with numerous benign implants throughout abdomen/pelvis producing large quantities of mucus

   iii. **Endometrioid** tumors: epithelial tumor with cells that resemble endometrium

   iv. **Brenner cell** tumors: uncommon solid epithelial tumors often with mucinous elements encased in cells resembling bladder transitional epithelium

   v. Clear **cell** tumors

3. **Sex cord-stromal** ovarian tumors (also called **gonadal stromal tumors**)

a. Functioning ovarian tumors: active endocrine-producing tumors of low malignant potential

   i. Most common after menopause

   ii. **Granulosa-theca cell** neoplasms

     (a) Produce estrogen, which manifests with **feminizing signs** (precocious puberty, irregular bleeding, postmenopausal bleeding, endometrial hyperplasia)

     (b) All granulosa tumors have potential for recurrence, even 20 years after removal

   iii. **Sertoli-Leydig cell** tumors: produce androgen, which manifest with **virilizing effects** (hirsutism, clitoromegaly, deepening of voice)

b. Fibroma: benign solid encapsulated tumor

   i. Can be associated with ascites and **Meigs syndrome** (ascites transversing lymphatics into pleural cavity and forming hydrothorax)

   ii. Combined with theca cells = **fibrothecoma**

4. Mixed ovarian neoplasms: contain multiple cell types

a. Cystoadenofibroma

b. Gonadoblastoma: seen in patients with dysgenic gonads (bilateral salpingo-oophorectomy indicated)

5. Evaluation: transvaginal ultrasonography, tumor markers

6. Management: surgical removal via laparoscopy/laparotomy due to risks of torsion, rupture, malignancy

a. Young women with unilateral benign neoplasms: cystectomy with preservation of normal ovarian tissue preferred

b. Postmenopausal women: bilateral salpingo-oophorectomy may be appropriate

E. **Adnexal torsion:** ovary/adnexa twists on its pedicle, obstructing normal blood flow

1. Acute severe pain can alternate with dull pain (intermittent torsion)

a. Obstructed venous flow increases pressure → edema and hemorrhage into mass

b. Obstructed arterial flow → necrosis

c. Ultrasound Doppler flow studies can detect lack of vascular flow

2. More likely when adnexa enlarged with mass/cyst

3. Untwist mass and remove cyst/pathology; necrotic ovary may have to be removed

---

Reproductive Tract Benign Conditions

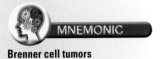

Brenner cell tumors
With **B**renner, think **b**ladder!

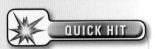

QUICK HIT

Because of the long-term (even after 20 years) recurrence risk of granulosa cell tumors, there is no such thing as a "benign" granulosa cell tumor.

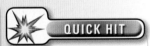

QUICK HIT

Because Meigs syndrome involves an ovarian mass, ascites, and even pleural effusion, the differential diagnosis will include any type of abdominal/pelvic malignancy.

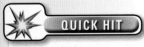

QUICK HIT

Ovaries are palpable on routine exam in only 50% of reproductive-age women. Women taking OCPs as well as premenarchal and postmenopausal women generally have ovaries too small to palpate.

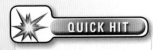

QUICK HIT

Adnexal torsion is a surgical emergency!

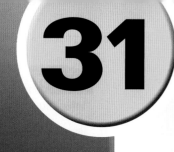
Vulvovaginitis and Sexually Transmitted Diseases

I. Vulvovaginal Ecosystem

A. Vulva: **keratinized**, stratified squamous epithelium
   1. Labia majora: hair follicles, sebaceous, sweat, and apocrine glands
   2. Labia minora: sebaceous, sweat, and apocrine glands

B. Vagina: **nonkeratinized**, stratified squamous epithelium
   1. Estrogen results in maturation of epithelial cells (occurs postpuberty)
   2. **Estrogen increases glycogen** levels, resulting in more lactobacilli growth
   3. Lactobacilli break down glycogen to lactic acid and production of hydrogen peroxide, which results in **normal vaginal pH of 3.5–4.7**
      a. Prepuberty: pH is 6–8 range
      b. Postmenopause: pH is 6–8 range
      c. Blood has pH of 7.34–7.45, so menses alters normal pH
      d. Semen has pH of 7.2–7.8, which favors anaerobe growth

C. Vaginal secretions
   1. Normal components
      a. Mucus from cervix
      b. Endometrial fluid
      c. Accessory gland exudates (Skene and Bartholin glands)
      d. Vaginal transudate (dependent on submucosal vascular supply)
      e. Microflora
         i. Lactobacilli
         ii. Aerobic bacteria
         iii. Anaerobic bacteria (5:1 anaerobic:aerobic)
      f. Exfoliated squamous cells (off-white color)
   2. Function: prevent dryness and irritation

II. Vulvovaginitis *(Table 31.1)*

A. Symptoms
   1. Itching
   2. Burning
   3. Irritation
   4. Abnormal discharge
   5. Abnormal odor

B. May be associated with reproductive consequences in pregnant and nonpregnant women

C. Differential diagnosis
   1. Bacterial vaginosis (BV) (22%–50% of symptomatic women)
   2. Vulvovaginal candidiasis (17%–39% of symptomatic women)
   3. *Trichomonas* infection (4%–35% of symptomatic women)
   4. Sexually transmitted infections (STIs)
      a. Gonorrhea
      b. Chlamydia
      c. Herpes simplex virus (HSV)
      d. Human papillomavirus (HPV)

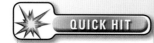

Because blood and semen increase the pH of the vagina, both of these can predispose women to an overgrowth of anaerobic bacteria (BV).

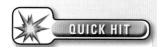

Leukorrhea is the term applied to heavier than normal, off-white discharge without any abnormality in pH or normal flora.

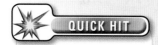

Asymptomatic women produce 1.5 g of vaginal fluid per day.

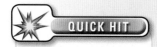

Vulvovaginitis is among the most common reasons for women to visit an ob/gyn.

TABLE 31.1 Common Vaginal Infections

Infection	Unique Symptoms	Diagnostic Criteria	Treatment
Bacterial vaginosis	Malodor Gray-white/yellow discharge	*3 of the following 4* 1. Clue cells 2. pH >4.5 3. Positive whiff test 4. Abnormal gray discharge	Metronidazole (oral or topical), clindamycin (oral or topical)
Vulvovaginal candidiasis	Itching Thick white discharge	Blastopores or pseudohyphae on wet mount OR Positive culture	Fluconazole (oral), synthetic imidazole (topical)
Trichomonas vulvovaginitis	Frothy discharge Dyspareunia/dysuria	Wet mount with *Trichomonas* and WBCs	Metronidazole (oral), tinidazole (oral)
Chlamydia	Irregular intermenstrual bleeding, discharge	NAATs most sensitive test	Doxycycline or azithromycin
Gonorrhea	Mucopurulent discharge	Culture, NAAT, or nucleic acid hybridization	Ceftriaxone or cefixime

NAAT, nucleic acid amplification test; WBC, white blood cell.

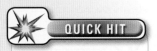

QUICK HIT

Chronic scratching causes lichen simplex chronicus, which results in hyperkeratosis, inflammation, and edema.

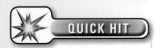

QUICK HIT

Among women with vaginitis, 70% remain undiagnosed.

    e. Syphilis
    f. Chancroid
    g. Granuloma inguinale
    h. Lymphogranuloma venereum
    i. Molluscum contagiosum
    j. Scabies
    k. Pubic lice
  5. Atrophic vaginitis (secondary to lack of estrogen)
  6. Dermatologic conditions
    a. Allergic
    b. Contact dermatitis
    c. Chemical dermatitis
  7. Chronic irritation (from scratching)
D. Evaluation (Table 31.2)
  1. Focused history
    a. Discharge characteristics
      i. Color
      ii. Consistency
      iii. Odor
    b. Symptoms and duration
      i. Itching
      ii. Irritation
      iii. Burning
      iv. Swelling
      v. Dyspareunia
      vi. Dysuria: when inflamed tissue is contacted by urine
    c. Associated urinary symptoms
      i. Dysuria
      ii. Frequency
      iii. Urgency
    d. Location of symptoms
    e. Relation to menstrual cycle
    f. Treatment history
    g. Self-treatment
      i. Douching
      ii. Over-the-counter preparations
      iii. Probiotics

TABLE 31.2 Diagnosis and Treatment of Physiologic Vaginal Secretions and Common Vaginal Infections

	Normal	Bacterial Vaginosis	Candidiasis	Trichomoniasis
Common symptoms	None	Discharge Odor that gets worse after intercourse; may be asymptomatic	Itching Burning Irritation Thick, white discharge	Frothy discharge Bad odor Dysuria Dyspareunia Vulvar itching and burning
Amount of discharge	Small	Often increased	Sometimes increased	Increased
Appearance of discharge	White Clear Flocculent	Thin, homogeneous Gray-green White Adherent	White Curdy "Cottage cheese–like"	Gray-green Frothy Adherent
Vaginal pH	3.8–4.2	>4.5	Normal	>4.5
KOH "whiff test" (amine odor)	Absent	Present (fishy)	Absent	Possibly present (fishy)
Microscopic appearance	Normal squamous epithelial cells Numerous lactobacilli	Increased white blood cells Decreased lactobacilli Many clue cells	Hyphae and buds	Normal epithelial cells Increased white blood cells Trichomonads
Treatment	N/A	Metronidazole (oral or topical) Clindamycin (oral or topical)	Topical synthetic imidazoles or oral fluconazole	Oral metronidazole or tinidazole

KOH, potassium hydroxide.

Vulvovaginitis and STDs

    h. Sexual history: predisposing factors
    i. Recent use of antiobiotics for another reason
    j. Diabetes
    k. Immunosuppression
    l. Douching
  2. Focused physical exam
    a. Visual inspection of external genitalia
    b. Speculum exam of vagina
  3. Laboratory tests
    a. Vaginal pH
    b. Amine (whiff) test: potassium hydroxide (KOH) releases fishy odor (amines) from anaerobic bacteria
    c. Wet mount (saline)
    d. KOH microscopy (lysis of cell membranes but not yeast hyphae)
    e. DNA amplification tests

III. Bacterial Vaginosis

  A. Etiology
    1. Lack of hydrogen peroxide producing lactobacilli
    2. Overgrowth of anaerobic organisms
  B. Signs and symptoms
    1. Fishy odor
    2. Thin, gray or white to yellow discharge
    3. 25% patients also have vulvar irritation
    4. Discharge is adherent to vaginal wall
  C. Laboratory tests
    1. pH >4.5
    2. Wet mount
      a. **Clue cells** (Figure 31.1): epithelial cells with numerous bacteria attached to surface
      b. Increased white blood cells (WBCs)

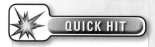

QUICK HIT

Because antibiotic therapy for something like a urinary tract infection (UTI) will also affect the normal vaginal microflora, women can be predisposed to developing an overgrowth of yeast.

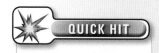

QUICK HIT

Bacteria that cause bacterial vaginosis are part of the normal vaginal flora.

FIGURE
31.1 Clue cell in a case of presumed bacterial vaginosis.

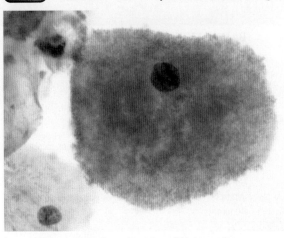

Innumerable coccobacilli cling to the surface of this intermediate squamous cell. (From Reichert R. *Diagnostic Gynecologic and Obstetric Pathology*. Baltimore: Lippincott Williams & Wilkins; 2011.)

    c. Loss of normal lactobacilli

    d. Bacteria clumps

  D. **Diagnostic criteria** (Amsel Criteria) (3 of following)

    1. Abnormal gray discharge

    2. **pH >4.5**

    3. Positive **"whiff" test**

    4. ≥20% of the epithelial cells are **clue cells**

  E. Treatment options

    1. **Metronidazole:** oral or topical

    2. **Clindamycin:** oral or topical

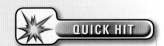

Candida albicans causes 90% of vulvovaginal candidiasis.

IV. Vulvovaginal Candidiasis

  A. Etiology

    1. Airborne fungi

    2. Yeast is commonly present in gastrointestinal (GI) tract

  B. Risk factors

    1. **Medical conditions**

      a. Pregnancy

      b. Diabetes

      c. Obesity

      d. Immunocompromised status

    2. **Medications**

      a. Corticosteroids

      b. Combination oral contraceptive agents (OCAs)

      c. Broad-spectrum antibiotics (kill normal microflora)

    3. **Environmental**

      a. Tight clothing or nonbreathing fabrics

      b. Persistent moisture

      c. Chronic use of panty liners

    4. **Cycle related:** vagina is most acidic after menses when in estrogen-only phase

  C. Signs and symptoms

    1. Vaginal/vulvar **itching**

    2. Vaginal/vulvar **burning**

    3. External dysuria

    4. Dyspareunia

    5. Erythema

      a. Can have intense erythema at introitus

      b. Vulva can be erythematous and even macerated

    6. Excoriations

    7. Odorless thick, white, and clumped discharge ("cottage cheese")

BOX 31.1

Classification of Vulvovaginal Candidiasis

Uncomplicated	Complicated
Sporadic or infrequent episodes	Recurrent episodes (4 or more per year)
Mild to moderate symptoms or findings	Severe symptoms or findings
Suspected *Candida albicans* infection	Suspected or proven non–*C. albicans* infection
Nonpregnant woman without medical complications	Women with diabetes, severe medical illness, immunosuppression, other vulvovaginal conditions
	Pregnancy

(Modified from Centers for Disease Control and Prevention. Sexually transmitted diseases treatment guidelines, 2002. *MMWR Recomm Rep.* 2002;51[RR-6]:1–78.)

D. Laboratory tests
1. **pH 4–5**
2. **Wet mount**
    a. Saline: hyphae visible
    b. KOH: hyphae resist KOH and are more easily seen
3. Culture
4. DNA amplification tests are specific and sensitive
E. Diagnostic criteria (1 of following)
1. Visualization of blastopores or pseudohyphae on wet mount or with KOH microscopy
2. Positive culture in a symptomatic woman
    a. Can then be classified as complicated or uncomplicated (Box 31.1)
    b. Latex agglutination test for non–*Candida albicans* strain (no pseudohyphae on wet prep)
3. Positive DNA amplification
F. Treatment options
1. **Topical synthetic imidazole** (cream or suppository)
2. **Oral fluconazole**
3. Recurrent infections
    a. Weekly therapy for 6 months effective in preventing recurrences
    b. Avoid early in pregnancy

V. *Trichomonas* Vulvovaginitis
A. **Flagellate protozoan** only in vagina, Skene ducts, male and female urethra
B. Transmitted via sexual contact or fomites
C. Associated with pelvic inflammatory disease (PID), endometritis, infertility, ectopic pregnancy, and preterm birth
D. Signs and symptoms
1. Vulvar itching/burning
2. Copious discharge with rancid odor
    a. Yellow-green color
    b. "**Frothy**" appearance
    c. **pH >4.5**
3. Dysuria
4. Dyspareunia
5. Petechia ("**strawberry**" patches) in upper vagina and cervix
E. Diagnosis
1. Wet mount
    a. **Motile *Trichomonas* organisms** (flagellated)
    b. WBCs
    c. Mature epithelial cells
2. DNA amplification test
3. Check for other sexually transmitted diseases (STDs) in women diagnosed with trichomoniasis

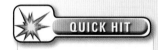

QUICK HIT

Trichomonas frequently coexists with bacterial vaginosis and other sexually transmitted infections (STIs) and facilitates HIV transmission.

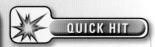

Trichomoniasis requires oral metronidazole therapy, whereas BV can be treated with either oral or topical metronidazole.

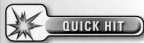

Test of cure means bringing the patient back after completion of therapy to exclude persistent or recurrent infection.

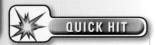

Patients should avoid alcohol when taking metronidazole to avoid a disulfiram-like reaction.

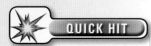

Postmenopausal women should always be asked about dyspareunia, because vaginal estrogen therapy will markedly alleviate symptoms.

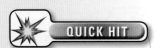

In postmenopausal women with symptoms of overactive bladder or frequent UTIs, local vaginal estrogen therapy can be very helpful.

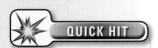

Systemic hormonal therapy is indicated only for vasomotor symptoms (hot flashes) that are affecting quality of life. Although systemic estrogen therapy effectively treats atrophic vaginitis, if that is the only indication for treatment, local vaginal therapy should be used.

F. Treatment
1. **Metronidazole** or tinidazole (oral)
2. Avoid unprotected intercourse
3. **Treat sexual partners**
4. Test of cure (TOC) in high-risk patients
5. **Treat during pregnancy**
   a. Pregnancy complications include premature rupture of membranes, preterm delivery, low birth weight
   b. Treatment may not prevent pregnancy complications

VI. Atrophic Vaginitis
A. Caused by lack of estrogen
1. Loss of cellular glycogen with resulting loss of lactic acid
2. **pH >4.7**
3. +/− Loss of elasticity resulting in narrowing and shortening of vagina
B. Risk factors
1. Postmenopausal women not on hormonal therapy
2. Surgical menopause not on hormonal therapy
3. Postpartum patients who are breastfeeding (very low estrogen state)
4. Hypoestrogenic states (hyperprolactinemia)
C. Signs and symptoms
1. Abnormal vaginal discharge
2. Dryness
3. Itching
4. Burning
5. Dyspareunia
6. Urinary symptoms
D. Treatment
1. Systemic estrogen therapy: oral, vaginal ring, transdermal patch, mist, lotion, gel or cream
2. Local vaginal estrogen therapy: suppository, cream, ring

VII. Desquamative Inflammatory Vaginitis
A. Peri- or postmenopausal women
B. Signs and symptoms
1. Purulent discharge
2. Exfoliation of epithelial cells with burning and erythema
3. Overgrowth of gram-positive cocci
4. pH >4.5
C. Treatment
1. Clindamycin cream applied daily
2. 14-day duration of treatment

VIII. Sexually Transmitted Diseases
A. General principles
1. Transmitted by oral, anal, or vaginal sex
2. STD assessment is a routine part of women's health care
3. 20%–50% have coexisting (multiple) infections; affected women should be tested for all infections
4. Complete physical assessment
   a. Inguinal region: evaluate for rashes, lesions, and adenopathy
   b. Vulva, perineum, and perianal region: evaluate for lesions, ulcerations, thickening, swelling
   c. Bartholin glands, Skene ducts, urethra
   d. Vagina and cervix: inspect for lesions and abnormal discharge
   e. Oral cavity and anal region: based on sexual history
5. Screening
   a. Indications
      i. Any patient who requests screening
      ii. High-risk sexual behavior

   iii. Sexually active patients age ≤25 years
      (a) Gonorrhea
      (b) Chlamydia
   iv. Pregnancy
      (a) Gonorrhea
      (b) Chlamydia
      (c) Syphilis
      (d) Hepatitis B and C
      (e) Human immunodeficiency virus (HIV)
   b. Screening tests
      i. Cervical: gonorrhea, chlamydia
      ii. Vaginal: *Trichomonas*
      iii. Serologies: HIV, hepatitis B and C, syphilis
6. Prevention
   a. Education
      i. Delay sexual activity
      ii. Limit number of partners
      iii. Condom use
      iv. Immunizations: HPV and hepatitis B
   b. Patient notification
      i. Evaluation of sexual partner
      ii. Expedited partner therapy: prescribing treatment for a patient's partner without evaluation (not permissible in all states)
   c. Reporting certain STDs to state health department (requirements vary by state)
B. *Chlamydia trachomatis*
   1. **Gram-negative obligate intracellular bacterium**
   2. Infects columnar epithelial cells (endocervix)
   3. If untreated, 40% will develop PID
   4. Responsible for nongonococcal urethritis and inclusion conjunctivitis
   5. Screen all sexually active women younger than age 25 years annually; screen those older than age 25 years based on risk factors
   6. Signs and symptoms
      a. **Asymptomatic** is most common
      b. **Mucopurulent cervicitis**, abnormal vaginal discharge, irregular intermenstrual bleeding, culture-negative urinary tract infection symptoms, post coital bleeding
      c. PID
   7. Diagnosis
      a. Culture: endocervical
      b. Enzyme immunoassay (EIA): endocervical
      c. Nucleic acid hybridization tests: endocervical
      d. Nucleic acid amplification tests (NAATs)
         i. Most sensitive
         ii. Endocervical or vaginal swab specimen
         iii. Urine screening is acceptable if no pelvic exam
   8. Treatment
      a. Antibiotics: **azithromycin or doxycycline**
      b. TOC
         i. For noncompliant patients or those who may have become reinfected
         ii. Retest 3–4 weeks posttreatment (antigen can remain present for several weeks)
      c. All women should be retested 3–12 months posttreatment
      d. Encourage abstaining from intercourse until patient and all partners have been treated
C. *Neisseria gonorrhoeae*
   1. **Gram-negative intracellular diplococcus**
   2. If untreated, can lead to PID

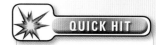

STDs are the most common cause of preventable infertility and have a strong association with ectopic pregnancy, pain, and strain on personal relationships.

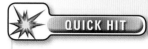

All women should be offered STD testing at every visit.

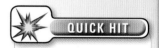

Many STDs can be asymptomatic and detectable only with comprehensive screening.

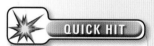

After HPV infection, chlamydia is the next most common STD.

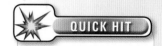

Asymptomatic and untreated chlamydial infection can lead to PID, ectopic pregnancy, chronic pelvic pain, and infertility.

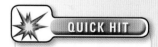

Because chlamydia and *Neisseria gonorrhoeae* infections frequently coexist, screening and/or treatment should always include both.

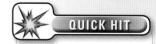

The highest rate of chlamydia and gonoccocal infections is in adolescents and young adults.

Vulvovaginitis and STDs

3. May facilitate HIV transmission
4. Infection can affect genital tract, pharynx, and rectum
5. Signs and symptoms
   a. May be asymptomatic
   b. Usually present 3–5 days postinfection
   c. Males
      i. Urethritis
      ii. Mucopurulent or purulent discharge
   d. Females
      i. Purulent discharge from urethra, Skene duct, cervix, vagina, or anus
      ii. Cervicitis
      iii. May coexist with Bartholin glands infection
      iv. Anal intercourse is not prerequisite to anal infection
6. Diagnosis
   a. Test endocervical, vaginal, or urine specimen
   b. Test by culture, NAAT, or nucleic hybridization
7. Treatment
   a. **Ceftriaxone or cefixime**
   b. Recent emergence of quinolone-resistant strains
   c. If chlamydia is not ruled out, treat for chlamydia as well

D. PID
1. Infection of upper genital tract after initial infection of cervix caused by spread along mucosal surfaces
2. Predominant organisms
   a. Chlamydia
   b. Gonorrhea
   c. Other organisms including staphylococci, streptococci, *Escherichia coli*, and anaerobes
3. Timing of infection relative to menstrual cycle is important: symptoms more likely to present right after cessation of bleeding
   a. Progesterone-dominant part of cycle has endocervical mucus that resists spread
   b. Oral contraceptives mimic progesterone-dominant part of cycle and therefore reduce risk for PID
4. Risk factors
   a. Prior PID
   b. 1st month after insertion of IUD
   c. Adolescence
   d. Multiple sexual partners
   e. Infection with any causative organisms
5. Signs and symptoms: nonspecific
   a. Cervical discharge
   b. Cervical motion tenderness
   c. Abdominal/adnexal/pelvic pain
   d. Fever
   e. Elevated WBCs
   f. Perihepatitis (**Fitz-Hugh-Curtis syndrome**)
      i. Inflammation leading to localized fibrosis and scarring of anterior liver to peritoneum
      ii. More often caused by chlamydial infection
   g. Tubo-ovarian abscesses (TOA)
      i. Acutely ill patients
      ii. Fevers, tachycardia, vomiting, severe pelvic and abdominal pain
6. Diagnosis of PID: clinical criteria
   a. *All of following are needed*
      i. Abdominal tenderness with/without rebound
      ii. Adnexal tenderness
      iii. Cervical motion tenderness

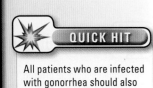

QUICK HIT

All patients who are infected with gonorrhea should also be tested for other STDs.

b. *1 or more of following is needed*
   i. Gram stain of endocervix positive for gram-negative intracellular dipococcic
   ii. Temperature ≥38°C
   iii. WBC >10,000
   iv. Pus on culdocentesis or laparoscopy
   v. Pelvic abscess on bimanual exam or sonogram
7. Treatment
   a. Hospitalization criteria
      i. Unable to exclude surgical emergency
      ii. Pregnancy
      iii. No response to oral antibiotics
      iv. Unable to tolerate oral intake
      v. TOA is present
      vi. Patient with severe illness
   b. Oral antibiotics unless hospitalized for intravenous (IV) antibiotic treatment
   c. TOA
      i. IV antibiotics
      ii. May require surgery or drainage by interventional radiology
      iii. If ruptured, mortality can approach 10% (*surgical emergency*)
   d. All women diagnosed with PID should be screened for other STDs

E. **Genital herpes**
   1. Caused by HSV: DNA virus
      a. HSV-1: more common with cold sores; can also be genital
      b. HSV-2: more common with genital lesions; can also be oral
         i. More likely to cause recurrence
         ii. Consider suppressive therapy
   2. Signs and symptoms
      a. 1st episode is most severe
         i. Flu-like syndrome
         ii. Neurologic involvement (2–3 days postinfection)
         iii. Resolution within 7–10 days
      b. Lesions are painful, vesicular, and ulcerated
      c. Location: vulva, vagina, cervix, perineum, perianal skin
      d. Urethral lesions or neurologic sequelae may lead to urinary retention
      e. Aseptic meningitis may occur 5–7 days postinfection
      f. Recurrent infections triggered by unknown stimuli
         i. Milder than primary infection
         ii. Persist for 2–5 days
      g. Most are asymptomatic
      h. Viral shedding can occur for up to 3 weeks after lesions appear
   3. Diagnosis
      a. Viral culture: very specific, but poor specificity
      b. Polymerase chain reaction (PCR)
      c. Detection of type-specific antibodies (HSV-1, HSV-2)
         i. Useful in patients with recurrent infections or atypical symptoms with HSV-negative culture; partner with herpes; clinical diagnosis without laboratory diagnosis
         ii. Can be false negative in first 3 weeks to 3 months after infection
   4. Treatment
      a. Antiviral drugs
         i. Decrease duration of viral shedding
         ii. Shorten symptomatic disease course if started immediately with onset of symptoms
         iii. Acyclovir, famciclovir, or valacyclovir
      b. Supportive therapy
         i. Keep lesion clean and dry
         ii. Analgesia
         iii. Foley catheter if urinary retention or severe dysuria

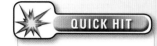

QUICK HIT

Treat all sexually active young women for PID without other cause of symptoms who present with uterine tenderness, adnexal tenderness, or cervical motion tenderness.

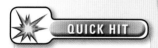

QUICK HIT

As many as 75% of primary herpes infections are unrecognized.

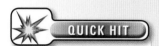

QUICK HIT

HSV migrates via nerve fibers and remains dormant in the dorsal root ganglia.

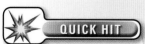

QUICK HIT

Antiviral treatment does not decrease likelihood of recurrence or long-term sequelae.

Vulvovaginitis and STDs

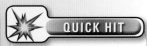

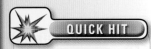

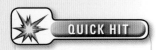

c. Episodic therapy for recurrent outbreaks
   i. Most effective when initiated at prodrome
   ii. Decreases duration of episode
   iii. For patients with infrequent symptomatic recurrences
d. Suppressive therapy
   i. Most effective for patients with frequent occurrences
   ii. For women with HSV-2 whose partner does not have HSV-2 (50% reduction in transmission)

F. **HPV**
1. Transmission
   a. Via contact with infected genital skin, mucous membranes, or body fluids from a person with HPV
   b. Most infections are transient, but persistence increases with age
   c. Sequelae may take years to develop in persistent infections
2. Multiple serotypes exist
   a. Low risk are commonly associated with genital condyloma (types 6, 11)
   b. High risk are generally associated with cervical dysplasia and cancer (types 16, 18)
3. Manifestations: most individuals are asymptomatic
4. Prevention
   a. Condoms helpful but not protective
   b. Vaccination approved for men and women ages 9–26 years
      i. Quadrivalent vaccine (types 6, 11, 16, 18)
      ii. Bivalent vaccine (types 16, 18)

G. **Condyloma accuminata** (genital or venereal warts)
1. Soft flesh growths that may arise on vulva, vagina, cervix, urethral meatus, perineum, anus, or oral cavity
2. Signs and symptoms
   a. Single or multiple lesions with few symptoms
   b. Spread by direct contact
   c. Common to have symmetric lesions across midline
3. Diagnosis
   a. Physical exam
   b. Confirmed by biopsy
4. Treatment
   a. Chemical treatment
   b. Cautery (electrical, cryo, laser ablation)
   c. Topical immunologic treatment (imiquimod cream)

H. Cervical dysplasia (cervical intraepithelial neoplasia [CIN]): see Chapter 48
I. Cervical cancer: see Chapter 48
J. **Syphilis**
1. *Treponema pallidum* (spirochete) is causative organism
2. Most common sites of entry are vulva, vagina, and cervix
3. Congenital syphilis may result from transplacental spread
4. Signs and symptoms
   a. Primary syphilis
      i. Chancre at site of entry 10–60 days postinfection
      ii. Chancre is firm with punched-out appearance and firm edges
      iii. Painless lesion
      iv. Chancre spontaneously heals in 3–6 weeks
      v. Negative serology testing at this stage
   b. Secondary syphilis
      i. 4–8 weeks after primary chancre
      ii. Skin rash on palms and soles that is red or brown and rough
      iii. Lymphadenopathy, fever, muscle aches, headache, weight loss, fatigue, and patchy hair loss
      iv. Condyloma lata: flat-topped papules that coalesce in moist areas
      v. Mucocutaneous patches: highly infective
      vi. Without treatment, this stage spontaneously resolves in 2–6 weeks

   c. Latent syphilis
      i. Early latent: infected within 1 year
         (a) Asymptomatic
         (b) Positive serology
      ii. Late latent – greater than 1 year or unknown duration
   d. Tertiary syphilis
      i. Transmission at this stage is only transplacental or via blood transfusion
      ii. Central nervous system, cardiovascular, ophthalmic, and auditory abnormalities
      iii. Gummas
         (a) Destructive, necrotic granulomatous lesions
         (b) 1–10 years after infection
5. Diagnosis
   a. Motile spirochetes on dark field microscopy
   b. Direct fluorescent antibody test from primary or secondary lesions or lymph nodes
   c. Presumptive diagnosis with nontreponemal tests
      i. Venereal Disease Research Laboratory (VDRL) test
      ii. Rapid plasma reagin
      iii. Automated reagin test
      iv. May be false positive in women with medical conditions unrelated to syphilis, e.g. systemic lupus erythematosis (SLE)
      v. *Many institutions now screen using syphilis IgG antibodies*
   d. Treponemal confirmatory test
      i. Fluorescent treponemal antibody-absorption (FTA-ABS) test
      ii. Microhemagglutination assay for *T. pallidum* antibodies (MHA-TP)
      iii. Will usually be positive for life regardless of treatment
   e. In cases of neurosyphilis, a VDRL is performed on spinal fluid
6. Treatment
   a. Intramuscular (IM) benzathine penicillin G (long-acting penicillin)
      i. Single treatment if <1-year duration
      ii. Weekly treatment for 3 weeks if late latent or unknown duration
   b. Followed by VDRL titers and exams at 3, 6, and 12 months
   c. Abstain from intercourse until lesions healed
   d. Tertiary requires IV therapy

K. **HIV and AIDS**
1. AIDS is advanced manifestation of HIV infection
2. HIV is caused by RNA retrovirus
   a. Targets helper T cells (CD4) and monocytes
   b. Depletion of CD4 cells is manifestation of infection
3. Two types of HIV
   a. HIV-1: most common in United States
   b. HIV-2: most common in West African countries
4. Virus is contacted by
   a. Intimate sexual contact
   b. Use of contaminated needles or blood products
   c. Perinatal transmission (mother to child)
5. Diagnosis
   a. Screening test is enzyme-linked immunosorbent assay (ELISA): test for HIV antibodies
   b. Confirmatory test: Western blot
6. Treatment
   a. Prevention
      i. Condoms
      ii. Safe sex practices
   b. Multiple drug therapies: highly active antiviral therapy (HAART)
      i. Nucleoside reverse transcriptase inhibitors (NRTIs)
      ii. Nonnucleoside reverse transcriptase inhibitors (NNRTIs)
      iii. Protease inhibitors

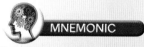

MNEMONIC

Treponemal confirmatory test
FTA-ABS = **ABS**olutely sure!

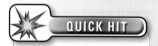

QUICK HIT

Confirmatory tests are not useful in cerebrospinal fluid because the antibodies do not cross the blood–brain barrier.

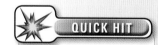

QUICK HIT

AIDS is one of the top five causes of death in reproductive-age women.

     c. Monotherapy is discouraged because of development of drug resistance

     d. Pregnancy

       i. Combination therapy

       ii. Zidovudine (AZT) in labor

       iii. Cesarean section in some situations

L. Less common STDs

  1. **Granuloma inguinale**

    a. Caused by sexual transmission of *Klebsiella granulomatis*

    b. Genital **ulcers**

      i. Vascular

      ii. Bleed on contact

    c. Diagnosis

      i. Clinical

      ii. Special stains or biopsy revealing Donovan bodies

      iii. Pseudo-buboes: granulomatous lesions just below skin (not true lymph nodes)

  2. **Lymphogranuloma venereum**

    a. Caused by *C. trachomatis* serotypes L1, L2, and L3

    b. Systemic infection

    c. If untreated, can cause **fistulas and abscess**

    d. Signs and symptoms

      i. If transmitted via vaginal intercourse

        (a) Genital **ulcers**

        (b) Inguinal and femoral **lymphadenopathy** (buboes)

      ii. If transmitted via anal intercourse

        (a) Genital ulcers

        (b) Anal bleeding, purulent anal discharge, constipation, and anal spasms

  3. **Chancroid**

    a. Painful genital **ulcer**

    b. Discrete outbreaks

    c. Cofactor for HIV transmission

    d. Caused by *Haemophilus ducreyi*

    e. Diagnosis is by PCR

  4. **Molluscum contagiosum**

    a. Highly contagious **pox virus** skin infection

    b. Can be transmitted via sexual contact

    c. Small, **painless raised papules**

      i. Genital region, inner thighs, buttocks

      ii. Central depression (**umbilication**)

    d. Resolve spontaneously in 6 months to 1 year

    e. Can be treated with topical agents or destruction techniques

  5. **Pubic lice** (*Pediculosis pubis*) "Crabs"

    a. Usually transmitted by sexual contact, bedding, or clothing

    b. Itching in pubic area soon after infection

    c. Lice or **nits detected on pubic hair**

    d. Treatment is with topical preparations

  6. **Scabies - Mites**

    a. Usually transmitted by sexual contact, bedding, or clothing

    b. Intense itching in pubic area – delayed after infection (secondary to antibody response)

    c. **Burrows** seen between fingers

    d. Treatment is with topical preparations

MNEMONIC

Remember: chancroid caused by *Haemophilus ducreyi* is a painful genital ulcer in comparison to the primary syphilis chancre (ulcer). You **do cry** with *H. ducreyi*!

Pelvic Support Defects, Urinary Incontinence, and Urinary Tract Infection

I. Pelvic Support Defects

A. Etiology

1. Damage to or weakening of normal pelvic support structures including muscle, fascia, or ligaments (**pelvic relaxation**)
2. Pelvic organ prolapse: occurs when loss of support allows descent through urogenital hiatus
   a. Uterus
   b. Paravaginal tissue
   c. Bladder wall
   d. Urethrovesical angle
   e. Distal rectum

B. Epidemiology

1. Race
   a. Rates are highest for Caucasian women
   b. Lower rates of prolapse seen in African Americans and Asians
2. Risk factors
   a. Birth trauma
      i. Prolonged labor
      ii. Large infants (macrosomia)
      iii. Operative delivery
   b. Chronic increases in intra-abdominal pressure
      i. Obesity
      ii. Chronic pulmonary disease (COPD, emphysema, cystic fibrosis)
      iii. Repetitive heavy lifting
      iv. Straining with constipation
      v. Ascites
      vi. Large pelvic tumors
   c. Tissue atrophy
      i. Aging
      ii. Menopause (hypoestrogenic state)
   d. Intrinsic tissue weakness (i.e., genetic)
   e. Prior pelvic surgery (e.g., hysterectomy)
   f. Smoking

C. Anatomy

1. Support provided by network of tissues
   a. Muscles (**levator ani**)
      i. Puborectalis
      ii. Pubococcygeus
      iii. Iliococcygeus
   b. Fascia
      i. Urogenital diaphragm
      ii. Endopelvic fascia

QUICK HIT

Visualize the anterior vaginal wall as a hammock. When the hammock is pulled tight, there is good support; when the hammock is slack, there is poor support.

QUICK HIT

Multiple organ involvement is common.

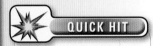

QUICK HIT

Most women who have pelvic support defects on physical exam (PE) are not symptomatic, and PE findings are not well correlated with specific pelvic relaxation symptoms.

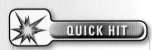

QUICK HIT

Pelvic support defects can have both medical and social implications.

    c. Ligaments
        i. Uterosacral ligaments
        ii. Cardinal ligaments (broad ligament)
  2. Pelvic compartments (characterize type of prolapse)
    a. Anterior
        i. Loss of support to urethra (**urethrocele**)
        ii. Descent of anterior vaginal wall in midline (**cystocele**)
        iii. Descent of anterior vaginal wall laterally (**paravaginal** defect)
    b. Posterior
        i. Loss of lateral support allowing rectum to bulge upward (**rectocele**)
        ii. Endopelvic fascia weakness of rectovaginal septum, allowing small bowel to create vaginal bulge (**enterocele**)
    c. Apical
        i. Compromise to cardinal ligaments and other supporting structures resulting in varying degrees of uterine prolapse
        ii. **Vaginal vault prolapse** occurs when vaginal tissues descend following hysterectomy
        iii. When cervix is beyond vaginal outlet, it is commonly referred to as **procidentia**

D. Clinical presentation
  1. History
    a. Symptoms vary with degree of prolapse and affected compartment; *patients are often asymptomatic*
    b. Physical complaints
        i. Pelvic pressure
        ii. Backache
        iii. Dyspareunia
        iv. Discomfort with walking or sitting
        v. Bleeding secondary to tissue ulceration
    c. Urinary symptoms
        i. Incontinence
        ii. Frequency
        iii. Hesitancy or using abdominal muscles to void
        iv. Incomplete emptying
        v. Recurrent urinary tract infections (UTIs)
    d. Bowel symptoms
        i. Constipation
        ii. Incomplete evacuation
        iii. Pain with defecation (dyschezia)
        iv. Incontinence (even just fecal soiling)
        v. Splinting (applying vaginal or perineal pressure with fingers to effect evacuation)
    e. Rare complications
        i. Ureteral obstruction
        ii. Bowel incarceration
        iii. Evisceration
  2. Physical exam
    a. Site-specific evaluation to identify the locations of prolapse within the pelvis and their severity
    b. Pelvic organ prolapse quantification (POP-Q) exam
        i. Standardized exam to assess support in each of the 3 anatomic compartments with straining
        ii. Provides a staging system based on the leading edge of prolapse (Figure 32.1)
  3. Differential diagnosis
    a. Anterior
        i. **Urethral diverticulum**
        ii. **Gartner duct** cyst (lateral vaginal wall)
        iii. **Skene gland** abscess (periurethral)

FIGURE 32.1 Schematic of the quantified pelvic organ prolapse (POP-Q) system.

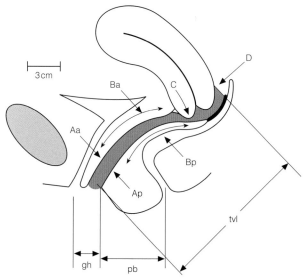

Six sites (*points Aa, Ba, C, D, Bp, Ap*), genital hiatus (*gh*), perineal body (*pb*), and total vaginal length are used to quantify the degree of pelvic organ prolapse. The vagina and hymenal ring are shown in *blue*. (From Callahan T, Caughey AB. *Blueprints: Obstetrics & Gynecology*, 5th ed. Baltimore: Lippincott Williams & Wilkins; 2009.)

b. Posterior
   i. **Bartholin gland** abscess
   ii. Obstructive lesions of the colon including lipoma, fibroma, and sarcoma
c. Apical
   i. Elongated cervix
   ii. Cervical polyp
   iii. Prolapsed fibroid
   iv. Neoplasms of cervix or endometrium
E. Treatment
   1. Nonsurgical
      a. Correction of associated problems such as chronic pulmonary dysfunction or constipation
      b. Weight loss
      c. **Kegel exercises**: physical therapy to strengthen the muscles of the pelvic floor
      d. Topical hormone treatment may improve estrogen-sensitive tissue quality and underlying vascularity
      e. **Pessary** (Figure 32.2)
         i. Mechanical silicone devices placed vaginally to compensate for loss of pelvic support
         ii. Useful for pregnant/postpartum women and those medically unfit for or unwilling to pursue elective surgery
         iii. Types (patients are individually fitted for size and type)
            (a) Supportive (e.g., ring)
            (b) Space-occupying (Gellhorn, donut)
         iv. Long-term use acceptable but should be monitored with routine removal and cleaning (every 6–12 weeks)
         v. Postmenopausal women may use vaginal estrogen to minimize complications
         vi. Complications
            (a) Vaginal erosions
            (b) Bleeding
            (c) Infection
            (d) Fistula formation

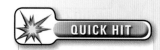

QUICK HIT

All patients should be offered conservative treatment options before proceeding to surgery.

FIGURE 32.2 Placement of a vaginal pessary to treat pelvic organ prolapse.

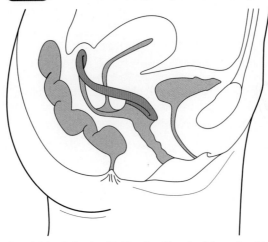

(From Callahan T, Caughey AB. *Blueprints: Obstetrics & Gynecology*, 5th ed. Baltimore: Lippincott Williams & Wilkins; 2009.)

2. Surgical
   a. Primary goal is to alleviate functional problems and restore anatomic support whenever possible
   b. Anterior prolapse
      i. **Anterior colporrhaphy** (anterior repair): plication of anterior endopelvic fascia in the midline
      ii. **Paravaginal repair:** reattachment of lateral vaginal sidewalls to the arcus tindineus fascia pelvis (white line)
   c. Posterior prolapse
      i. **Posterior colporrhaphy:** plication of the rectal fascia in the midline or at site-specific locations
      ii. Attachment of graft to repair fascial defect
   d. Uterine prolapse
      i. Hysterectomy may be performed abdominally, vaginally, or laparoscopically
      ii. After hysterectomy, vaginal cuff is suspended/attached (see below)
   e. Apical prolapse: approach is often dictated by severity of the prolapse; skill of the surgeon; and patient characteristics including age, weight, lifestyle, and surgical history
      i. **Uterosacral ligament** suspension
         (a) Suspension of vaginal cuff to bilateral uterosacral ligaments. Can be approached either vaginally or abdominally
         (b) Rate of ureteral obstruction as high as 11%
      ii. **Sacrospinous ligament** suspension
         (a) Suspension of vaginal cuff to sacrospinous ligament running from sacrum to ischial spine; typically unilateral on patient's right side
         (b) Performed vaginally
         (c) Risk of pudendal artery or sciatic nerve injury
      iii. **Sacral colpopexy**
         (a) Suspension of vaginal cuff to anterior longitudinal ligament overlying sacral promontory using mesh secured to anterior and posterior vaginal walls
         (b) Acute risks include bowel or iliac vessel injury, hemorrhage from middle sacral vessels, or small-bowel obstruction associated with mesh in immediate post-op period
         (c) Risk of mesh exposure/erosion ~3%–4%, typically presenting as vaginal spotting, discharge, odor, or dyspareunia
      iv. **Colpocleisis**
         (a) Obliteration of vaginal cavity using permanent suture placed in concentric purse-string fashion to reduce prolapse and close vaginal cavity

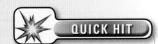

QUICK HIT

It is not uncommon to have multiple defects; when a patient has both a rectocele and a cystocele, the surgical procedure is referred to as an "A & P repair."

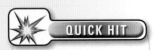

QUICK HIT

Surgical repair of prolapse can occasionally result in urinary incontinence in a patient who did not demonstrate any before.

(b) Advantage: Vaginal approach allows for reduction in complications and shorter operative time for medically complicated patients

(c) Disadvantage: Patients are no longer able to have vaginal intercourse

v. **Enterocele repair**

(a) Prolapse due to weakness in vaginal walls, which typically allows for prolapse of small bowel into "hernia sack" of peritoneum

(b) Repair can be accomplished either vaginally or abdominally and involves isolation and ligation of sack with reinforcement of surrounding tissue to prevent recurrence

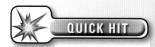

It is often difficult to differentiate between a high rectocele and an enterocele, and only surgery can make a definitive diagnosis.

II. Urinary Incontinence

A. Definition

1. Involuntary loss of urine for any reason, which can be clinically demonstrated and is socially or functionally problematic

2. Types of incontinence

   a. **Stress**

   b. **Urge** (detrusor overactivity, overactive bladder, detrusor dysynergia, spastic bladder)

   c. **Mixed** (a + b above)

   d. **Overflow**

B. **Stress urinary incontinence:** loss of urine associated with increases in intra-abdominal pressure (coughing, sneezing, laughing) in absence of detrusor contraction

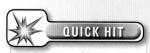

Most women experience some urinary incontinence in their lifetime.

1. Etiology

   a. Most often due to compromise in anterior vaginal wall and endopelvic fascia, which supports bladder neck and urethra

      i. Increased intra-abdominal pressure is transmitted unevenly to bladder and urethra

      ii. Results in elevated pressures within bladder relative to urethra and subsequent urine loss

   b. **Intrinsic sphincter deficiency (ISD):** urethral sphincter mechanism weakness causing incontinence even when pressures are equally distributed between bladder and urethra

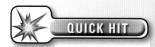

ISD can be visualized as the urethra being a rigid pipe allowing urine to leak with any pressure.

2. Risk factors

   a. Factors that affect pelvic support to bladder neck

      i. Vaginal childbirth

      ii. Aging

      iii. Genetic weakness intrinsic to tissue

   b. Factors that result in chronic increases in intra-abdominal pressure

      i. Chronic coughing (COPD, pulmonary disease)

      ii. Obesity

      iii. Work-related chronic lifting

      iv. Constipation

   c. Factors that cause sphincter weakness

      i. Prior surgery or scarring

      ii. Neurologic denervation (stroke, trauma, surgical injury, diabetes, Multiple Sclerosis)

      iii. Poor tissue coaptation (e.g., related to hypoestrogenic state)

3. Evaluation

   a. History (Table 32.1)

      i. Characterization of situations in which leaking occurs

         (a) Frequency and volume of leaking

         (b) Awareness of leaking events

         (c) Use of absorbent products

         (d) Duration and severity of problem over time

         (e) Any previous interventions

      ii. Voiding diary

Pelvic Support Defects

TABLE **32.1** **Genuine Stress Incontinence Versus Detrusor Instability Symptom Comparison**

Symptom	Genuine Stress Incontinence	Detrusor Instability
Precipitating factor	Cough, lift, exercise position change	Preceding unexpected position change
Timing of leakage	Immediate	Delayed
Amount of leakage	Small → large	Large
Voluntary inhibition	Frequently	Possibly
Urgency, frequency	Occasionally	Yes
Nocturia	Rarely	Yes
Spontaneous remissions	No	Occasionally

From *Glass' Office Gynecology*, 6th edition. Baltimore: Lippincott Williams & Wilkins, 2005.

b. Physical exam
  i. Evaluation of pelvic support to all compartments using POP-Q
  ii. Basic neurologic exam
    (a) Assess sensory perception: soft versus sharp touch
    (b) Presence of normal bulbocavernosus and anal wink reflexes
  iii. Gross assessment
    (a) Estrogen status of tissue
    (b) Presence of tenderness
    (c) Scarring or rigidity of anterior vaginal wall or urethra secondary to prior surgery
  iv. Q-tip test: placement of lubricated cotton swab in urethra at level of urethrovesical junction
    (a) With patient straining (causing descent at bladder neck) in lithotomy position, position of swab is measured from horizontal
    (b) Angle of >30° from horizontal indicates compromise of normal support and "hypermobility" to bladder neck, typically associated with stress incontinence (Figure 32.3A,B)
c. Laboratory testing
  i. Urinalysis
  ii. Urine culture to rule out infection
d. Urodynamic testing
  i. Voiding volume and post-void residual to assess emptying function
  ii. Voiding diary: record of voiding frequency, volumes, incontinence episodes, and fluid intake (volume and type) can help characterize incontinence and identify maladaptive behaviors (e.g., frequent small voids or excessive caffeine intake)
  iii. Office stress test
    (a) Bladder is filled using a catheter up to 300 mL, and patient is asked to cough once
    (b) Leakage simultaneous with cough is consistent with stress incontinence
    (c) Can be done in supine or standing position (Figure 32.4)
  iv. Multichannel urodynamics
    (a) Catheter transducers to measure pressure are placed in bladder and vagina or rectum to measure intravesicular and intra-abdominal pressure respectively
    (b) Bladder is filled through catheter, and patient reports
      (i) First sensation of filling (50–150 mL)
      (ii) First urge to void (200–300 mL)
      (iii) Strong urge to void (300–500 mL)
      (iv) Capacity (500–600 mL)

FIGURE
32.3 Cotton Swab Test.

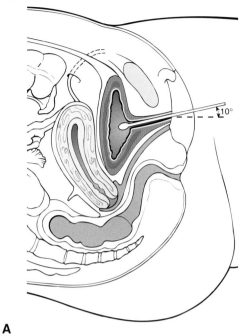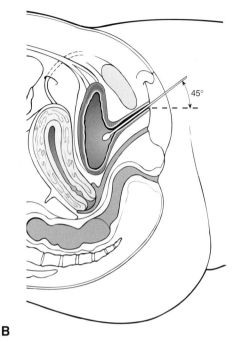

A   **B**

(A) During the cotton swab test, a swab is placed in the urethra to the bladder neck. Normal movement of the urethrovesical junction (UVJ) with Valsalva (straining) should be less than 30°. **(B)** When pelvic relaxation results in hypermobility of the bladder neck, there is a large change (30°–60°) of the UVJ with Valsalva (straining). (From Callahan T, Caughey AB. *Blueprints: Obstetrics & Gynecology*, 5th ed. Baltimore: Lippincott Williams & Wilkins; 2009.)

    (c) Stress testing with cough or Valsalva used to identify leaking from urethra at specific levels of pressure

    (d) Strength of urethral sphincter can be assessed by pulling catheter transducer across sphincter muscle (i.e., maximal urethral closure pressure)

    (e) Patient voids with catheters present, providing information on bladder contractility, abdominal straining with voiding, and emptying function

FIGURE
32.4 "Poor man's cystometrogram" for office evaluation of bladder filling function.

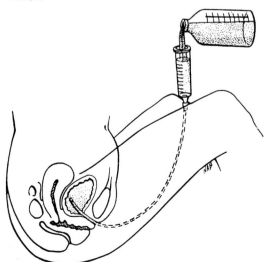

With the patient in sitting or standing position with a catheter in the bladder, the bladder is filled by gravity by pouring sterile water into the syringe (no more than 100 mL/min). A rise in the fluid level associated with urgency or leakage is suggestive of detrusor instability. (Used with permission from *Glass' Office Gynecology*, 6th edition. Baltimore: Lippincott Williams & Wilkins, 2005.)

v. Cystoscopy: Direct visualization of urethra and bladder may identify potential causes for incontinence including
(a) Bladder lesions
(b) Foreign bodies or stones
(c) Fistulas
(d) Diverticula
(e) Other urethral abnormalities
4. Treatment
a. Lifestyle modifications
i. Weight loss
ii. Caffeine/alcohol reduction and fluid management
iii. Smoking cessation
b. Physical therapy
i. Pelvic floor muscle training (Kegel) to increase muscle strength and voluntary control over muscles associated with maintaining continence
ii. Training aids
(a) Biofeedback systems
(b) Weighted vaginal cones
(c) Electrical muscle simulation units
c. Intravaginal devices
i. Pessaries
(a) Useful for patients who are unwilling or medically unable to pursue surgical correction
(b) Low risk and noninvasive
ii. Urethral plugs or caps temporarily block flow of urine, but these devices must be removed to allow for voiding
d. Surgery (Figure 32.5A–C)
i. **Retropubic resuspension**
(a) Use of sutures placed into vaginal tissue lateral to bladder neck to suspend and stabilize urethra and prevent stress-induced leaking as a result of hypermobility
(b) Typically performed via laparotomy or laparoscopy
ii. **Suburethral sling**
(a) Placement of either autologus (rectus fascia, fascia lata) or graft material (synthetic mesh, porcine, cadaveric) beneath urethra to provide support and to externally compress urethral lumen and prevent leaking
(b) Typically performed through vaginal incision
iii. **Bulking agent** therapy
(a) Injection of material transurethrally or periurethrally via cystoscopy into tissue adjacent to bladder neck
(b) Traditionally most effective for individuals with ISD and normal anatomic support
(c) Second-line intervention for patients who have failed previous surgical correction or have multiple medical comorbidities
iv. Surgical complications
(a) Acute (intraoperative)
(i) Bladder injury
(ii) Urethral injury
(iii) Unrecognized bowel or large vessel injury with sling placement
(b) Postoperative
(i) Voiding dysfunction ranging from poor emptying to complete retention
(ii) Mesh erosion
(iii) De novo detrusor overactivity
C. **Urge urinary incontinence** or **detrusor overactivity**
1. Definition
a. Involuntary loss of urine associated with uninhibited detrusor contraction
b. Often associated with strong urge to void

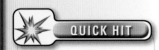

QUICK HIT

A loss of 7%–8% of total body mass index (BMI) in obese patients has been shown to improve incontinence profiles.

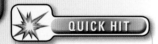

QUICK HIT

Both retropubic suspension and sling procedures have documented efficacy for the treatment of stress incontinence.

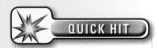

QUICK HIT

One of the most common types of retropubic suspension is called the "Burch procedure."

FIGURE
32.5 Surgical procedures for the treatment of incontinence.

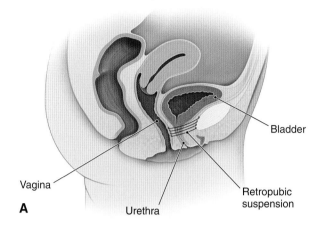

Bladder

Vagina

Retropubic
suspension

A

Urethra

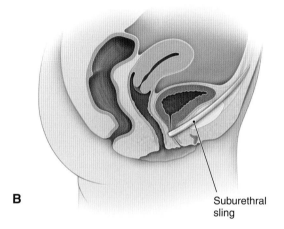

B

Suburethral
sling

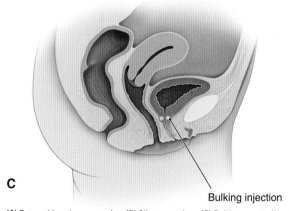

C

Bulking injection

(A) Retropubic colposuspension. **(B)** Sling procedure. **(C)** Bulking agents. (Used with permission from the American College of Obstetricians and Gynecologists.)

    c. Volume of loss can be large or small

    d. Subjective sense of sudden urgency

    e. Voiding frequently with or without leaking

2. Etiology

    a. *Most often idiopathic*

    b. Predisposing factors

       i. Bladder irritants

       ii. Bladder stones

       iii. Bladder cancers

       iv. UTIs

       v. Urethral diverticula

3. Chronic disorders that affect nervous system

    a. Strokes

    b. Diabetes with peripheral sequelae

    c. Multiple sclerosis

    d. Parkinson disease

    e. Alzheimer disease

3. Risk factors

    a. Aging

    b. Lower genital atrophy associated with lack of estrogen

    c. Prior pelvic surgery, particularly surgery for stress incontinence

    d. Smoking

    e. Obesity

    f. Chronic medical conditions as noted previously

    g. Medications (e.g., diuretics, psychotropics)

4. Evaluation

    a. History

       i. Characterize situations in which leaking occurs

       ii. Symptoms

         (a) Frequency of urination

         (b) Nocturia

         (c) Voiding difficulty

         (d) Hematuria

       iii. History of prior pelvic surgery

    b. Physical exam

       i. Evaluation of pelvic support to all compartments using POP-Q, with particular attention to anterior compartment for any condition which might impair emptying function or cause obstruction

         (a) Anterior prolapse

         (b) Hyperangulation of bladder neck from prior surgery

       ii. Basic neurologic evaluation

         (a) Assess sensory perception: soft *versus* sharp touch

         (b) Presence of normal bulbocavernosus and anal wink reflexes

    c. Laboratory testing

       i. Urinalysis

       ii. Culture to rule out infection

    d. Urodynamic testing

       i. Void and post-void residual to assess emptying function

       ii. Voiding diary

         (a) Voiding frequency

         (b) Volumes

         (c) Incontinence episodes

         (d) Fluid intake (volume and type)

       iii. Office urodynamic testing: as bladder is filled by gravity with a catheter, any rise in fluid level in filling bag associated with onset of urgency is indicative of uninhibited detrusor contraction (see Figure 32.4)

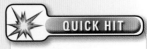

QUICK HIT

Urodynamic testing is typically less useful for the evaluation of urge incontinence as compared to stress incontinence.

    iv. Multichannel urodynamics

      (a) Inappropriate detrusor contractions can be seen as rises in true bladder pressure during filling or resting stages of study; patients will often describe sense of urgency

      (b) Leaking may also be present with uninhibited contractions

4. Treatment

  a. Behavioral modifications

    i. Kegel exercises

    ii. Relaxation techniques

    iii. Biofeedback and psychotherapy

    iv. Avoidance of recognized bladder irritants

      (a) Caffeine

      (b) Alcohol

      (c) Some foods

    v. Fluid restriction in evening

    vi. Bladder training: establishing voiding schedule that is gradually lengthened over time to increase interval between voids, increase voided volumes, and improve bladder control

  b. Pharmacotherapy: first-line therapy designed to suppress involuntary detrusor contractions while improving muscle relaxation and bladder storage

    i. **Anticholinergics** (e.g., oxybutynin) suppress unwanted bladder contractility

    ii. **Antimuscarinics** (e.g., tolterodine, trospium, and solifenacin) provide both anticholinergic and smooth muscle relaxant effects that primarily target bladder smooth muscle but may result in side effects at unintended target organs such as gut, salivary gland, and eyes

    iii. **Tricyclic antidepressants** (e.g., imipramine): have both anticholinergic (detrusor relaxation) and α-adrenergic (urethral sphincter contraction) properties, which help decrease leaking and increase bladder capacity

  c. Nerve stimulation: second-line therapy for individuals unresponsive to or unable to tolerate pharmacotherapy

    i. Sacral nerve stimulation: direct stimulation of S3 sacral nerve root with implanted generator can be effective for urinary frequency, urgency, and unobstructed poor emptying

    ii. Posterior tibial nerve stimulation

      (a) Indirect stimulation of bladder via posterior tibial nerve

      (b) Uses acupuncture needle and handheld generator, performed in ambulatory setting

  d. Surgery: no effective surgical interventions

III. Urinary Tract Infections

A. Definition

  1. Condition in which urinary tract is infected with pathogen, resulting in inflammation

  2. Should be differentiated from other conditions

    a. **Bacteriuria**: presence of bacteria in urine

    b. **Cystitis**: inflammation to bladder; may be bacterial or nonbacterial

    c. **Pyelonephritis**: Bacterial infection involving renal parenchyma and pelvi-calyceal system accompanied by bacteriuria

B. Etiology

  1. Most often result of ascending infection secondary to bacteria commonly associated with digestive tract

  2. Females are at greater risk given shorter length of urethra

  3. Common bacterial pathogens

    a. *Escherichia coli* (most common)

    b. *Pseudomonas*

    c. *Proteus*
    d. *Klebsiella*
    e. *Enterococcus*
    f. *Enterobacter*
  4. Yeast: diabetics or immunosuppressed
  5. Occasional infections from hematogenous or lymphatic spread
C. Risk factors
  1. Premenopausal
    a. Sexual activity
    b. Systemic diseases: diabetes mellitus, sickle cell
    c. Congenital anatomic abnormalities (ureteral stricture, urethral stenosis)
    d. Diaphragm contraception or spermicide use
    e. Renal calculi
    f. Obesity
    g. Medical conditions requiring indwelling or repetitive bladder catheterization
  2. Postmenopausal
    a. Vaginal atrophy
    b. Incomplete bladder emptying due to prolapse or surgical procedures for incontinence
    c. Poor hygiene
    d. Type 1 diabetes mellitus
    e. Lifetime history of UTIs
D. Evaluation
  1. History
    a. Acute bacterial cystitis
      i. Urinary frequency
      ii. Urgency
      iii. Dysuria
      iv. Small voided volumes
      v. Suprapubic discomfort
      vi. Hematuria
    b. Acute pyelonephritis
      i. Fever
      ii. Chills
      iii. Flank pain
      iv. Variable urinary symptoms
      v. Nausea/vomiting
  2. Physical exam
    a. Signs of systemic infection (fever, arthralgias)
    b. Costovertebral angle tenderness (CVAT)
  3. Laboratory testing
    a. Urine dipstick testing has both good sensitivity and specificity
      i. Leukocyte esterase
      ii. Nitrites
      iii. Blood
    b. Microscopic evaluation
      i. Pyuria (10 leukocytes per high power field)
      ii. Bacteria
    c. Urine culture to isolate organism and colony count
      i. Colony counts $>10^5$ CFU/mL considered positive
      ii. Typing and sensitivity testing directs antibiotic intervention
      iii. First morning midstream collection most sensitive
    d. Complicated infections
      i. Urodynamics
      ii. Cystourethroscopy
      iii. Radiologic imaging

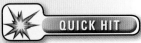

QUICK HIT

Elderly patients with UTIs may have very limited symptoms other than mental status changes and incontinence.

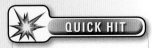

QUICK HIT

In patients with pyelonephritis, consider the presence of renal calculi.

E. Treatment
1. Acute cystitis
    a. Efficacy of 3 days of therapy is equivalent to 7 days, with exception of nitrofurantoin
    b. Commonly used agents include trimethoprim with or without sulfamethoxazole, nitrofurantoin, and quinolones
    c. Increasing resistance to amoxicillin and first-generation cephalosporins
    d. Urinary analgesics such as phenazopyridine may be useful for short-term relief of dysuria
    e. Aggressive hydration results in frequent emptying and dilution of bacterial counts; acidification of urine may also be useful
2. Acute pyelonephritis
    a. Outpatient management is reasonable for healthy, clinically stable patients who can tolerate oral medication
    b. Hospitalization should be considered for unreliable, unstable, or elderly patients
    c. Antibiotic selection is similar to that for cystitis, although treatment course is 14 days
3. Recurrent infections
    a. Defined as 2 infections in 6 months or 3 infections in 1 year
    b. Differentiate between recurrent infection caused by same organism following adequate therapy (**relapse**) and (**reinfection**), which is either the same organism with negative intervening culture or new organism
    c. Antibiotic selection is as outlined previously
    d. Management should include evaluation and modification of possible risk factors
    e. For frequent infections, antibiotic prophylaxis has been shown to be effective when taken daily or postcoitally if intercourse is thought to be causative factor

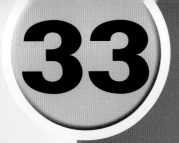

33 Endometriosis

I. Definition

A. Endometrial **glands and stroma** in extrauterine site(s)

B. Hormonally responsive, similar to endometrium within uterus

C. **Adenomyosis:** form of endometriosis in which endometrial tissue is found within myometrium

II. Incidence

A. Estimates of incidence vary widely
1. 5%–15% of women in general population
2. 12%–32% of women undergoing laparoscopy for pain
3. 21%–48% of women undergoing workup for infertility

B. Increasing incidence may reflect increasing awareness and diagnostic surgeries

III. Risk Factors

A. Reproductive age
1. May begin in adolescence, although usually later
2. Rare in menopause

B. Nulliparity
1. Can result in infertility
2. Often improves during and after pregnancy

C. Family history
1. Women with 1st-degree relative with endometriosis have 7- to 10-fold increased risk
2. Multifactorial inheritance pattern

IV. Theories of Pathogenesis

A. **Sampson theory:** retrograde menstruation
1. Endometrial tissue carried through tubes into peritoneal cavity
2. Accounts for high incidence of endometriosis when uterine outflow tract obstruction present (e.g., imperforate hymen)

B. **Halban theory:** lymphovascular dissemination
1. Endometrial cells carried through lymphovascular channels to remote body parts
2. Accounts for endometriosis occasionally found in head, chest cavities

C. **Meyer theory:** coelomic metaplasia
1. Totipotential cells in peritoneal lining transform into endometrium
2. Accounts for development of endometriosis in some women without uterus

D. Direct implantation
1. Endometriosis implants in spaces exposed to endometrial tissue
2. Accounts for the occurrence of endometriosis in Cesarean delivery scars, episiotomies

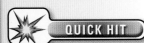

Unlike endometriosis, adenomyosis occurs more often in parous women, later in reproductive years.

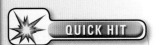

Women who have had severe symptoms of endometriosis in their reproductive years will have marked improvement in menopause, because estrogen no longer stimulates the endometrial epithelium.

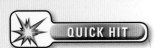

During pregnancy, high levels of progesterone counter the high levels of estrogen, thereby inhibiting endometrial epithelium stimulation.

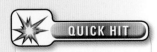

Family history is a risk factor for endometriosis.

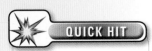

Insofar as most women have some retrograde menstruation at some time, underlying immunologic factors may allow endometriosis to implant in some women and not others.

V. Presentation

A. Symptoms: very variable, but "cyclic" (e.g., exacerbated during menses)
1. **Dysmenorrhea**
   a. Hallmark of endometriosis
   b. Usually progressive, with pain lasting longer over time
2. **Dyspareunia**: typically deep as opposed to entry pain
3. **Chronic pelvic pain**: secondary to pelvic adhesions
4. **Dyschezia**: particularly with implants in cul-de-sac or rectovaginal septum
5. **Infertility**
   a. More common in women with endometriosis
   b. May be result of scarring that distorts or occludes tubes
   c. Even without fibrosis, inflammatory mediators may inhibit conception
6. **Menorrhagia**: particularly if adenomyosis is also present
7. May be completely asymptomatic

B. Differential diagnosis
1. Dysmenorrhea
   a. Primary: prostaglandin mediated
   b. Secondary: fibroids, endometrial polyps
2. Chronic pelvic pain may be gynecologic or from other organs
   a. Gynecologic: chronic pelvic inflammatory disease, ovarian adhesions
   b. Gastrointestinal: inflammatory bowel disease, irritable bowel syndrome
   c. Urologic: interstitial cystitis
   d. Neuromuscular: fibromyalgia, neuropathic pain
3. Deep dyspareunia
   a. Pelvic adhesive disease
   b. Retroverted uterus
   c. Ovarian cysts

C. Disease location (Table 33.1)
1. Usually found in most dependent areas of peritoneal cavity (Figure 33.1)
   a. Posterior cul-de-sac, uterosacral ligaments, ovaries, tubes, uterus
   b. Less common: rectosigmoid, other intestine, bladder, vagina

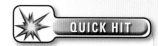

QUICK HIT

The classic symptoms of endometriosis include progressive dysmenorrhea and deep dyspareunia.

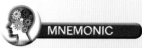

MNEMONIC

3 Ds of enDometriosis
Dysmenorrhea
Dyspareunia
Dyschezia

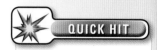

QUICK HIT

The degree of symptoms does not correspond with the amount of disease present.

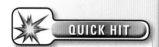

QUICK HIT

The four most common etiologies for **secondary dysmenorrhea** are endometriosis, adenomyosis, leiomyomas, and endometrial polyps.

Endometriosis

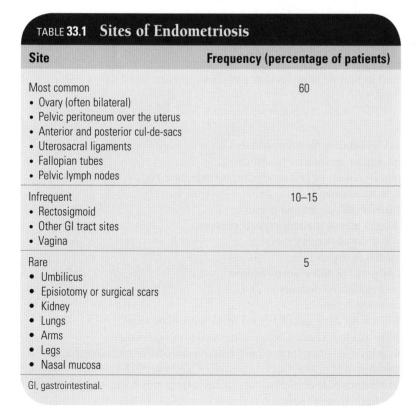

TABLE 33.1 Sites of Endometriosis	
Site	**Frequency (percentage of patients)**
Most common • Ovary (often bilateral) • Pelvic peritoneum over the uterus • Anterior and posterior cul-de-sacs • Uterosacral ligaments • Fallopian tubes • Pelvic lymph nodes	60
Infrequent • Rectosigmoid • Other GI tract sites • Vagina	10–15
Rare • Umbilicus • Episiotomy or surgical scars • Kidney • Lungs • Arms • Legs • Nasal mucosa	5

GI, gastrointestinal.

Endometriosis

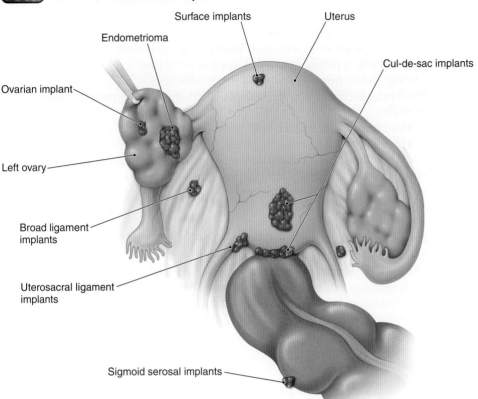

FIGURE 33.1 Location of endometriosis implants.

Surface implants

Uterus

Endometrioma

Cul-de-sac implants

Ovarian implant

Left ovary

Broad ligament implants

Uterosacral ligament implants

Sigmoid serosal implants

(From Beckmann CRB, Ling FW, et al. *Obstetrics and Gynecology*, 7th ed. Philadelphia: Lippincott Williams & Wilkins; 2014.)

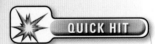

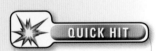

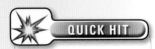

> **QUICK HIT**
>
> The clue to suspect endometriosis in remote sites is the "cyclic pattern" to the symptoms, such as recurrent pneumothorax only during menses.

> **QUICK HIT**
>
> Most women with endometriosis have a completely normal exam.

> **QUICK HIT**
>
> The classic powder burn lesions are due to repetitive cycles of bleeding and accumulation of hemosiderin in macrophages.

2. May form a cyst within ovary, called **endometrioma**
   a. Endometrioma often called "**chocolate cyst**" because of appearance of contents (i.e., old blood)
   b. Densely adherent to surrounding ovarian stroma and adjacent pelvic structures
3. Rarely found in remote sites such as umbilicus, pleura, nasal cavity

VI. Diagnosis

A. Examination
   1. **Uterosacral nodularity**: best appreciated on rectovaginal exam
   2. Tenderness and/or nodularity in cul-de-sac
   3. Fixed uterus or adherent pelvic structures; may have retroverted uterus secondary to adhesions
   4. Adnexal mass if endometrioma present
   5. Enlarged **boggy** uterus if adenomyosis present
B. Visualization at time of surgery
   1. Highly variable in appearance
      a. Brown or gray "**powder burn**" lesions
      b. Dark red "mulberry" lesions
      c. Clear or white lesions
      d. Cysts filled with dark red or brown fluid "chocolate cysts"
   2. Reactive fibrosis often creates dense adhesions around lesions
   3. Peritoneal "windows" may form where reactive fibrosis retracts overlying peritoneum
   4. Extent and severity of lesions also vary greatly, from tiny focus to widespread involvement and "frozen" pelvis

C. Biopsy of suspected lesions
  1. Biopsy should be performed of any suspicious lesion
  2. 2 or more of following features required for pathologic confirmation
    a. Endometrial epithelium (**glands**)
    b. Endometrial **stroma**
    c. **Hemosiderin-laden macrophages**
  3. Adenomyosis usually only confirmed after hysterectomy
D. Other modalities may be helpful in diagnosis
  1. Ultrasound or computed tomography useful only in diagnosing endometrioma
  2. Magnetic resonance imaging may detect adenomyosis or deeply infiltrating lesions
  3. CA-125 frequently elevated when endometriosis is present but not specific enough to be of diagnostic use
E. Staging
  1. 1996 Revised American Society for Reproductive Medicine Classification provides uniform system for describing findings
  2. Documents extent and severity of both implants and adhesions
  3. Useful to compare treatment outcomes in research; less useful in clinical management

VII. Treatment

A. Choice depends on patient circumstances
  1. Presenting symptoms and severity
  2. Location and severity
  3. Desire for future childbearing
B. Expectant management
  1. Patients attempting to conceive
  2. Usually resolves with menopause (atrophy of endometrium)
  3. Reasonable for mild symptoms, close to menopausal age
  4. Nonsteroidal anti-inflammatory drugs (NSAIDs) useful for pain and dysmenorrhea
C. Hormonal therapies
  1. **Combination contraceptives** (estrogen + progestin)
    a. May be given orally, vaginally, or transdermally
    b. Constant opposition of estrogen by progestins leads to atrophy
    c. Often used *continuously* with no break so as to cause amenorrhea
      i. Decreases number of menstrual cycles and, therefore, dysmenorrhea
      ii. Breakthrough bleeding: common side effect
  2. **Continuous progestins**
    a. Administered as intramuscular injection, subcutaneous implant, or orally
    b. Induces endometrial atrophy by preventing estrogenic proliferation
    c. Suppresses gonadotropin release, which inhibits ovarian steroidogenesis and therefore estrogen production
    d. Low estrogen may contribute to decreased bone mineral density (BMD) with long-term use
    e. Intrauterine device with progestin may cause endometrial atrophy, but without systemic effects, to extrauterine implants
  3. Danazol
    a. Weak androgen: suppresses pituitary hormone release
    b. Induces endometrial atrophy and amenorrhea
    c. Long-term use limited by side effects
      i. Androgenic
        a. Acne
        b. Oily skin
        c. Hirsutism
        d. Deepening of voice
      ii. Hypoestrogenic vasomotor symptoms: vaginal atrophy
      iii. Degree of side effects increases with increasing dose
    d. Infrequently used due to better alternatives

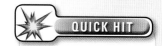

Reliable diagnosis of endometriosis depends on confirmation by tissue biopsy, insofar as appearance alone is often misleading.

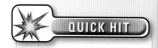

Hysterectomy with bilateral oophorectomy is most likely to be curative but is also the most radical approach.

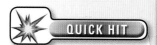

All hormonal therapies share the goal of inducing endometrial atrophy by suppressing estrogen stimulation of endometrial proliferation.

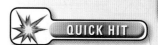

Combined oral contraceptive therapy in conjunction with NSAIDs are the first-line treatment for dysmenorrhea.

Endometriosis

Endometriosis

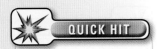

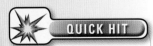

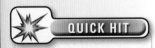

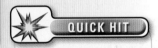

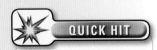

4. **Gonadotropin-releasing hormone agonists (GnRH agonist)**
   a. Induce "**chemical menopause**" by completely suppressing pituitary hormones
   b. Have similar effect to surgically removing ovaries
   c. Hypoestrogenic side effects but no androgenic side effects
      i. Hot flashes
      ii. Vaginal atrophy
      iii. Decreased libido
      iv. Occasional breakthrough bleeding
   c. Use is limited by expense, side effects, and decrease in BMD, especially with long-term use
   d. Hypoestrogenic side effects can be mitigated with concurrent use of low dose progestin (termed "**add-back**" **therapy**)
D. Surgical treatment
   1. Conservative surgery: usually laparoscopic
      a. Conserves childbearing potential
      b. Ablation of endometriotic lesions
         i. May use laser or cautery
         ii. Most effective for superficial lesions
      c. Excision of lesions
         i. Success depends on complete excision of lesion
         ii. Difficult because implants often deeper than appreciated
      d. Lysis of adhesions
         i. May be helpful when pain is due to adhesions
         ii. Adhesions will recur unless underlying problem addressed
      e. Success rates
         i. Depend on how completely lesions are destroyed and extent of disease
         ii. ~1/3 will need additional surgery within 5 years
   2. Extirpative surgery: usually reserved for patients who have failed medical management and conservative surgery or in those who no longer desire reproductive capability
      a. Bilateral salpingo-oophorectomy
         i. Induces permanent menopause
         ii. Theoretically curative because it eliminates hormonal stimulation
         iii. Some additional hormonal stimulation may persist through peripheral aromatization of adrenal androgens
         iv. Unilateral oophorectomy may be considered if only 1 ovary involved and endometriosis completely resected
      b. Hysterectomy
         i. May be done concurrently to resect all endometriotic lesions
         ii. Curative for adenomyosis
      c. Success rate
         i. 10% have persistent or recurrent symptoms even after hysterectomy and bilateral oophorectomy
         ii. Possible that symptoms were not related to endometriosis

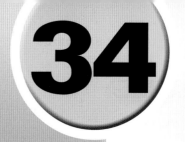

I. Dysmenorrhea

A. Definition

1. Painful menstruation preventing a woman from performing normal activities or affecting quality of life

2. May be accompanied by other symptoms: diarrhea, nausea and vomiting, headache

B. Classification

1. **Primary (1°):** excess prostaglandins (PGs), which increase uterine contractions (Table 34.1)

   a. Etiology: excess PG production in endometrium

     i. $F_{2\alpha}$: uterine—smooth muscle contractions

     ii. $F_{2\alpha}$: extrauterine—nausea, vomiting, diarrhea

     iii. E_2: vasodilator and inhibits platelet aggregation

   b. Symptoms

     i. Recurrent, spasmodic, central, lower abdominal pain

     ii. Typically first 1–3 days of menstruation

     iii. Can radiate to back – especially if retroverted uterus

   c. Assessment

     i. Eliminate any identifiable cause

     ii. Physical exam and pelvic exam are normal

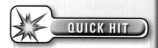

QUICK HIT

Because dysmenorrhea occurs only when the patient is bleeding, pain that is not related to uterine bleeding is *not* dysmenorrhea.

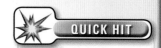

QUICK HIT

Primary dysmenorrhea usually occurs after the first 3–6 menstrual periods (which are usually anovulatory).

QUICK HIT

Progesterone increases prostaglandin production in the uterus.

TABLE 34.1	Comparison of Primary and Secondary Dysmenorrhea	
	Primary Dysmenorrhea	**Secondary Dysmenorrhea**
Etiology	Excess prostaglandins (PGF₂α and PGE₂) in endometrium	Clinically identifiable cause (see Table 34.2)
Incidence	Late teens to early 20s Declines with age	Later in reproductive years Increases with age
Symptoms	Spasmodic, colicky, diffuse lower abdominal and suprapubic pain first 1–3 days of menses Dyspareunia generally absent ±Nausea, vomiting, diarrhea, fatigue, headache, and/or backache	Aching pain starts before, becomes worse during, and persists after menses Dyspareunia often present Symptoms associated with underlying cause (see Table 34.2)
Exam	Normal	Consistent with cause (see Table 34.2)
Investigations	Physical and pelvic exam	Directed at suspected cause (see Table 34.2)
Therapy	NSAIDs Topical heat, exercise, psychotherapy Oral contraceptives → anovulation Rarely, presacral neurectomy in refractory cases	Treatment of underlying cause Analgesics as symptomatic treatment Oral contraceptives help in some cases (e.g., endometriosis, adenomyosis)

NSAIDs, nonsteroidal anti-inflammatory drugs.

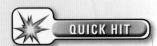

QUICK HIT

Primary dysmenorrhea is an appropriate diagnosis when no other clinically identifiable cause is apparent.

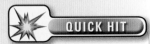

QUICK HIT

A patient with primary dysmenorrhea can appear pale and "shocky," but the abdomen is soft and non-tender, and the pelvic exam is normal.

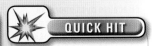

QUICK HIT

If patient does not have a response to NSAIDs, then diagnosis of primary dysmenorrhea needs reevaluation.

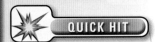

QUICK HIT

Childbearing does not affect incidence of either primary or secondary dysmenorrhea.

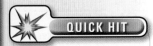

QUICK HIT

Because the uterus is smooth muscle, it is either relaxed or contracted. If there is a polyp or leiomyoma within the endometrial cavity, the uterus will try to "cramp" it out, resulting in dysmenorrhea.

d. Treatment
    i. Nonsteroidal anti-inflammatory drugs (NSAIDs) inhibit prostaglandin production and therefore provide exceptional pain relief
    ii. Topical heat
    iii. Exercise
    iv. Psychotherapy
    v. Reassurance (lack of other pathology)
    vi. **Oral contraceptive pills (OCPs)**: decrease prostaglandin production and decrease amount of bleeding through atrophy of endometrium
    vii. In rare circumstances, presacral neurectomy
2. **Secondary (2°)**: clinically identifiable cause within uterus, uterine wall, or outside uterus (Table 34.2)
    a. Etiology: structural abnormalities or disease processes
        i. **Endometriosis** (ectopic endometrial tissue outside uterus) (see Chapter 33)
        ii. **Adenomyosis** (endometrial tissue growing into myometrium) (see Chapter 33)
        iii. **Adhesions** in peritoneal cavity
        iv. **Pelvic inflammatory disease (PID)** (see Chapter 31)
        v. **Leiomyomas** – especially submucosal location
        vi. Endometrial **polyps**
        vii. Cervical **stenosis**: outflow obstruction
        viii. Uterine synechae (adhesions) in endometrial cavity (**Asherman syndrome**): outflow obstruction
    b. Symptoms
        i. Often begins in later reproductive years
        ii. Typically cramping pain before, during, and after menstruation
        iii. Often history will reflect chronic progressive increase in amount of pain across time
    c. Assessment
        i. Directed at identifying possible causes
        ii. Pelvic exam
            (a) Asymmetry or irregularities of uterus (fibroids)
            (b) Restricted uterine mobility (endometriosis or adhesions)
        iii. Cultures for gonorrhea/chlamydia

TABLE **34.2** **Common Causes, Associated Symptoms, Exam Findings, and Possible Investigations of Secondary Dysmenorrhea**

Underlying Cause	Associated Symptoms	Physical Exam Findings	Investigation
Endometriosis	Infertility	Painful nodules in cul-de-sac and restricted motion of uterus	Laparoscopy
Adenomyosis	Heavy menstruation	Tender, symmetrically enlarged boggy uterus	Pelvic ultrasonography/MRI
Uterine leiomyomata	Heavy menstruation, anemia	Enlarged uterus with irregular contour and rubbery consistency	Pelvic ultrasonography
Infection or past infection	Fever, chills, nausea	Cervical motion tenderness or thickening and tenderness of adnexa with restricted motion of uterus	Cervical cultures Laparoscopy
Pelvic adhesions		Restricted motion of uterus	Laparoscopy
Endometrial polyps	Menorrhagia	Polyp may be visible at external cervical os	Pelvic ultrasound Sonohysterography Hysteroscopy

MRI, magnetic resonance imaging.

iv. Imaging such as pelvic ultrasound

v. **Sonohysterography** ([SHG] also called **saline infusion sonohysterography** [SIS]): saline used to distend endometrial cavity (see Chapter 40)

vi. Diagnostic surgery: **hysteroscopy** or **laparoscopy**

d. Treatment

i. Directed at underlying etiology

ii. Combination OCPs: decrease bleeding and cramping

iii. Continuous progesterone therapy (pills, injectable, subcutaneous implant)

iv. Hysterectomy is definitive therapy if other management fails

II. Chronic Pelvic Pain

A. Definition: **noncyclic pain** lasting for more than 6 months that localizes to anatomic pelvis, anterior abdominal wall at or below the umbilicus, lumbosacral back, or buttocks and is of sufficient severity to cause functional disability or lead to medical care

B. Etiology (Box 34.1)

1. Gynecologic, gastrointestinal (GI), urologic, musculoskeletal, psychiatric, others

2. Common causes include endometriosis, PID, irritable bowel syndrome (IBS), interstitial cystitis, and adhesions

3. Some cases may have multiple causes, whereas others have no clear etiology

C. Assessment: often requires a multidisciplinary approach

1. History

a. Description and timing of symptoms

b. Thorough medical, surgical, menstrual, and sexual history

c. Home and work status, social and family history

d. Sleep disturbances, other signs of depression

e. Past history of physical or sexual abuse, rape

f. Past or current history of intimate partner violence

2. Physical exam to detect underlying cause

a. General physical exam

b. Abdominal exam

i. Ability to reproduce pain/severity/location

ii. Masses

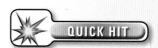

QUICK HIT

SHG provides the ability to identify intracavitary masses or distortions of the endometrial cavity such as caused by a submucosal leiomyoma.

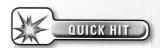

QUICK HIT

Physical examination in dysmenorrhea is directed at finding possible causes of secondary dysmenorrhea. Exam in primary dysmenorrhea should be normal.

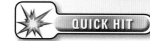

QUICK HIT

The main distinction between dysmenorrhea and chronic pelvic pain is the cyclical nature of dysmenorrhea, insofar as it only occurs with bleeding.

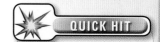

QUICK HIT

Among women ages 18–50 years, 15%–20% have chronic pelvic pain >1 year.

Dysmenorrhea and Chronic Pelvic Pain

BOX 34.1

Causes of Chronic Pelvic Pain

Gynecologic
Endometriosis
Uterine leiomyomata
Adenomyosis
Endometrial polyps
Intrauterine device (IUD)
Adhesions
Infection (PID)
Ovarian remnant syndrome
Pelvic congestion syndrome
Adnexal cysts
Pelvic malignancies
Pelvic relaxation/prolapse

Gastrointestinal
Irritable bowel syndrome
Inflammatory bowel disease
Carcinoma
Hernia
Diverticular disease

Recurrent partial bowel obstruction
Abdominal angina
Constipation

Urologic
Interstitial cystitis
Chronic/recurrent cystourethritis
Urethral syndrome
Urethral diverticulum
Carcinoma of bladder
Ureteral obstruction
Urolithiasis
Pelvic kidney

Musculoskeletal
Nerve entrapment
Iliohypogastric and other neuropathies
Trigger points
Myofascial pain
Fibromyalgia

Osteoporosis
Spondylosis
Spondylolisthesis
Degenerative changes
Scoliosis and kyphosis
Tumors and inflammation
Coccydynia
Spinal injuries
Congenital anomalies

Psychiatric
Somatization
Depression
Anxiety
Personality disorders
Posttraumatic Stress Disorder

Others
Porphyria
Connective tissue diseases
(e.g., SLE)

SLE, systemic lupus erythematosus. (Modified from Berek JS, ed. *Berek & Novak's Gynecology*, 14th ed. Philadelphia: Lippincott Williams & Wilkins; 2007:517.)

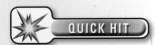

QUICK HIT

Many of the conditions that cause secondary dysmenorrhea may cause chronic pelvic pain.

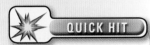

QUICK HIT

Of patients who undergo laparoscopy for chronic pelvic pain, 1/3 will have no identifiable cause.

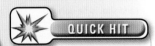

QUICK HIT

History of childhood sexual or physical abuse is highly correlated with severity of symptoms.

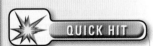

QUICK HIT

Patients with chronic pelvic pain offer a therapeutic challenge.

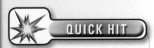

QUICK HIT

One of the challenges of chronic pelvic pain is managing the patient's pain without narcotics or other drugs with an addictive potential.

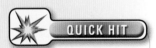

QUICK HIT

Analgesics and follow-up visits should be on a fixed time schedule, rather than as needed, to avoid enhancing pain behavior.

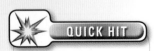

QUICK HIT

Both continuous progesterone and combination contraceptives (progesterone continuously opposing estrogen) lead to atrophy of endometrial tissue.

iii. Exclude hernias
iv. Search for myofascial trigger points
c. Pelvic exam
d. Rectovaginal exam
3. Investigations for suspected underlying cause
a. Cervical cultures for suspected infection
b. Imaging ultrasonography, magnetic resonance imaging, computed tomography (USG/MRI/CT) for suspected uterine leiomyomata, adenomyosis, adnexal masses
c. Laparoscopy for suspected endometriosis and cases with unclear etiology
d. Hysteroscopy
e. Cystoscopy
f. Colonoscopy
D. Conditions associated with chronic pelvic pain (see Box 34.1)
1. **Endometriosis** (see Chapter 33)
2. **PID** (see Chapter 31)
a. 18%–35% subsequently develop chronic pelvic pain
b. May be due to chronic inflammation, adhesions, and psychosocial factors
3. **IBS**
a. 50%–80% of women with chronic pelvic pain
b. Rome II criteria: abdominopelvic pain ≥12 weeks in 12 months and not explained by other diseases and have at least 2 of the following:
i. Relieved by defecation
ii. Change in bowel movement frequency (diarrhea or constipation)
iii. Change in form of stool (loose/watery/mucous/pellet-like)
4. **Interstitial cystitis (IC)**
a. Chronic inflammation of bladder characterized by pelvic pain, urinary urgency and frequency, and dyspareunia
b. Due to disruption of glycosaminoglycan layer coating bladder mucosa
c. Investigations include cystoscopy, bladder hydrodistention, and intravesical potassium sensitivity test
5. Myofascial pain syndromes and hernias
6. Inflammatory bowel disease
7. Renal nephrolithiasis
8. Chronic pain of unknown etiology
E. Therapy
1. General rules
a. Therapy should be directed to underlying cause
b. Strong patient–doctor relationship is critical
c. Multidisciplinary approach with consultation of psychiatrists, psychologists, social workers, physical therapists, gastroenterologists, anesthesiologists or chronic pain specialists, orthopedists, urologists, sexual therapists, and others as needed
d. Often, goal of treatment is improving quality of life rather than elimination of pain altogether
2. Suppression of ovulation: can be either therapeutic modality or diagnostic tool
a. Extended regimen or continuous **combination OCPs** (see Chapter 27): minimizes number of episodes of bleeding and therefore dysmenorrhea
b. **Continuous progesterone** (pills, Depo-Provera injection, subcutaneous progestin implant)
c. **GnRH agonists:** lead to complete suppression of ovarian function and menopausal-like state
3. IBS
a. Refer to gastroenterologist for further evaluation
b. Use food diary to identify and eliminate etiologic foods
c. Limit caffeine, alcohol, fatty foods, and gas-producing vegetables
d. Treatment based on predominant symptoms
i. Constipation: fiber and lactulose
ii. Diarrhea: antidiarrheals
iii. Gas pain and cramping: antispasmodics (dicyclomine or hyoscyamine)

4. IC
   a. Eliminate caffeine, alcohol, artificial sweeteners, and acidic foods
   b. Intravesical instillation of dimethyl sulfoxide (DMSO)
   c. Oral antihistamines, tricyclic antidepressants, and pentosan polysulfate (glycosaminoglycan analogue)
5. Surgery: only after exclusion of nongynecologic causes
   a. Laparoscopy with lysis of adhesions or destruction of endometriotic implants
   b. Hysterectomy is very effective for pain originating from uterus
   c. Bilateral salpingo-oophorectomy (BSO) may be necessary, especially with cyclic pain
6. Alternate modalities
   a. Transcutaneous electrical nerve stimulation (TENS)
   b. Biofeedback
   c. Nerve blocks, presacral neurectomy, ablation of uterosacral ligaments, sacral nerve root stimulator implants

F. Follow-up
1. Monitor for success of treatment and complications of therapy
2. Reevaluate patients started on OCPs at 2 and 6 months

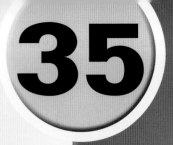

35 Breast Disorders

I. Anatomy

A. Modified sebaceous gland containing glands, milk ducts, connective tissue, fat
B. Architecture: 12–20 lobes
1. Secretory cells arranged in alveolar pattern
2. Secretory cells surrounded by myoepithelial cells
3. Glands drain into collecting milk ducts coalescing in major ducts leading to nipple
C. More glandular/lobular tissue in upper outer quadrant
D. Age differences
1. Younger women: mainly glandular
2. Older women: glands involute, replaced by fat
3. *Involution accelerated by menopause*
E. Congenital anomalies
1. Absence of breast
2. Accessory breast tissue along "**milk lines**" extending from axilla to groin
3. Extra nipples (**polythelia**) more common than true accessory breasts (**polymastia**)
F. Blood supply
1. Internal mammary artery
2. Lateral thoracic artery
3. Thoracodorsal artery
4. Thoracoacromial artery
5. Intercostal perforating arteries
G. Lymphatic drainage
1. Superficial and deep nodal chains in trunk and neck
2. Axilla, deep to pectoralis, caudal to diaphragm
H. Sensitivity to hormones
1. **Estrogen** responsible for growth of adipose tissue and lactiferous ducts
2. **Progesterone** stimulates lobular growth and alveolar budding

II. Evaluation of Breast Signs and Symptoms

A. Patient history
1. Most common complaints: pain and concern about mass
2. 6% of patients with complaint (most commonly, mass) have cancer
3. Important information: location, duration, how discovered, nipple discharge, size, relation to menstrual cycle
4. Also ask about risk factors (Box 35.1)
B. Physical examination
1. Include both breasts, axillae, chest wall
2. Follicular phase of menstrual cycle
3. If no dominant mass, risk factors can help determine need for referral or repeat exam in 3 months or imaging
C. Diagnostic testing (Figure 35.1)
1. Mammography
a. Can detect lesion 2–3 years before being palpable
b. Lesions <1 cm can be seen

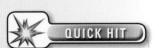

QUICK HIT

Disproportionate distribution of glandular tissue accounts for why breast cancer most commonly arises in the upper outer quadrant.

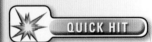

QUICK HIT

Breast tissue is very sensitive to hormonal changes, especially the glandular cells.

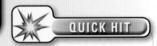

QUICK HIT

The best time to perform a physical breast examination is during the follicular phase of the menstrual cycle.

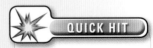

QUICK HIT

Mammography X-ray can detect lesions 2–3 years before they are palpable on physical examination.

BOX 35.1

Risk Factors for Breast Cancer

- Age
- Personal history of breast cancer
- History of atypical hyperplasia (ductal or lobular) on past biopsies
- Inherited genetic mutations
- First-degree relatives with breast or ovarian cancer diagnosed at an early age
- Early menarche (age <12 years)
- Late cessation of menses (age >55 years)
- No term pregnancies
- Late age at first live birth (>30 years)
- Never breastfed
- Alcohol consumption
- Recent oral contraceptive use
- Use of hormone therapy
- Personal history of endometrial, ovarian, or colon cancer
- Jewish heritage

(From Beckmann CRB, Ling FW, et al. *Obstetrics and Gynecology*, 7th ed. Baltimore: Lippincott Williams & Wilkins; 2014.)

FIGURE 35.1 Workup of dominant, indeterminate, or suspicious breast mass.

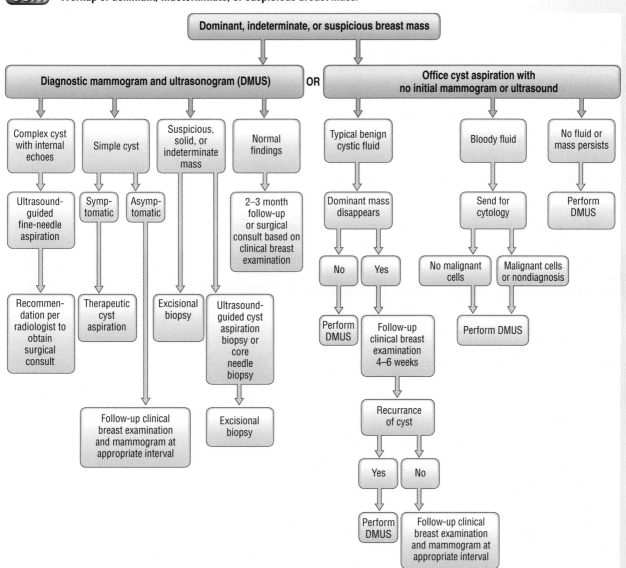

(From Pruthi S. Detection and evaluation of a palpable breast mass. *Mayo Clin Proc.* 2001;76[6]:641–647.)

Breast Disorders

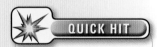

QUICK HIT

Lobular carcinoma is more difficult to detect with routine screening mammography.

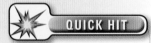

QUICK HIT

In women age <40 years, ultrasonography is the recommended initial modality to evaluate a breast mass because of dense breast tissue.

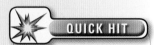

QUICK HIT

A negative FNA result should not be considered definitive if mammographic or clinical findings are suspicious.

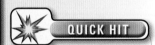

QUICK HIT

FNA provides a cellular specimen for cytologic evaluation, whereas a core needle biopsy provides a tissue specimen for histologic evaluation.

c. Suspicious findings include densities, microcalcifications, and architectural distortion

d. **Screening** mammography
   i. 2 craniocaudal and 2 mediolateral images
   ii. Typical radiation dose = 0.3 cGy
   iii. Standard reporting system: **Breast Imaging Reporting and Data System (BI-RADS)** (Table 35.1)

e. **Diagnostic** mammography
   i. Done to supplement abnormal screening mammogram
   ii. Woman age >40 years complaining of mass, even if not palpable on physical exam
   iii. Contralateral breast should also be imaged if mass is clinically apparent

2. Ultrasonography
   a. Useful in young women and others with dense breast tissue
   b. Can differentiate between solid and cystic lesion
   c. Used as guide for core-needle biopsies with palpable mass

3. Magnetic resonance imaging (MRI)
   a. Increasingly used for screening/early detection in very–high-risk women
   b. Use for screening limited by cost, lack of standardized technique, inability to detect microcalcifications

4. Fine-needle aspiration biopsy (FNAB or FNA)
   a. Useful to determine if palpable mass is simple cyst
   b. Local anesthesia, 22–24-gauge needle
   c. Clear aspirated fluid does not need pathologic evaluation
      i. Disappearance of mass with aspiration is reassuring, with follow-up in 4–6 months
      ii. If mass reappears, diagnostic mammography and ultrasonography indicated
   d. Bloody fluid needs pathologic evaluation, diagnostic mammography, ultrasonography
   e. Negative result not necessarily definitive

5. Core-needle biopsy (14–16-gauge needle)
   a. For use in larger solid masses to obtain a tissue diagnosis
   b. To obtain 3–6 samples, ~2 cm long

TABLE 35.1	American College of Radiology Breast Imaging Reporting and Data System (BI-RADS)	
BI-RADS Classification	**Summary Recommendations**	**Explanation**
0	Need additional imaging evaluation	Mammogram with a lesion that needs additional imaging such as spot compression films, magnifications, or additional views
1	Negative	Breast appears normal
2	Benign findings	Negative mammogram but interpreter wishes to describe a finding
3	Probably benign finding	Mammogram with a lesion highly likely to be benign; follow-up is suggested to establish mammographic stability
4	Suspicious abnormality	Concerning lesion with a definite probability of being malignant; recommend biopsy
5	Highly suggestive of malignancy	Lesion with a high probability of being cancer—appropriate referral to a breast surgeon is needed
6	Known biopsy-proven malignancy	Appropriate action should be taken

(From Beckmann CRB, Ling FW, et al. *Obstetrics and Gynecology*, 7th ed. Baltimore: Lippincott Williams & Wilkins; 2014.)

III. Benign Breast Disease

A. **Mastalgia** (breast pain, **mastodynia**): 3 general types
  1. Cyclic mastalgia
     a. During luteal phase, with resolution at onset of menses
     b. Usually bilateral, involving upper outer quadrants
  2. Noncyclic mastalgia
     a. Etiologies include tumors, mastitis, cysts, history of breast surgery, idiopathic
     b. Some medications as cause: hormones, antidepressants, antihypertensives
     c. Direct trauma: can lead to localized fat necrosis
  3. Nonmammary pain
     a. Chest wall trauma
     b. Fibromyalgia
     c. Rib fractures
     d. Costochondritis
     e. Angina
  4. Treatment
     a. Nonpharmacologic treatments: fitted brassiere/sports bra, weight reduction, regular exercise
     b. Medical treatment
        i. Danazol, bromocriptine and gonadotropin-releasing hormone agonist (GnRHa), and selective estrogen receptor modulators (SERMs) (e.g., tamoxifen)
        ii. For cyclic mastalgia: extended duration oral contraceptive pills (OCPs) and depot medroxyprogesterone acetate can help
     c. Reduction mammoplasty

B. Nipple discharge
  1. Usually benign, but can be early sign of endocrinopathy or cancer
  2. Color, consistency, bilaterality can help with determining cause
     a. Nonspontaneous, nonbloody, bilateral: suggests fibrocystic changes or **ductal ectasia** (dilation of mammary ducts, periductal fibrosis, inflammation)
     b. Green, yellow, brown, sticky: also associated with fibrocystic changes or ductal ectasia
     c. Milky, often spontaneous
        i. Physiologic: associated with childbearing
        ii. Hormonal: hyperprolactinemia, hypothyroidism
        iii. Medications: combination OCPs, tricyclic antidepressants, and psychotropics
        iv. Neurologic: chest wall surgery
     d. Purulent: associated with mastitis or breast abscess
     e. Bloody, unilateral
        i. Intraductal papilloma, intraductal carcinoma, invasive ductal carcinoma
        ii. Requires ductography and ductal excision

C. Benign breast masses (3 general types)
  1. Nonproliferative lesions
     a. **Fibrocystic changes**
        i. Dilation of lobules that can rupture and cause fibrosis
        ii. **Adenosis:** increased number of glands with lobular growth
     b. **Fibroadenoma:** Most common tumor in late teens to early 20s
        i. Solid, round, rubbery, mobile on exam
        ii. Can enlarge (especially in pregnancy)
     c. Lactational adenomas due to exaggerated hormone response in lactating women
  2. **Proliferative** lesions **without atypia** (epithelial hyperplasia without atypia)
     a. Seen on mammography, not usually associated with mass
     b. 4 general types
        i. **Epithelial hyperplasia:** excess number of cell layers (beyond the usual myoepithelial and luminal layers)
        ii. **Sclerosing adenosis:** fibrosis with distortion and compressing of epithelium

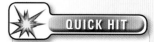
QUICK HIT

Danazol is the only U.S. Food and Drug Administration (FDA)–approved medication for mastalgia, but it has significant side effects.

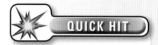
QUICK HIT

GnRH agonists have side effects that limit their widespread use.

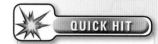
QUICK HIT

Tamoxifen should only be used for severe cases of mastalgia unresponsive to other treatments because it is associated with increased risk of endometrial hyperplasia, deep vein thrombosis, hot flashes, and vaginal bleeding.

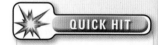
QUICK HIT

Although nipple discharge is usually benign, it can be an early sign of endocrinopathy or cancer.

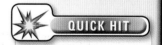
QUICK HIT

Bloody, unilateral nipple discharge requires ductography and ductal excision.

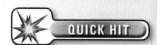
QUICK HIT

Fiberoptic ductoscopy (FDS) is a newer technique that allows direct visualization of ducts as well as ductal cell sampling.

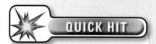
QUICK HIT

Nonproliferative lesions have a relative risk of 1.0 of developing invasive breast cancer.

Breast Disorders

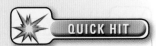

Proliferative lesions without atypia have a relative risk of 1.5–2.0 of developing invasive breast cancer.

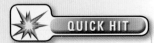

Proliferative lesions with atypia have a relative risk of 4.0–5.0 of developing invasive breast cancer.

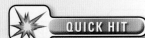

LCIS has a relative risk of 7.0–11.0 of developing breast cancer.

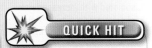

LCIS and DCIS should be excised, following which radiation therapy or use of SERMs can reduce risk of developing invasive cancer.

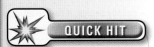

Although 90% of in situ carcinoma is of the ductal variety, LCIS has a higher chance of being multifocal, including the contralateral breast.

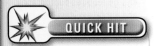

Breast cancer is second only to skin cancer as the most common malignancy in women. There were 230,400 new cases and 39,500 deaths in 2011.

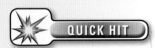

Increased incidence of breast cancer is related to greater prevalence and access to screening and therefore earlier detection of in situ lesions.

      iii. **Complex sclerosing adenosis:** tubules trapped in dense stroma; mimics carcinoma

      iv. **Papillomas:** intraductal growths within major lactiferous ducts between ages 30 and 50 years with serous or serosanguineous drainage

3. **Proliferative** lesions with **atypia**

   a. Ductal epithelial hyperplasia with cytologic atypia: 5-fold increase risk

   b. Lobular hyperplasia with cytologic atypia

4. **In situ lesions:** malignant cells replace normal lining of ducts or lobules, but basement membrane remains intact; 10-year risk of developing invasive carcinoma = 5%

   a. **Ductal carcinoma in situ (DCIS)**

   b. **Lobular carcinoma in situ (LCIS):** obliteration of gland lumens with neoplastic cells

IV. Breast Cancer

A. Overview

  1. #2 most common cancer in women; lifetime risk = 1:8

  2. #2 leading cause of cancer-related deaths in women; lifetime risk = 1:28

  3. Increasing incidence

  4. Decreasing mortality

  5. Characteristics of malignant breast mass

    a. Size >2 cm

    b. Immobile

    c. Poorly defined margins (not circumscribed)

    d. Firm

    e. Skin dimpling

    f. Nipple retraction or redness/itching/scaliness of areola (**Paget disease**)

    g. Ipsilateral lymphadenopathy

    h. Bloody nipple discharge

  6. Growth rate thought to be constant from origin

  7. On average, takes 5–7 years to become palpable

B. Risk factors

  1. Age: single greatest risk factor (except for gender)

    a. Risk increases with age

    b. Most cancers occur after age 50 years

  2. Race: Caucasians at greater risk than Hispanics, Asians, or African Americans

  3. Family history: 1st-degree relative (parent, sibling, offspring) confers greater risk

  4. Genetic predisposition

    a. *BRCA1* genetic mutation

      i. On 17q21 chromosome

      ii. Linked to 50% of early-onset breast cancers and 90% of hereditary ovarian cancers

    b. *BRCA2* genetic mutation

      i. On 13q12–13 chromosome

      ii. Associated with 35% early breast cancers; much lower risk of ovarian cancer than BRCA1

  5. Reproductive and menstrual history

    a. Early menarche (before age 12 years) and late menopause (after age 55 years)

    b. Delayed childbearing and nulliparity

  6. Radiation exposure

    a. Takes 5–10 years after exposure for cancer to develop

    b. Radiation therapy: such as for Hodgkin disease or enlarged thymus gland

    c. No significant increased risk for cumulative radiation dose <20 cGy

  7. Breast changes

    a. Dense breast tissue may be risk factor but clearly makes palpation and imaging more difficult

    b. Prior breast biopsy revealing atypical hyperplasia or in situ carcinoma

8. Other
   a. Overweight after menopause
   b. Alcohol consumption
9. 75% of patients with breast cancer have no identifiable risk factor
10. Personal history of invasive carcinoma: risk of developing 2nd invasive carcinoma in remaining breast or contralateral breast = 1% per year for premenopausal women and 0.5% per year for postmenopausal women

C. **Gail model:** breast cancer risk assessment tool
   1. Developed by National Cancer Institute to estimate risk for next 5 years and lifetime (up to age 90 years)
   2. Falsely increased in patients with multiple biopsies and limited value in patients with 2nd-degree relatives with breast cancer
   3. 7 factors used: history of LCIS/DCIS, age, menarche, age at 1st childbirth, number of 1st-degree relatives with breast cancer, history of breast biopsy, race/ethnicity
   4. High risk = 5-year risk exceeds 1.7%; possible candidate for prophylactic therapy
      a. Chemoprevention with SERMs (tamoxifen or raloxifene)
      b. Prophylactic mastectomy

D. Three histologic types of breast cancer (Table 35.2)
   1. Ductal: 75%–80% of breast cancers
      a. DCIS (stage 0)
      b. Infiltrating ductal carcinoma
   2. Lobular: more often bilateral/multicentric
      a. LCIS (stage 0)
      b. Infiltrating lobular carcinoma
   3. Nipple (**Paget disease**)
      a. Starts as intraductal carcinoma and presents as superficial skin lesion similar to eczema (3% of cases)
      b. Essentially 100% association with underlying breast carcinoma

E. Staging
   1. **TNM** system (American Joint Committee on Cancer)
      a. Characteristics of primary **T**umor
      b. Involvement of regional lymph **N**odes
      c. Presence of distant **M**etastases
   2. In addition to stage, receptor status is important prognostic factor
      a. Expression of estrogen or progesterone receptors positively affects prognosis
      b. Overexpression of **HER2/neu** (or c-erb-B2) oncogene confers poor prognosis (present in 20%–30% of invasive ductal cancers)

F. Spread by local infiltration, lymphatic, and hematogenous routes
   a. Lymphatic spread
      i. Mainly to axillary nodes
      ii. Supraclavicular spread only after axillary involvement

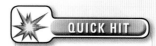
QUICK HIT Decreasing mortality from breast cancer is due to earlier diagnosis and improvement in treatment.

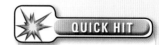
QUICK HIT Women of Ashkenazi Jewish descent have a higher prevalence of both BRCA gene mutations.

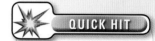
QUICK HIT Between ages 40 and 49 years, a woman has a 1.4% chance of developing breast cancer; between ages 60 and 69 years, that risk increases to 3.7%.

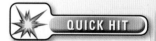
QUICK HIT Strong family history or breast cancer diagnosed before age 40 years should lead to genetic evaluation for *BRCA1* or *BRCA2* mutation.

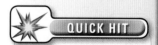
QUICK HIT Women who drink 2–4 alcoholic beverages per week have a 30% greater risk of dying from breast cancer than do women who never consume alcohol.

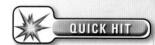
QUICK HIT Of patients with breast cancer, 75% have no identifiable risk factor.

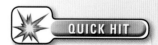
QUICK HIT The American Joint Committee on Cancer classifies most breast malignancies into three histologic categories according to their cells of origin: ductal, lobular, or nipple.

TABLE 35.2 Major Differences Between Ductal Carcinoma In Situ (DCIS) and Lobular Carcinoma In Situ (LCIS)

	DCIS	LCIS
Structure involved	Ducts	Lobules
Type of subsequent cancer	Ductal	Ductal or lobular
Breast at risk for invasive cancer	Ipsilateral breast	Either breast
Laterality	Unilateral	Often bilateral
Number of sites of origin	Unicentric	Multicentric

(From Beckmann CRB, Ling FW, et al. *Obstetrics and Gynecology*, 7th ed. Baltimore: Lippincott Williams & Wilkins; 2014.)

TABLE 35.3	**Treatment of Breast Cancer by Stage**	
Stage	**Surgery**	**Adjuvant Treatment**
0	DCIS: Breast-conserving surgery OR total mastectomy LCIS: Prophylactic mastectomy	With or without radiation and/or tamoxifen Observation or tamoxifen as alternatives to surgery
I	Breast-conserving surgery OR modified radical mastectomy OR sentinel lymph node biopsy followed by surgery	Radiation, chemotherapy, hormone therapy
II	Breast-conserving surgery OR modified radical mastectomy OR sentinel lymph node biopsy followed by surgery	Radiation, chemotherapy, hormone therapy
IIIA	Breast-conserving surgery OR modified radical mastectomy OR sentinel lymph node biopsy followed by surgery	Radiation, chemotherapy, hormone therapy
IIIB	Breast-conserving surgery OR total mastectomy (after chemotherapy)	Chemotherapy pre-op, radiation/hormone therapy post-op
IIIC	(Operable) Breast-conserving surgery OR modified radical mastectomy OR sentinel lymph node biopsy followed by surgery	Radiation, chemotherapy, hormone therapy
IIIC	(Inoperable) Breast-conserving surgery OR total mastectomy (after chemotherapy)	Chemotherapy pre-op, radiation/hormone therapy post-op
IV	Breast-conserving surgery OR total mastectomy (after chemotherapy)	Chemotherapy pre-op, radiation/hormone therapy post-op

Breast Disorders

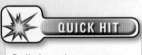

Radiation + lumpectomy has outcomes comparable to radical mastectomy.

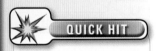

Breast reconstruction should be an option for all women who desire it.

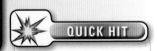

The most important prognostic indicator of breast cancer is axillary lymph node status.

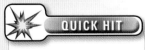

Evaluation of breast mass in pregnancy should *not* be delayed until after pregnancy.

b. Hematogenous spread mainly to lungs and liver; also bone, brain, ovaries, pleura, adrenals
c. Local spread to skin (blockage of skin lymphatics causes lymphedema and thickening of skin (**peau d'orange**) — inflammatory breast cancer
  i. 1%–5% of all breast cancers
  ii. Most are invasive ductal carcinomas
  iii. Stage III or IV at diagnosis
  iv. Median age of 57 compared to 62 for other types of breast cancer
  v. More common in African American women (median age 54)
G. Treatment (Table 35.3)
  1. Risks of cancer: both local/regional (including lymph nodes) and systemic
  2. Surgical management aimed at local control
    a. Lumpectomy (breast conservation surgery)
    b. Mastectomy (removal of all breast tissue, nipple areolar complex, preservation of pectoralis muscles)
    c. Modified radical mastectomy also removes axillary lymph nodes
  3. Radiation
    a. In conjunction with lumpectomy or partial mastectomy for early stages
    b. In conjunction with mastectomy for late stages
    c. Can be given if breast reconstruction has taken place
  4. Adjuvant (systemic) therapy used in all stages regardless of lymph node status
    a. Chemotherapy that kills cancer cells
    b. Hormonal therapy (e.g., tamoxifen) acting as estrogen antagonists
      i. Used to treat estrogen receptor–positive cancer
      ii. Typically used for 5 years
    c. Aromatase inhibitors: prevent estrogen production
      i. Used to treat estrogen receptor–positive cancer
      ii. Extend survival in metastatic cancer cases
    d. Trastuzumab (Herceptin) used in cases of HER2/neu overexpression
  5. Breast reconstruction: can take place immediately or be delayed
    a. Implants
    b. Surgical flaps (e.g., using rectus muscle)
    c. Microvascular reconstructive surgery

H. Recurrence: most occur within 1st 5 years

I. Prognosis: status of axillary lymph nodes most important prognostic indicator; also related to age and stage of disease

V. Breast Cancer in Pregnancy

A. 1 in 3,000 pregnancies; 3% of all breast cancers

B. Delayed diagnosis due to difficulty in palpating

C. Treatment similar to nonpregnant patients

    1. Surgical management is same

    2. Postoperative radiation delayed until after pregnancy

    3. For patients with nodal metastases, adjuvant chemotherapy can potentially be given in 2nd and 3rd trimester

D. Prognosis not much worse than nonpregnant cancer

VI. Screening Guidelines

A. Recommendations vary among professional organizations

B. Breast self-examination recommended by American College of Obstetricians and Gynecologists (the College) but not by U.S. Preventive Services Task Force (USPSTF)

C. Clinical breast examination supported (annually after age 40 years, every 3 years from ages 20–39 years)

D. Mammography value increases with age

    1. Yearly after age 50 years agreed upon, but controversial before then: every 1–2 years between ages 40 and 49 years

    2. Women with inherited genetic mutations: cancers missed 50% of time with mammography screening only

        a. MRI recommended as supplement to mammography

        b. Screening should start at age 25 years or 5–10 years before age of diagnosis in youngest 1st-degree relative

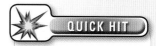

QUICK HIT

There is no reason to advise against subsequent pregnancy if there is no evidence of breast cancer recurrence.

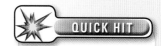

QUICK HIT

Breast cancer screening includes self-exam, clinical exam, and mammography.

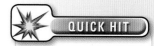

QUICK HIT

In women with inherited genetic mutations (such as *BRCA1* or *BRCA2*), breast cancer screening should start at age 25 years or 5–10 years before age of diagnosis in the youngest first-degree relative with breast cancer.

Breast Disorders

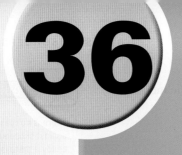

36 Gynecologic Procedures

I. Genital Tract Biopsy

A. Vulvar biopsy (punch biopsy of skin of vulva)
  1. Indication: any new lesion, lesion started changing color or size
  2. Technique: 3–5-mm circular hollow device removes small disk of tissue (punch) under local anesthesia

B. Vaginal biopsy
  1. Indication: any visible lesion, Bartholin gland duct cyst, or abscess (especially age >40 years)
  2. Technique: biopsy forceps; topical anesthesia as needed

C. Cervical biopsy
  1. Indications
    a. Abnormal Pap smear (cervical cytology)
    b. Any grossly abnormal lesion (even with negative Pap)
  2. Technique
    a. Colposcopy (see the following) is used to identify area to biopsy
    b. Biopsy forceps; no anesthesia needed
    c. Silver nitrate or Monsel solution used for hemostasis

D. Endometrial biopsy
  1. Indication (see also Chapter 40)
    a. Any woman with abnormal uterine bleeding (AUB) age ≥40 years
    b. AUB at any age with risk factors for endometrial neoplasia
      i. Chronic anovulation
      ii. Obesity
      iii. Tamoxifen therapy
    c. AUB age <40 years if medical management has failed
    d. Any bleeding in postmenopausal woman
  2. Techniques
    a. Pipelle
      i. Plastic cannula aspirates tissue by creating small negative pressure; no need for anesthesia
      ii. Sensitivity of diagnosing endometrial cancer = 97.5%
    b. Dilatation (or dilation) and curettage (D&C)
      i. After dilating cervix, scrape endometrial cavity under anesthesia
      ii. Also used for incomplete/missed/elective abortion
    c. Pelvic ultrasound: can be used to determine endometrial stripe (EMS) thickness
      i. EMS ≤4 mm in postmenopausal woman excludes pathology
      ii. EMS >4 mm in postmenopausal woman is abnormal and requires tissue evaluation
    d. Saline infusion sonohysterography ([SHG] see XII.5 for description): useful to image endometrial cavity (e.g., polyps and submucosal leiomyomas)

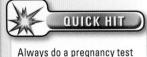

QUICK HIT

Always do a pregnancy test for women of reproductive age before the endometrial biopsy.

Gynecologic Procedures

II. Colposcopy

A. Special binocular lens to magnify cervix

B. Identifies precancerous or cancerous lesions in woman with abnormal Pap smear

C. Special stains applied to cervix
1. 5% **acetic acid**: dysplastic areas turn white because of high protein content
2. **Lugol solution** (strong iodine): glycogen in normal squamous cells turns black, and areas of dysplasia fail to take up stain

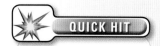

QUICK HIT

Colposcopy is indicated after any abnormal Pap smear or in women with a negative Pap smear but who are persistently high-risk human papillomavirus (HPV) positive.

III. Cervical Cone Biopsy (Conization)

A. Removing transformation zone with part of endocervical canal in it; cone-shaped specimen

B. Indications
1. High-grade cervical dysplasia on either Pap smear or cervical biopsy (both diagnostic and therapeutic)
2. Discrepancy between Pap smear and cervical biopsy (unexplained abnormal Pap)
3. Unsatisfactory colposcopy exam (not being able to visualize entire cervical lesion or entire transformation zone)
4. Endocervical neoplasia on biopsy or endocervical curettage
5. Colposcopy with lesion suspicious for invasive cancer
6. Cervical biopsy revealing microinvasion: need cone biopsy to exclude invasion somewhere else on cervix

C. Techniques
1. **Cold knife cone (CKC)**: using scalpel to remove cone-shaped specimen under anesthesia
2. **Loop electrosurgical excision procedure (LEEP)**: using monopolar energy on semicircular wire to remove cone-shaped specimen (also called **large loop excision of transformation zone [LLETZ]**); can be done in office with local anesthesia

D. Comparison and complications
1. Neither superior in diagnosis or treatment of cervical dysplasia
2. Long-term possible complications of either is cervical stenosis or cervical insufficiency (incompetence)

IV. Hysteroscopy

A. Indications (see Chapter 40)
1. View and remove endometrial or endocervical polyps
2. Adhesiolysis for intrauterine adhesions (Asherman syndrome)
3. Remove submucosal leiomyomas (uterine fibroids)
4. Placing permanent sterilization devices (metal coils) in fallopian tubes (Essure™ procedure)
5. Inspection prior to endometrial ablation
6. For diagnosis and evaluation of AUB

B. Technique
1. Introduce camera with fiberoptic light source into endometrial cavity with help of distention material such as fluid or gas to visualize cavity
2. Diagnostic hysteroscopy can be done in office setting; operative hysteroscopy is done in operating room under anesthesia

V. Cryotherapy

A. Indications: mild cervical dysplasia, vulvar or vaginal condyloma

B. Technique: destroys tissue by freezing with probe

C. Destructive procedure only (i.e., in contrast to LEEP where tissue specimen is generated for pathologic examination and margins of specimen are examined)

VI. Laser

A. Indications: vulvar or vaginal condyloma, vulvar or vaginal intraepithelial neoplasia, vulvar dermatologic disorders

Gynecologic Procedures

B. Technique: vaporizes tissue by light beam using 1 of following sources
   1. CO_2
   2. Yttrium aluminum garnet (YAG)
   3. Argon
   4. Potassium titanyl phosphate (KTP)
C. Destructive procedure only (no tissue specimen)

VII. Pregnancy Termination

A. Planned interruption of pregnancy
   1. Missed abortion (early fetal demise)
   2. Anembryonic gestation (no fetal pole present, just empty sac)
   3. Incomplete abortion (spontaneous but incomplete passage of products of conception leading to heavy bleeding)
   4. Hydatidiform mole or partial mole
   5. Elective or secondary to fetal anomalies
B. Techniques
   1. Surgical
      a. Suction curettage: after dilating cervix, negative pressure applied to curette in intrauterine cavity to evacuate products of conception
      b. D&C: manually scraping uterine cavity
      c. **Dilatation and evacuation:** 2nd-trimester abortion technique; removing products of conception in small pieces through partially dilated cervix
   2. Medical
      a. Vaginal misoprostol
      b. Vaginal misoprostol + mifepristone tablet orally
      c. Misoprostol and mifepristone tablets, both orally

VIII. Endometrial Ablation

A. Indications
   1. Women with menorrhagia who no longer desire future fertility
   2. Endometrial biopsy done prior to rule out endometrial neoplasia (hyperplasia)
   3. Success rates after ablation measured with 2 parameters: amenorrhea rate (generally 30%) and patient satisfaction rate (majority of women experience less bleeding)
B. Techniques (none clearly superior)
   1. **Thermal balloon:** 5-mm probe with attached balloon introduced into uterine cavity then expanded with heated fluid to conform to cavity
   2. **Cryoablation:** 5.5-mm probe with liquid nitrogen coolant introduced into endometrial cavity until ice ball forms
   3. Bipolar **radiofrequency** ablation: 7.5-mm probe opened inside endometrial cavity like umbrella to draw endometrium to device
   4. **Microwave** ablation: 8.8-mm probe delivers microwave energy to endometrial cavity
   5. **Hydrothermal** ablation: heated saline is introduced into endometrial cavity under direct visualization to observe cavity change from red to white
   6. **Electrosurgical** ablation
      a. Rollerball device desiccates endometrium under direct visualization
      b. Fan-shaped metal device expanded within endometrial cavity, and electrical current applied simultaneously
C. Complications: endometritis, uterine perforation, surrounding organ damage, instrument malfunctions
D. Contraindications
   1. Women planning future pregnancies
   2. Endometrial cavity measures >10 cm
   3. Endometrial neoplasia
   4. Intracavitary fibroid >3 cm or cavity significantly distorted

IX. Hysterectomy

A. General
1. >600,000 hysterectomies performed annually in United States
2. Hysterectomy-related mortality is 1/1,000

B. Reasons for hysterectomy
1. 43% for symptomatic leiomyomata
2. 20% endometriosis
3. 20% pelvic organ prolapse
4. 17% other, including malignancies

C. Indications
1. Abnormal bleeding refractory to medical management
2. Pelvic pain and dysmenorrhea refractory to medical management
3. Endometriosis that has failed other therapy
4. Tubo-ovarian abscess that fails medical treatment
5. Persistent or recurrent cervical intraepithelial neoplasia 2 or 3 after LEEP/CKC
6. Patients with uterine prolapse (**procidentia**)
7. Endometrial **hyperplasia with atypia** and endometrial carcinoma
8. Uterine leiomyosarcoma or endometrial stromal sarcoma
9. Selected cervical and ovarian cancer cases

D. Complications
1. Most frequent is pelvic infection from vaginal flora
2. Ureteral injury
3. Bladder injury or vesicovaginal fistula
4. Bowel injury or rectovaginal fistula
5. Bleeding
6. Anesthesia-related complications
7. Intra- or postoperative thromboembolic events

E. Terminology
1. **Total hysterectomy:** removing uterus and cervix
2. **Subtotal hysterectomy (supracervical hysterectomy):** removing uterus but preserving cervix and its attachments (uterosacral ligaments)
   a. Shortens surgical time and decreases blood loss
   b. Less risk of ureteral or bladder injury
   c. Risk of cervical cancer in the future is still present
   d. Some patients can still have vaginal bleeding
   e. No evidence that this improves sexual function
3. **Simple hysterectomy:** removing uterus and cervix only (also a **total hysterectomy**), but term used to differentiate from "radical" (see the following)
4. **Radical hysterectomy:** removing uterus and cervix and surrounding tissue
   a. Depending on type, removing more of uterosacral ligament, cardinal ligament (toward lateral pelvic wall), parametrium, upper part of vagina
   b. Required in certain types of gynecologic cancers; most commonly for cervical carcinoma
5. Hysterectomy + **bilateral salpingo-oophorectomy (BSO):** removing uterus, cervix, along with both fallopian tubes and ovaries
   a. **Elective oophorectomy:** during hysterectomy, removing normal-looking ovaries to prevent future ovarian cancer
   b. **Incidental oophorectomy:** during hysterectomy, pathology is found in ovaries, necessitating removal
6. **Cesarean hysterectomy:** during Cesarean delivery, hysterectomy may become necessary for following indications
   a. Uterine rupture and inability to repair defects
   b. Laceration of uterine vessels and inability to control bleeding
   c. **Placenta previa** and inability to remove placenta
   d. **Placenta accreta** (placenta growing deep into myometrium)
   e. Placental abruption and inability to control bleeding

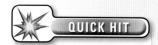

QUICK HIT

Patients with adenomyosis commonly do not respond to medical therapies and opt for hysterectomy.

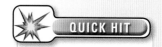

QUICK HIT

Any woman age >40 years with abnormal vaginal bleeding requires endometrial biopsy before hysterectomy to rule out malignancy.

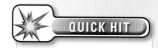

QUICK HIT

Hysterectomies are classified as "clean-contaminated surgery cases" because the vaginal cuff has to be opened to remove the cervix or the surgery is done through the vagina; therefore, prophylactic antibiotic treatment is always indicated 30 minutes before the incision.

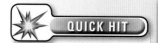

QUICK HIT

Patients often *incorrectly* think that "total" or "complete" hysterectomy means that tubes and ovaries are also removed.

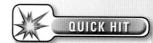

QUICK HIT

The lifetime risk of ovarian cancer is 1/70 women.

Gynecologic Procedures

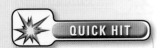

QUICK HIT

A vertical skin incision is done whenever the diagnosis is uncertain because it provides the maximum amount of exposure (e.g., pelvic mass that may be an ovarian malignancy).

f. **Uterine atony** that has not responded to medical therapy
g. Cervical cancer diagnosed during pregnancy

F. Classification: based on surgical approach
1. **Abdominal hysterectomy (total abdominal hysterectomy [TAH])**: 66% of hysterectomies done with abdominal incision (i.e., either midline vertical or transverse incision)
2. **Vaginal hysterectomy (total vaginal hysterectomy [TVH])**: 22% of hysterectomies done with all-vaginal approach
   a. Preferred for mobile and minimally enlarged uterus and in pelvic prolapse cases
   b. Not preferred for very large uterus, adnexal masses, or when pelvic adhesions are likely (e.g., endometriosis)
   c. If BSO is planned, ovaries can be removed vaginally about 90% of the time
   d. Postoperative recovery is shorter because no abdominal incision
3. Minimally invasive hysterectomies: 12% of hysterectomies done with minimally invasive surgery (MIS) techniques
   a. Number quickly increasing as technology improves and more surgeons receive specialized training
   b. At start of procedure, carbon dioxide is used to distend peritoneal cavity to gain better visualization and provide enough room to manipulate instruments
   c. Laparoscopic hysterectomies: performed by introducing pencil-size trocars into abdominal cavity to free uterus, which can either be removed vaginally or morcellated into small pieces and removed via abdominal trocars

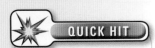

QUICK HIT

Because of superior visualization with 3-D technology and increased manual dexterity, many cases that formerly would not have been eligible for laparoscopic procedures can now be done with the robot to achieve a minimally invasive approach.

   i. **Total laparoscopic hysterectomy (TLH)**: uterus freed, uterine artery ligated, and vaginal cuff closed laparoscopically
   ii. **Laparoscopic-assisted vaginal hysterectomy (LAVH)**: uterus freed, uterine artery ligated laparoscopically or vaginally, and cuff closed vaginally
   iii. **Robotic hysterectomy (RH)**: after laparoscopic trocars are introduced into abdomen, robotic arms are connected to trocars, and surgery is done by surgeon sitting at console (away from patient); can be done as TLH or completed vaginally
4. Comparison of approaches (Table 36.1): meta-analyses of different approaches have shown that vaginal route should be 1st choice if patient is appropriate candidate

X. Preoperative Evaluation

A. Workup
1. Detailed history and physical examination to assess surgical risk and medical comorbidities
2. Endometrial biopsy
3. Pap smear
4. Pregnancy test

TABLE 36.1	Comparisons of Routes of Hysterectomy		
Comparative Factor	**Abdominal Hysterectomy**	**Vaginal Hysterectomy**	**Laparoscopic Hysterectomy**
Operating time	Average	Least	Longest
Hospital stay	3 days	Overnight/same day	Overnight/same day
Recovery	Long	Short	Short
Blood loss	Most	Less	Least

5. Laboratory tests
   a. Complete blood count to correct anemia or diagnose possible thrombocytopenia
   b. Creatinine for diabetic or hypertensive patients
   c. Coagulation studies if indicated
   d. Selected cases may require preoperative intravenous (IV) pyelogram, mammography (MMG), pulmonary function tests, colonoscopy, cystoscopy
6. Electrocardiography (Echo) in patients with history of heart disease or risk factors
7. Chest film for smokers and those suspected to have pulmonary disease
8. Imaging studies (if abnormal uterine anatomy or adnexal pathology): ultrasound, computed tomography (CT) scan, or magnetic resonance imaging (MRI)

B. Informed consent should include
1. Risks, benefits, and planned outcomes
2. Alternatives to planned procedure
3. Documentation of completion of childbearing especially before hysterectomy cases
4. Discussion of risks and benefits of prophylactic oophorectomy
5. Discussion of possible intraoperative incidental findings and how to approach them
6. All questions need to be answered to patient's satisfaction
7. Document whether patient will accept blood products; if so, explain risks involved with transfusion (e.g., fever, transfusion reaction, heart failure, hepatitis, human immunodeficiency virus, West Nile virus)

C. Review current medications
1. Nonsteroidal anti-inflammatory drugs, acetylsalicylic acid
   a. Decrease thromboxane A_2 production, which increases intraoperative bleeding
   b. Stop these medications 1 week before surgery
2. Vitamin E: stop 14 days before surgery to prevent intraoperative bleeding
3. Chronic steroid users will need stress doses of steroids before surgery
4. If patient is on β-blockers, they should be continued on day of surgery

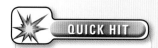

QUICK HIT

Preoperative discussions need to include contingency plans. For example, a patient with secondary dysmenorrhea refractory to medical management may want to keep her ovaries if there is no extrauterine pathology, but may want to have a BSO if endometriosis is found at the time of surgery.

XI. Postoperative Evaluation

A. Starts with operative note
1. Pre- and postoperative diagnosis
2. Type of anesthesia
3. Procedures performed
4. Detailed description of entire operation
5. Estimated blood loss
6. Amount and type of fluid including blood products/colloid given
7. Intraoperative urine output
8. Intraoperative findings
9. Specimens sent to pathology
10. Complications
11. Patient's condition at end of procedure

B. Postoperative orders
1. Name of surgery team and service
2. Vital signs and IV fluid monitoring orders
3. Foley catheter and output monitoring instructions
4. Diet, physical activity, incentive spirometry, deep vein thrombosis (DVT) prophylaxis
5. Necessary labs
6. Resume medications that patient was on prior to surgery

C. Postoperative complications
1. Common: fever (2 oral temperatures ≥38°C at 4-hour intervals), urinary tract infection, surgical site drainage/bleeding/infection, skin separation, hemorrhage, pneumonia, ileus

Gynecologic Procedures

2. Rare: wound evisceration, bowel perforation, urinary tract injury, DVT, pulmonary embolism, abscess, sepsis, fistulas, anesthetic reactions

XII. Imaging Studies

A. Ultrasound
1. Uses high-frequency sound waves to identify abdominal and pelvic anatomy
2. Also differentiates between solid and fluid-filled masses
3. **Transvaginal ultrasound**
   a. Higher frequency, shorter depth of penetration
   b. Better visualization of cervix, uterus, and adnexa
4. **Transabdominal ultrasound**
   a. Increased depth of penetration
   b. Better visualization of pelvic masses extending into abdomen
5. **SHG**
   a. 7 French balloon catheter introduced through cervix into uterine cavity then 10–20 mL of sterile saline injected through catheter under direct transvaginal ultrasound
   b. Evaluates size and shape of endometrial cavity
   c. Allows identification of mass-occupying lesions within endometrial cavity (e.g., endometrial polyps or submucosal leiomyomata)

B. CT scan
1. Provides constructed cross-sectional images with or without enhancement of oral and/or IV contrast agents
2. More frequently used in gynecologic oncology cases to evaluate for abdominal metastasis, enlarged lymph nodes, renal function, and patency of ureters or to plan field of radiation therapy

C. MRI: based on magnetic characteristics of atoms and molecules in area of interest, useful to distinguish different types of tissue (e.g., ovaries *versus* uterus)

D. Breast imaging (see Chapter 35)

E. Hysterosalpingography
1. Technique: radio-opaque dye injected through cervix, and using fluoroscopic imaging, can follow contrast medium into endometrial cavity and fallopian tubes to ascertain whether dye spills into peritoneal cavity (patent tubes)
2. Indications
   a. Infertility evaluations to assess tubal patency
   b. Evaluate size and shape of endometrial cavity
   c. Intrauterine adhesions

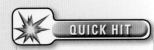

QUICK HIT

Ultrasound is a very cost-effective technique and the most commonly used imaging in obstetrics and gynecology.

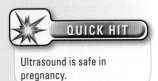

QUICK HIT

Ultrasound is safe in pregnancy.

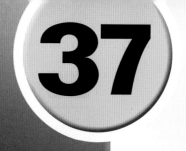

Sexual Function and Dysfunction

I. Sexual Problems

A. Prevalence = up to 40% in U.S. women

B. Important predictor of quality of life for men and women

C. Physicians must be able to identify sexual dysfunction and either treat or refer to subspecialist for management

D. Very dependent on cultural, societal, and personal health and psychological factors

E. Approach must be nonthreatening, nonjudgmental; good physician–patient relationship is paramount

F. Determinants of healthy sexuality are complex
  1. Intrapersonal factors
     a. Sense of self as sexual being
     b. Overall health status
     c. General perception of well-being
     d. Quality of previous sexual experiences
  2. Interpersonal factors
     a. Partner's intrapersonal factors
     b. Duration and quality of relationship
     c. Communication styles
     d. Ongoing life events and stressors

G. Sexual identity
  1. Genotype
  2. Phenotype
  3. Gender identity: early childhood
  4. Sexual orientation: can vary across time or be bisexual

II. Normal Sexual Response

A. Masters and Johnson (1966) (Figure 37.1): 4-stage model (with desire = 5 stages)
  1. Desire
     a. Spontaneous
     b. Characterized by fantasies
     c. Genital tingling
     d. Overall receptiveness to sexual activity
  2. Excitement/arousal
     a. Pelvic, vulvar, and vaginal vasocongestion
     b. Vaginal lubrication
     c. Vaginal lengthening and dilatation
     d. Increased clitoral length and diameter
     e. Increased heart rate, blood pressure, and respiration
     f. Generalized flushing
     g. Nipple engorgement
     h. Increased muscle tension might be noted
  3. Plateau
     a. Maintenance of high level of arousal as orgasm approaches
     b. Intensity of arousal is highly variable

FIGURE
37.1 **Male and female sexual response patterns.**

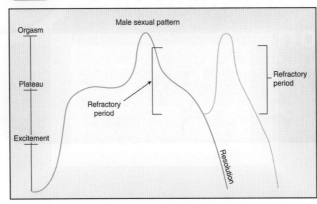

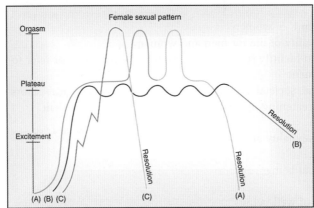

There are three female patterns shown. (*A*) Steady progression to plateau stage is followed by intense orgasm; subsequent orgasms may occur; resolution is slower. (*B*) Slower progression to plateau stage is followed by minor surges toward orgasm, causing prolonged pleasurable feelings without definitive orgasm; resolution is slowest. (*C*) Rapid progression to plateau stage with some peaks and dips; one intense orgasm follows with rapid resolution. This most closely resembles the male pattern. (From Taylor CR, Lillis C, et al. *Fundamentals of Nursing: The Art and Science of Nursing Care*, 6th ed. Philadelphia: Lippincott Williams & Wilkins; 2008.)

4. Orgasm
   a. Increased vasocongestion and muscle tension
   b. Rhythmic, involuntary contractions of outer 1/3 of vagina and pelvic floor
5. Resolution
   a. Gradual return to unstimulated anatomy and physiology
   b. Outcome of experience strongly motivates desire to repeat
B. Basson intimacy-based model (2005) (Figure 37.2)
   1. Primary motivation is often to be "closer" to partner
   2. Desire and arousal overlap
   3. Spontaneous desire common early in relationships or after absence
   4. Related to menstrual cycle and highly variable
   5. Spontaneous desire may be lacking or follow onset of arousal
   6. May become desirous of sexual activity *after* arousing stimuli are noted
   7. When positive experiences occur, motivation to continue to repeat activity increases as in positive feedback loop
   8. Orgasm not necessary for satisfaction for some women
C. Both models note complex interplay of biologic, physiologic, and psychological factors dependent on cultural, societal, and personal factors

III. Physiology of Female Sexual Response
A. General
   1. Complex interactions not yet clearly defined
   2. Some augment and others impede various stages in sexual response cycle

FIGURE 37.2 Negative and positive feedback loops on sexual function.

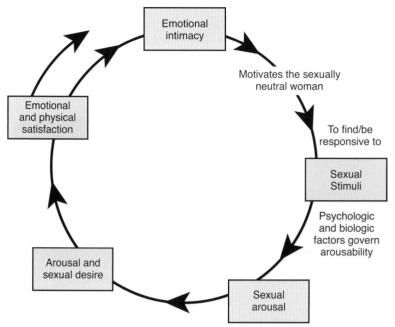

(From Basson R. Female sexual response: the role of drugs in the management of sexual dysfunction. *Obstet Gynecol.* 2001;98:350–359.)

B. Components
   1. Mental sexual excitement
   2. Vulvar congestion
   3. Pleasure from stimulation causing vulvar engorgement
   4. Vaginal congestion
   5. Pleasure from stimulation to congested vaginal walls
   6. Increased and modified lubrication
   7. Vaginal nonvascular smooth muscle relaxation
   8. Pleasure from stimulating nongenital areas of body (other erogenous zones)
   9. Somatic changes (increased activity of autonomic system)
      a. Increased blood pressure
      b. Increased heart rate
      c. Increased muscle tone
      d. Increased respiratory rate
      e. Increased temperature from energy output
C. Mediators
   1. Positive effects through 5-hydroxytryptamine (5-HT) 1A and 2C
      a. Norepinephrine
      b. Dopamine
      c. Oxytocin
      d. Serotonin
   2. Negative effects through other receptors
      a. Serotonin
      b. Prolactin
      c. γ-Aminobutyric acid (GABA)
   3. Parasympathetic-mediated vasodilatation
      a. Nitric oxide (NO)
      b. Acetylcholine
      c. Vasoactive intestinal peptide (VIP)
   4. Also present in genital tissues
      a. Neuropeptide Y (NPY)
      b. VIP
      c. Calcitonin gene-related peptide (CGRP)
      d. Substance P

5. Estrogen: important for vaginal tissue health
   a. Thickness of squamous epithelium
   b. Underlying vascularity
6. Testosterone: contributes to sexual desire
   a. Serum levels not predictive of effect (can be used for monitoring therapy)
   b. Response to exogenous testosterone not predictable

IV. Definitions of Sexual Dysfunction *(Table 37.1)*

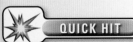

QUICK HIT

Each sexual dysfunction definition becomes a "disorder" *only* when the symptom *causes marked distress or interpersonal difficulty.*

TABLE 37.1 Types of Female Sexual Dysfunction

	Disorder	Description
Sexual desire disorders	Hypoactive sexual desire disorder	Absence or deficiency of sexual fantasies/thoughts or desire for or receptivity to sexual activity
	Sexual aversion disorder	Aversion to and avoidance of genital sexual contact with partner
Sexual arousal disorders	Female sexual arousal disorder	Inability to attain or maintain adequate lubrication/swelling response of sexual excitement
Orgasmic disorders	Female orgasmic disorder	Delay in or absence of orgasm after a normal sexual excitement phase
Pain disorders	Dyspareunia	Genital pain associated with sexual intercourse
	Vaginismus	Involuntary contraction of the perineal muscles preventing vaginal penetration

(Data from the American Psychiatric Association. *Diagnostic and Statistical Manual of Mental Disorders: DSM-IV-TR,* 4th rev ed. Washington, DC: American Psychiatric Association; 2000.)

V. Factors That Affect Sexual Function

A. Depression
   1. ~1/3 of women presenting with sexual dysfunction are clinically depressed
   2. Depression itself causes reduced sexual desire and response
   3. Selective serotonin reuptake inhibitors (SSRIs) and antidepressants that activate other 5-HT and GABA receptors (e.g., benzodiazepines): may have negative impact on
      a. Sexual desire
      b. Sexual arousal
      c. Ability to reach orgasm
   4. Antidepressants that activate dopaminergic, noradrenergic, and 5-HT1A and 5-HT2C receptors (e.g., bupropion, aripiprazole): may have positive effect on sexual response
   5. Least likely to interfere with sexual response
      a. Nefazodone
      b. Mirtazapine
      c. Venlafaxine
      d. Bupropion
      e. Aripiprazole
      f. Buspirone

B. Menopausal status
   1. Estrogen deficiency
      a. Direct effect on vulvar and vaginal tissues: leads to atrophy of epithelium and reduced blood supply
         i. Vaginal dryness
         ii. Dyspareunia

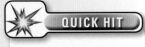

QUICK HIT

Bupropion (Wellbutrin) is often the drug of choice to treat depression in a woman who is also concerned about the impact of treatment on sexual function.

BOX 37.1

Medical Risk Factors for Sexual Disorders

Depression, with or without antidepressants
Breast cancer that required chemotherapy
Radical hysterectomy for cancer of the cervix
Multiple sclerosis
Hypertension
Diabetes
Sexual abuse

(From Beckmann CRB, Ling FW, et al. *Obstetrics and Gynecology*, 7th ed. Baltimore: Lippincott Williams & Wilkins; 2014.)

   b. Indirect effect on mood
   c. Treatment of estrogen deficiency
      i. Systemic estrogen or estrogen + progestin therapy will reverse these lower genital tract changes
      ii. For women who do not require systemic therapy for vasomotor symptoms, topical therapy will correct vaginal atrophy (see Chapter 32)
   2. Testosterone is significantly reduced after menopause (surgical or natural)
C. Medical conditions commonly affecting sexual response: thorough history and physical examination to rule out underlying or concurrent medical conditions (Boxes 37.1 and 37.2)
D. Medications commonly affecting sexual response (Box 37.3)
E. Psychological factors affecting sexual response
   1. Effect cannot be overstated
   2. Continuous and changing modulation of sexual stimuli with direct effect on how (or if) that stimuli is interpreted

BOX 37.2

Conditions Commonly Affecting Sexual Response

Conditions associated with loss of adrenal androgen production and/or loss of estrogen production
• Bilateral salpingo-oophorectomy
• Chemotherapy-induced menopause
• Gonadotropin-releasing hormone–induced menopausal symptoms
• Premature ovarian failure
• Oral estrogen therapy (may cause androgen insufficiency)
• Oral contraceptives (may cause androgen insufficiency)
• Addison disease
• Hypopituitary states
• Hypothalamic amenorrhea
• Chronic renal failure
• Chronic cardiac failure
• Chronic neurologic conditions
• Chronic renal disease
• Arthritis
• Hyperprolactinemia
• Hypothyroid and hyperthyroid states

Conditions interfering with autonomic function +/− somatic genital nerve function
• Diabetes mellitus
• Multiple sclerosis
• Spinal cord injury
• Radical pelvic surgery
• Post Guillain–Barré syndrome

(From Beckmann CRB, Ling FW, et al. *Obstetrics and Gynecology*, 7th ed. Baltimore: Lippincott Williams & Wilkins; 2014.)

BOX 37.3

Medications Commonly Affecting Sexual Response

- Codeine-containing analgesics
- Alcohol (chronic abuse)
- Cyproterone acetate
- Medroxyprogesterone (high doses)
- Some β-blockers used for hypertension or migraine prevention
- Anticonvulsants taken for epilepsy (but not necessarily for other conditions)
- Combination oral contraceptives (via increase in sex hormone–binding globulin)
- Selective estrogen receptor modulators (such as raloxifene, tamoxifen, and phytoestrogens)

(From Beckmann CRB, Ling FW, et al. *Obstetrics and Gynecology*, 7th ed. Baltimore: Lippincott Williams & Wilkins; 2014.)

---

    3. Direct influence on woman's motivation to seek or respond to those stimuli
    4. Stress or distractions will drastically reduce woman's motivation and ability to respond and can completely shut down sexual arousal
  F. Reproduction-related risk factors (Box 37.4)

VI. Screening for Sexual Dysfunction *(Box 37.5)*
  A. Concerns often missed by health care providers
  B. Indication to patient that clinician cares and understands importance of this aspect of overall health
  C. Patient–clinician relationship must establish mutual trust and respect
  D. Confirm confidentiality of patient–clinician discussions
  E. Environment must be conducive to open discussion without distractions
  F. Nonthreatening and nonjudgmental (must include awareness of clinician's own biases)
  G. Use simple terms, visual aids (drawings or models), and treat as any other medical problem with open discussion
  H. Use "partner" instead of husband; use "sexual activity" instead of "intercourse"
  I. Interview should be done with patient clothed

VII. Factors to Consider When Establishing Diagnosis *(Figure 37.3)*
  A. Duration
    1. Lifelong (primary)
    2. Acquired (secondary)
  B. Situation
    1. Specific to certain set of circumstances (partner, place, sexual position, relationship to menstrual cycle)
    2. Generalized/global (with all partners, locations, or alone)

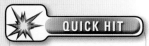

QUICK HIT

Healthy sexuality promotes physical and emotional well-being.

QUICK HIT

Satisfaction with sexual function should routinely be addressed during preventative health maintenance exams because patients will often be reluctant to bring these issues up on their own.

BOX 37.4

Reproductive Issues as Risk Factors for Sexual Disorders

- Healthy pregnancy
- Complicated pregnancy where intercourse and orgasm are precluded
- Postpartum considerations
- Recurrent miscarriage
- Therapeutic abortion
- Infertility
- Perimenopause
- Natural menopause
- Premature menopause (idiopathic and iatrogenic)
- Use of oral contraceptives

(From Beckmann CRB, Ling FW, et al. *Obstetrics and Gynecology*, 7th ed. Baltimore: Lippincott Williams & Wilkins; 2014.)

BOX 37.5

Basic Screening Questions

"Are you sexually active?"

"Are you sexually satisfied?"

"Do you think your partner is satisfied?"

"Do you have questions or concerns about sexual functioning?"

(From Beckmann CRB, Ling FW, et al. *Obstetrics and Gynecology*, 7th ed. Baltimore: Lippincott Williams & Wilkins; 2014.)

C. Orgasm
   1. Coital or noncoital
   2. Clitoral or vaginal
   3. Psychological or physiologic
   4. Of varying importance for women and not necessarily a requirement for sexual satisfaction

VIII. Treatment *(Box 37.6)*
   A. Depends on diagnosis (Table 37.2)
   B. Therapeutic interview and education is essential (and may be all that is required)
   C. Referral may be necessary

FIGURE 37.3 Algorithm for establishing a diagnosis of female sexual dysfunction.

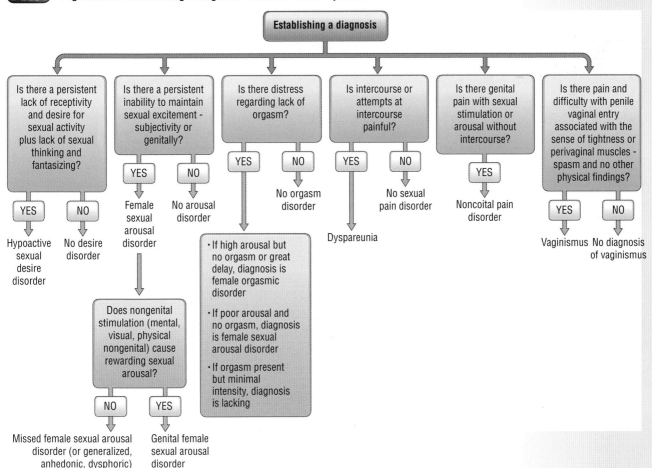

(From Beckmann CRB, Ling FW, et al. *Obstetrics and Gynecology*, 7th ed. Baltimore: Lippincott Williams & Wilkins; 2014.)

BOX 37.6

Primary Care Treatments for Sexual Dysfunction

The decision to refer a patient depends on a number of factors, including:

- Expertise of the obstetrician/gynecologist
- Complexity of the sexual dysfunction
- Presence or absence of partner sexual dysfunction
- Availability of a psychologist, psychiatrist, or sex therapist
- Motivation of the patient (and partner) to undergo more detailed assessments before therapeutic interventions

More detailed assessments and management may be available from:

- Physicians with extra training and expertise in sexuality (e.g., psychiatrists, family practitioners, gynecologists, urologists)
- Psychologists
- Sex therapists and abuse counselors
- Physiotherapists (regarding hypertonic pelvic muscle–associated dyspareunia
- Relationship counselors
- Support groups (e.g., for women with past histories of breast cancer, women with vulvar vestibulitis syndrome–associated chronic dyspareunia, women with interstitial cystitis–associated dyspareunia)

(From Beckmann CRB, Ling FW, et al. *Obstetrics and Gynecology*, 7th ed. Baltimore: Lippincott Williams & Wilkins; 2014.)

TABLE 37.2 Treatment Options for Female Sexual Dysfunction

Disorder	Treatment Options	Important Notes
Hypoactive sexual desire disorder (HSDD)	<ul><li>Therapeutic interview</li><li>Psychotherapy</li><li>Sex therapy</li><li>Marital therapy</li><li>Hormones</li><li>Neuromodulators and antidepressants</li></ul>	<ul><li>No FDA-approved treatment for HSDD</li><li>Estrogen</li><li>Androgens</li><li>Progesterone</li><li>Dopamine/serotonin agonist/antagonists</li><li>Must monitor closely if using medications</li></ul>
Sexual aversion disorder	<ul><li>Cognitive behavioral therapy (CBT)</li><li>Systematic desensitization</li><li>Referral to psychiatrist</li></ul>	<ul><li>Can be quite severe</li><li>May be related to history of sexual abuse</li></ul>
Female sexual arousal disorder	<ul><li>Sensate focus (focus on sexually arousing stimuli)</li><li>Estrogen</li><li>Lubricants</li><li>Nitric oxide precursors</li></ul>	<ul><li>Important component is clitoral stimulation</li><li>Understanding own body is essential</li><li>Communication with partner is key</li><li>Consider reducing medications (e.g., SSRIs)</li></ul>
Female orgasmic disorder	<ul><li>Masturbation</li><li>CBT to decrease anxiety</li><li>Systematic desensitization</li><li>Clitoral stimulators</li></ul>	<ul><li>A reflex noted at the peak of arousal</li><li>Distraction can shut down responses</li><li>Closely linked to arousal disorders</li></ul>
Dyspareunia	<ul><li>Treat underlying condition such as atrophy, urogenital prolapse, endometriosis, infection, fibroids, musculoskeletal pain, bowel pathology, bladder pain</li></ul>	<ul><li>Compassionate understanding required</li><li>If chronic, may lead to vaginismus</li></ul>
Vaginismus	<ul><li>Retraining pelvic floor muscles</li><li>Physiotherapy</li><li>Increase sense of control</li></ul>	<ul><li>Can be primary cause of dyspareunia or secondary to underlying condition</li></ul>

FDA, U.S. Food and Drug Administration; SSRIs, selective serotonin reuptake inhibitors.

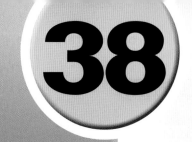

Sexual Assault and Domestic Violence

I. Sexual Assault

A. Description
   1. Any genital, oral, or anal penetration using force or without consent (including with an object)
   2. In vast majority of sexual assault cases, the victim knows the perpetrator
   3. Prevalent in all age, racial/ethnic, and socioeconomic groups

B. Types
   1. Acquaintance rape
   2. Date rape: forced sexual acts, includes situations where victim cannot give consent (asleep, alcohol/drugs)
   3. Statutory rape: sexual intercourse with a minor under a state-specified age (regardless of consent)
   4. Marital rape: 8%–15% of women; often occurs in conjunction with physical abuse
   5. Stranger rape
   6. Aggravated criminal sexual assault: criteria met when
      a. Weapons are used
      b. Physical violence is inflicted
      c. Lives endangered
      d. Victim is older than 60 years of age, physically handicapped, or mentally retarded
      e. Act is committed in relationship to another felony

C. Prevalence
   1. Difficult to determine precisely (majority of sexual assault goes unreported)
   2. Best estimates suggest that *1 in 6 women* sexually assaulted in their lifetime; 1 in 5 women in college are sexually assaulted
   3. 365,000 women sexually assaulted annually in United States
   4. Women ages 16–19 years report the highest rate of sexual victimization

D. Consequences (high risk for short- and long-term mental and physical health problems)
   1. Physical
      a. Sexually transmitted infections
      b. Unintended pregnancies, limited access to prenatal care, increased risk for miscarriages, stillbirths, preterm delivery, and low-birth-weight babies
      c. Chronic pelvic pain
      d. Dysmenorrhea
      e. Menstrual cycle disturbances
      f. Sexual dysfunction
   2. Somatic complaints
      a. Generalized pain
      b. Headaches
   3. Mental/behavioral
      a. Coping mechanisms depleted
      b. Symptoms consistent with posttraumatic stress disorder (PTSD) (or rape trauma)
         i. Acute phase: hours and days after the assault
            (a) Intense anxiety, depression, mood swings, anger, fear
            (b) Disturbances in sleep and appetite

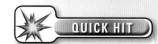

QUICK HIT

Given the prevalence, all women should be screened by their obstetrician–gynecologist (ob/gyn) for a history of sexual assault.

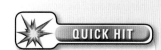

QUICK HIT

Girls ages 16–19 years are four times more likely than the general population to be victims of rape, attempted rape, or sexual assault.

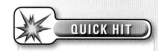

QUICK HIT

It is important to remember that there is no uniform response to trauma (none, some, or all of those discussed in "Consequences" (section D).

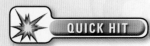

Victims of sexual assault often display an inability (not willful) to think clearly or remember things such as past medical history.

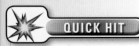

Obtaining informed consent from a victim of sexual assault is not only a legal requirement but also allows the patient to perceive that she is regaining control of her body and circumstances.

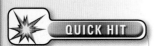

Sexual assault victims should be encouraged to come immediately to a medical facility and be advised not to bathe, douche, urinate, defecate, wash out her mouth, clean her fingernails, smoke, eat, or drink.

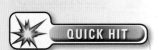

The patient should be encouraged, in a supportive, nonjudgmental manner, to talk about the assault and her reactions. This, however, does not obviate the need for follow-up care with trained counselor or psychologist.

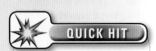

To assess mental (e.g., suicidality) and physical (e.g., evidence of pelvic infection) health, sexual assault victims should be contacted within 24–48 hours of initial treatment.

ii. Delayed or organization phase: months to years after the assault
    (a) Flashbacks, reliving the event, intrusive images, and nightmares
    (b) Physical reactions (panic, shaking, palpitations, chills)
    (c) Avoidance of reminders
    (d) Hyperarousal (hypervigilance, irritability, sleep disturbances, lack of concentration)
    (e) Disassociation (zoning out; losing conscious awareness of the present)
    (f) Heightened risk for alcohol and drug abuse
E. Care for patients/victims
  1. See Table 38.1 for initial management of emotional, medical, and forensic issues
  2. Details of sexual assault
    a. Location, timing, nature of assault
    b. Use of force, weapons, drugs
    c. Loss of consciousness
    d. Information about assailant
      i. Ejaculation?
      ii. Use of condom or lubricant?
  3. See Table 38.2 for testing and medical prophylaxis

TABLE 38.1 Physician's Role in Evaluation of Sexual Assault Patients

Emotional Issues	Medical Issues	Legal Issues
Obtain informed consent (helps woman regain control of her body and circumstances)	Assess and treat all injuries	Document details of sexual assault (location, timing, nature; use of force, weapons, or substances; loss of consciousness; ejaculation, use of condom or lubricant)
Perform exams with chaperone or support person present	Complete general physical examination	Document injuries Follow directions on forensic specimens kit
Support person should be provided to stay with the patient to provide advocacy and a sense of safety and security	Obtain past gynecologic history (menstrual history, contraception, date of last consensual sex, infections)	Collect samples in accordance with local protocol (pubic hair, fingernail scrapings, vaginal secretion and discharge samples, saliva, blood-stained articles)
Provide for counseling and refer for psychosocial needs	Obtain baseline serologic tests for Hep B, HIV, and syphilis (RPR) Screen for STDs and provide antibiotic prophylaxis for all adult patients Offer emergency contraception	Identify presence or absence of sperm and make appropriate slides Report to authorities as required Ensure security of "chain of evidence" (specimens in the protective custody of health professional until turned over to a legal representative) Encourage patient to work with police Results of forensic evaluation usually not provided to physician

Note: Check if your clinic has prepackaged rape kits and access to a sexual assault response team. Any disturbance to the chain of evidence may damage prosecution. If available, physicians should seek the assistance of specially trained medical personnel.
Hep B, hepatitis B; HIV, human immunodeficiency virus; RPR, rapid plasma reagin; STDs, sexually transmitted diseases.

TABLE 38.2 Testing and Medical Prophylaxis for Sexual Assault Patients

Sexually Transmitted Infections	Prophylaxis
Gonorrhea Chlamydia Trichomoniasis Bacterial vaginosis	Ceftriaxone, 125 mg intramuscularly in a single dose + Metronidazole, 2 g orally in a single dose + Azithromycin, 1 g orally single dose OR Doxycycline, 100 mg twice daily orally for 7 days *Testing for gonorrhea, chlamydia, and trichomoniasis should be done at initial examination. If vaginal discharge, malodor, and itching are present, examination for bacterial vaginosis and candidiasis should be conducted.*
Syphilis	Routine prophylaxis is not currently recommended. *Serologic tests should be conducted at initial evaluation and repeated 6, 12, and 24 weeks after the assault.*
Hepatitis B	Postexposure hepatitis B vaccination (without hepatitis B immune globulin) administered at time of initial examination if not previously vaccinated. Follow-up doses should be administered at 1–2 months and 4–6 months after first dose. *Serologic tests should be conducted at initial evaluation.*
Human immunodeficiency virus (HIV)	<72 hours postexposure with an individual known to have HIV, 28-day course of highly active antiretroviral therapy (HAART). Consultation with an HIV specialist is recommended. <72 hours postexposure to an individual of unknown HIV status, or >72 hours postexposure, individualized assessment *Serologic tests should be conducted at initial evaluation and repeated 6, 12, and 24 weeks after the assault.*
Herpes	Routine prophylaxis is not currently recommended but should be individualized if there is a report of a genital lesion on assailant. A 7–10-day course of acyclovir, famciclovir, or valacyclovir may be offered. However, there are no data on the efficacy of this treatment.
Human papillomavirus (HPV)	There is no preventive treatment recommended at this time.
Pregnancy	Emergency contraception *First dose should be given within 72 hours of the assault.*
Injuries	Tetanus toxoid booster, 0.5 mL intramuscularly, if more than 10 years since last immunization.

(Adapted from Workowski KA, Levine WC; Centers for Disease Control and Prevention. Sexually transmitted diseases treatment guidelines 2002. *MMWR Recomm Rep.* 2002;51[RR-6]:1–78; Smith OK, Grohskopf LA, Black RJ, et al. Antiretroviral postexposure prophylaxis after sexual, injection-drug use, or other nonoccupational exposure to HIV in the United States: recommendations from the U.S. Department of Health and Human Services. *MMWR Recomm Rep.* 2005;54[RR-2]:1–20; and Holmes M. Sexually transmitted infections in female rape victims. *AIDS Patient Care STDS.* 1999;13[12]:703–708.)

4. Documenting gynecologic history
   a. Menstrual history
   b. Contraception history
   c. Date of last consensual sexual experience
   d. Obstetric history
   e. History of infections
5. Follow-up care
   a. Within 24–48 hours: phone contact or follow-up evaluation
      i. Address emotional problems (e.g., suicidal ideation, cognitive dysfunction)
      ii. Address physical problems
      iii. Inquire about delayed physical problems (e.g., pelvic infections may not present immediately)
   b. 1 week
      i. Review patient's progress and address unresolved and new problems
      ii. Assess mental health, including risky behavior such as substance use
      iii. Refer to long-term counseling if needed

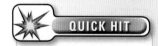

QUICK HIT

Be sure that any specimens collected are kept in a health professional's possession or control until turned over to an appropriate legal representative ("chain of evidence").

     c. 6 weeks
       i. Complete physical exam
       ii. Repeat cultures for sexually transmitted diseases (STDs), repeat rapid plasma regain (RPR)
       iii. Assess mental health and refer accordingly
     d. 12–18 weeks
       i. Repeat HIV titers
       ii. Assess mental health and refer accordingly

II. Child Sexual Assault (CSA)

A. Description
1. Any physical contact with a child for sexual gratification
2. Important to know the identity of the perpetrator to prevent further victimization
3. Exam generally done by a pediatrician or health care provider with particular skill set (beyond skills of most general gynecologists)
4. Ob/gyn often consulted to treat injury to the pelvic floor
5. Many cities have multidisciplinary trained teams

B. Immediate signs (consequences)
1. Mental/behavioral
  a. Night terrors
  b. Anger, embarrassment, guilt, self-blame
  c. Clingy and fearful
  d. Changes in sleeping and eating habits
  e. Sexual acting out
  f. Change in school functioning
  g. Regressive behavior (e.g., enuresis, encopresis, throwing temper tantrums)
2. Physical
  a. Recurrent somatic complaints (stomachaches, headaches)
  b. Vaginal pain
  c. Painful urination (dysuria)
  d. Rectal bleeding (hematochezia)
  e. Vaginal erythema, discharge, or bleeding

C. Evaluation
1. Establish rapport
2. Creating a safe and comfortable environment is essential
3. Care should be taken to reduce the number of times interviewed (statements should be recorded verbatim; consider recording interview)
4. Note specific names child uses for genitalia
5. If within 72 hours, focus on collection of forensic evidence (however, <10% reported within this time frame)

D. Management
1. Assess and attend to injuries
2. Treatment of STDs
3. Prevention of pregnancy
4. Protection against further abuse
5. Psychological support for the patient and family (provide long-term counseling for victim and family)
6. More extensive penetration injuries require thorough radiologic imaging and/or examination under anesthesia

E. Reporting
1. Be knowledgeable about state reporting requirements
2. **Health care professionals required to report any suspicion of child abuse**
3. Reporting of child abuse in good faith is immune from prosecution

III. Domestic Violence

A. Description
1. Domestic violence: violence within the context of family (parents, siblings, relatives) or intimate (boyfriend/girlfriend, spouse) relationships

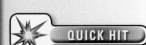

> **QUICK HIT**
>
> Ninety percent of CSA involves a parent, family member, or family friend.

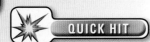

> **QUICK HIT**
>
> Only a small portion of children referred for medical evaluation have abnormal examinations.

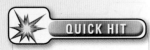

> **QUICK HIT**
>
> The lifetime prevalence of IPV = 25%.

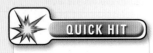

> **QUICK HIT**
>
> Many violent relationships are characterized by bidirectional violence (where both members of the couple are violent toward each other).

TABLE 38.3 Indicators of Physical Abuse in Domestic Violence

Area of Injury	Descriptions
Head and neck	Bruises; abrasions; strangle marks; black eye; broken nose, orbital ridge, or jaw; pulled hair, permanent hearing loss, lacerations
Trunk	Evidence of blunt trauma; bruises; fractured collarbones and ribs
Skin	Multiple lesions in various stages of healing; rug rash, abrasions, burns, bites
Extremities	Evidence of restraint; muscle strains; spiral fractures; rope or restraint burns; crescent moon–shaped fingernail marks

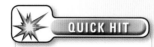

QUICK HIT

Psychological abuse may be as or more traumatic than physical violence.

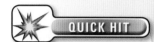

QUICK HIT

Younger and low-income women are disproportionately affected by IPV.

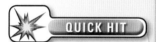

QUICK HIT

American Medical Association (AMA) and American College of Obstetricians and Gynecologists (ACOG) recommend screening every patient for violence as part of a routine health checkup.

2. Intimate partner violence (IPV) is between current or former partners (includes male-to-female and female-to-male as well as lesbian, gay, bisexual, and transgendered relationships)
3. Pregnant women at heightened risk of being abused

B. Presentation
  1. Physical violence: hitting, slapping, kicking, choking
  2. Psychological/emotional abuse: excessive jealousy, threatening, name calling, controlling, monitoring, economic restrictions, isolating from friends and family
  3. Sexual abuse: see previous
  4. Reproductive coercion: preventing access to or use of birth control methods

C. Consequences
  1. Physical
    a. See Table 38.3 for a description of acute injuries
    b. Somatic complaints, chronic pain
  2. Mental/behavioral
    a. Low self-esteem
    b. Stress
    c. Psychopathology (PTSD, depression, anxiety, panic disorders)
    d. Substance abuse

D. Indicators and clinical clues of abuse
  1. Women and men from all age groups, religions, ethnic/racial groups, socioeconomic status, educational backgrounds, and sexual orientations
  2. Unexplained, multiple, and recurring injuries
  3. Somatic complaints with no known cause
  4. Poor compliance, hostility, passivity, minimal responses
  5. Psychopathology
  6. Self-destructive, often high-risk behaviors
  7. Increased use of health care system
  8. Partner is overly attentive, almost always present, and answers for patient

E. Screening and management
  1. Always interview patient about IPV in private
  2. Funneling technique
    a. "Tell me about your relationship with your partner."
    b. "All couples get into arguments . . . what happens when you and your partner fight at home?"
  3. Work on safety/exit plan with patient (pack an emergency kit in case you have to leave suddenly, with money, keys, medicines, changes of clothes, important documents [health insurance cards, birth certificates, driver's license, court papers or orders])

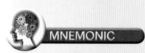

MNEMONIC

RADAR
Remember to ask about IPV.
Ask directly: "At any time, has a partner hit, kicked, hurt, or frightened you?"
Document information about suspected or actual IPV.
Assess for safety and red flags (weapons, substance use, escalating violence, children present, perpetrator threatening suicide, stalking).
Review options with your patients, and know about referral options (e.g., shelters, support groups, legal advocates). Suggest patient calls from your office.

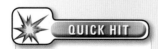

QUICK HIT

Leaving a violent relationship is often the most dangerous time.

Sexual Assault and Domestic Violence

Reproductive Endocrinology and Infertility

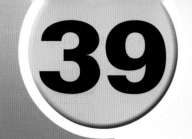

Puberty

I. Puberty

A. Series of neuroendocrine and physiologic events that results in development of secondary sex characteristics, menarche, and ovulation

B. Onset of puberty is determined by
1. Genetic factors (including race) (Table 39.1)
2. Geographic location
3. Nutritional status
4. Excessive exercise
5. Psychological factors

II. Neuroendocrine

A. Fetal physiology
1. Initially, gonadotropins (follicle-stimulating hormone [FSH] and luteinizing hormone [LH]) are produced by pituitary; this peaks at 20 weeks' gestation
2. Fetal hypothalamic–pituitary–ovarian (HPO) axis is suppressed by maternal estradiol

B. Newborn physiology
1. Most estradiol in fetus is maternal and placental in origin
2. At birth, maternal and placental estradiol levels drop
3. Negative feedback of estradiol on pituitary is lost; gonadotropins (FSH and LH) are produced
4. FSH and LH peak by age 3 months and decrease until age 4 years
5. Estradiol levels are low within 1 week of birth and remain low until puberty

C. Childhood physiology
1. HPO axis remains suppressed
2. Called the "gonadostat"

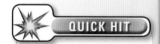

QUICK HIT

Clinically, the effect of maternal estrogens on the newborn can be seen as scant vaginal bleeding.

TABLE 39.1	Ethnicity and Onset of Puberty		
	Mean Age (Years)		
Event	**African Americans**	**Mexican Americans**	**Caucasians**
Thelarche	9.5	9.8	10.3
Pubarche	9.5	10.3	10.5
Menarche	12.3	12.5	12.7

(From American College of Obstetricians and Gynecologists. *Precis, An Update in Obstetrics and Gynecology: Reproductive Endocrinology*, 3rd ed. Washington, DC: American College of Obstetricians and Gynecologists; 2007; Wu T, Mendola P, Buck GM. Ethnic differences in the presence of secondary sex characteristics and menarche among U.S. girls: the Third National Health And Nutrition Examination Survey, 1988–1994. *Pediatrics*, 2002;110[4]:752–757. Reproduced with permission.)

FIGURE 39.1 Adrenarche/pubarche.

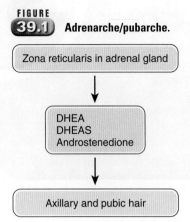

3. Suppression due to 2 factors
   a. LH and FSH levels are low despite low levels of estradiol; gonadostat has not yet developed negative feedback effect of estradiol
   b. Intrinsic central nervous system (CNS) suppression of hypothalamic gonadotropin-releasing hormone (GnRH) secretion
D. **Adrenarche** (Figure 39.1)
   1. First neuroendocrine change associated with puberty
   2. Starts ages 6–8 years
   3. Zona reticularis in the adrenal gland produces sex steroids
      a. Dehydroepiandrosterone sulfate (DHEA-S)
      b. DHEA
      c. Androstenedione
   4. Rise in adrenal androgens causes growth of axillary and pubic hair = pubarche
   5. Adrenarche occurs independent of gonadarche (HPO axis)
E. **Gonadarche** (Figure 39.2)
   1. Begins around age 8 years
      a. Gonadostat becomes sensitive to the negative feedback of estradiol
      b. Low estradiol levels decrease negative feedback on GnRH production, permitting pulsatile GnRH production
      c. CNS less effective at inhibiting hypothalamic GnRH production

FIGURE 39.2 Gonadarche.

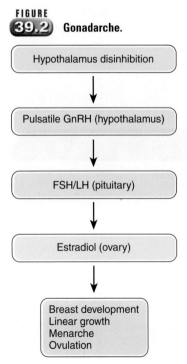

2. Nocturnal GnRH pulsatile release begins from the hypothalamus
3. Gradually GnRH pulsatile secretion occurs throughout the 24-hour day
4. Pulsatile hypothalamic GnRH secretion causes FSH/LH secretion from the pituitary
5. FSH/LH secretion causes ovarian follicular maturation and estradiol production
6. Estradiol causes secondary sex characteristics to develop

III. Somatic Changes

A. Physical changes of puberty include development of secondary sex characteristics and linear growth
B. Changes occur in a specific order (Figure 39.3)
C. 1> = Beginning of growth spurt
   1. Thelarche
   2. Pubarche
   3. Peak growth velocity
   4. Menarche
D. **Thelarche:** breast bud development (Figure 39.4)
   1. Usually 1st phenotypic sign of puberty
   2. Happens around age 10 years
   3. Stages of breast development are called Tanner stages (Table 39.2)

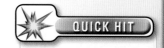

QUICK HIT

The beginning of the growth spurt precedes thelarche by about 1 year; however, it usually goes unnoticed.

Puberty

FIGURE
39.3 Basic principles of menstrual function.

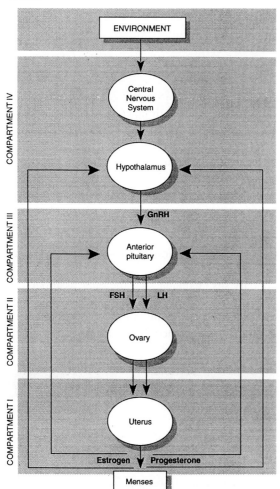

The hypothalamic–pituitary–ovarian axis can be segmented into distinct compartments; each is necessary for normal menstrual function. (From Bourgeois FJ. *Obstetrics & Gynecology Recall*, 3rd ed. Philadelphia: Lippincott Williams & Wilkins; 2008.)

Puberty

FIGURE
39.4 Tanner stages of thelarche and pubarche.

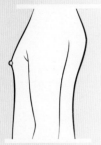 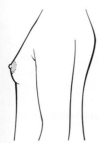 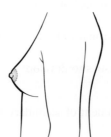 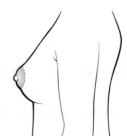 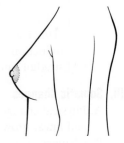

1. Prepubertal   2. Breast bud   3. Breast elevation   4. Areolar mound   5. Adult contour

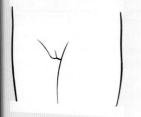 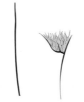 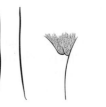 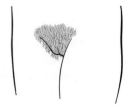

1. Prepubertal   2. Presexual hair   3. Sexual hair   4. Mid-escutcheon   5. Female escutcheon

(From Callahan T, Caughey AB. *Blueprints Obstetrics & Gynecology*, 5th ed. Baltimore: Lippincott Williams & Wilkins; 2009.)

    E. **Pubarche**
        1. Development of axillary and pubic hair
        2. Happens around age 11 years
        3. May precede thelarche in African American girls
    F. Peak growth velocity
        1. Happens around age 12 years
        2. Increased estradiol stimulates production of growth hormone and somatomedin C, which promotes growth
    G. **Menarche**
        1. Average age in United States is older than 12 years
        2. Initial cycles are typically irregular and anovulatory

IV. Precocious Puberty
    A. More common in girls than boys
    B. Two types
        1. Heterosexual: development of secondary sex characteristics opposite of anticipated phenotypic sex
        2. Isosexual: development of secondary sex characteristics the same as anticipated phenotypic sex
          a. Complete: entire pubertal process happens, culminating in menarche
          b. Incomplete: only a single secondary sex characteristic appears

QUICK HIT

Menarche usually occurs about 2.5 years after breasts bud.

QUICK HIT

Evaluate for precocious puberty when secondary sexual characteristics present before age 6 years in African American girls and age 7 years in Caucasian girls.

TABLE **39.2**	**The Tanner Stages of Breast Development**
Stage 1	Preadolescent: elevation of papilla only
Stage 2	Breast bud stage: elevation of breast and papilla, areolar enlargement
Stage 3	Further enlargement of breast and areola without separation of contours
Stage 4	Projection of areola and papilla to form a secondary mound
Stage 5	Mature stage: projection of papilla only as areola recesses to breast contour

BOX 39.1

Treatment Goals in Precocious Puberty

Arrest pubertal changes
Address psychological concerns
Attain adult stature

C. **Heterosexual precocious puberty**
  1. Caused by elevated androgens
  2. Sources of androgen production
     a. Virilizing tumors—very rare in childhood
     b. Congenital adrenal hyperplasia ([CAH] see also Chapter 41)
        i. Defect in 21-hydroxylase enzyme leads to increased androgen precursor and decreased glucocorticoid
        ii. Treatment includes replacement of glucocorticoid and possible surgical correction of ambiguous genitalia
        iii. Nonclassical or late-onset CAH presents with premature pubarche
D. **Complete isosexual precocious puberty** (Box 39.1)
  1. Risks
     a. Identifying underlying potentially life-threatening etiology
     b. Affected children at risk for psychological problems and sexual abuse
     c. Initially taller than age-matched peers, but with early epiphyseal closure, at risk for short stature as adults
  2. Central or true isosexual precocious puberty (HPO dependent)
     a. Activation of HPO axis
     b. Responds to GnRH stimulation test since HPO is activated
     c. Etiologies
        i. Idiopathic
           (a) Most common (75%)
           (b) Treatment with GnRH agonist
        ii. CNS (10%)
           (a) May present first with neurologic symptoms
           (b) Evaluation includes brain magnetic resonance imaging (MRI)
           (c) Infection: meningitis/encephalitis/abscess
           (d) Increased intracranial pressure: hydrocephalus
           (e) Head trauma
           (f) CNS tumors
           (g) Neurofibromatosis
           (h) Granulomatous disease: sarcoidosis/tuberculosis
  3. Peripheral (or pseudoisosexual) precocious puberty (HPO independent)
     a. Does not respond to GnRH stimulation test
     b. Results from increased estrogen levels
     c. Etiologies
        i. Ingestion of exogenous hormones: hormone therapy, oral contraceptives
        ii. Advanced hypothyroidism
        iii. Adrenal neoplasm
        iv. Ovarian neoplasm
           (a) Rare sex cord tumor with annular tubules that secrete estrogen
           (b) Treatment is surgical removal
        v. **McCune-Albright syndrome** (5%)
           (a) Isosexual precocious puberty
           (b) Polyostotic fibrous dysplasia and associated bone fractures
           (c) Café au lait spots
           (d) Adrenal hypercortisolism
        vi. Peutz-Jeghers syndrome

E. Incomplete isosexual precocious puberty
   1. Precocious thelarche
      a. Appearance of breast buds only
      b. May be unilateral
      c. Monitor for other signs of pubertal change
      d. Bone age normal
      e. No intervention required
   2. Precocious pubarche
      a. Appearance of axillary and/or pubic hair only
      b. Monitor for other signs of pubertal change
      c. Bone age normal
      d. No intervention required

V. **Delayed Puberty/Primary Amenorrhea** *(Box 39.2; see Chapter 40)*

BOX 39.2

When to Evaluate Pubertal Delay

No thelarche age ≥13 years
No menarche age ≥15 years
No menarche ≥4 years after thelarche

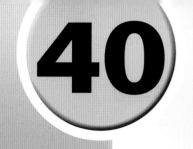

Amenorrhea and Abnormal Uterine Bleeding

I. Overview of the Menstrual Cycle

A. Normal cycle characteristics
1. Length of cycle: 21–35 days (average of 28 days)
2. Cycle duration: 3–7 days
3. Volume of menstrual flow: 20–60 mL
4. Regularity is predictive of ovulatory cycles

B. Hormones (Figure 40.1)
1. Hypothalamic
a. **Gonadotropin-releasing hormone (GnRH)** is secreted in a pulsatile manner and controls gonadotropin release
2. Gonadotropins (released from anterior pituitary)
a. **Luteinizing hormone (LH)**
b. **Follicle-stimulating hormone (FSH)**

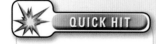

FIGURE 40.1 Hormonal feedback regulation (−ve indicates inhibitory effects; +ve stimulatory effects).

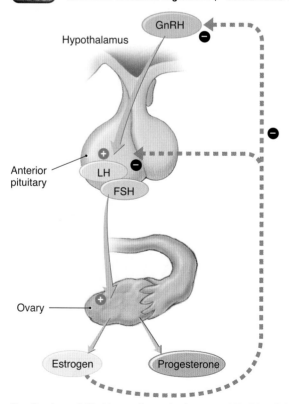

(From Premkumar K. *The Massage Connection Anatomy and Physiology*. Baltimore: Lippincott Williams & Wilkins; 2004.)

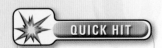

QUICK HIT

Terminology: *Gonadotropic* refers to the levels of gonadotropins (FSH and LH); *gonadism* refers to the levels of ovarian (sex) hormones (estradiol).

3. Ovarian
   a. Estrogen (as estradiol)
   b. Progesterone
C. Phases (Figure 40.2)
   1. Follicular phase
      a. Days 1–14 (**onset of menses until ovulation**)
      b. **Increase in FSH** stimulates growth of ovarian follicles; **1 dominant follicle develops** and matures, increasing estradiol production
      c. Also called **proliferative phase** because estrogen induces endometrial growth and thickening

FIGURE 40.2 Menstrual cycle.

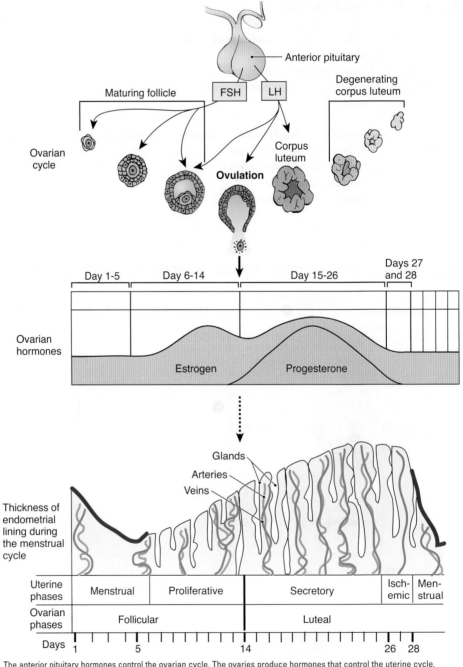

The anterior pituitary hormones control the ovarian cycle. The ovaries produce hormones that control the uterine cycle. (From Klossner NJ, Hatfield N. *Introductory Maternity and Pediatric Nursing.* Philadelphia: Lippincott Williams & Wilkins; 2005.)

2. Ovulation
   a. Estrogen levels increase
   b. **Rapid LH surge** causes follicular rupture and oocyte release within 30–36 hours
3. **Luteal phase**
   a. Days 14–28 (ovulation until onset of menses)
   b. Also called **secretory phase** because increase in progesterone induces endometrial gland secretion
   c. Granulosa and theca interna cells line follicular wall and form corpus luteum (CL), which secretes estrogen and progesterone
      i. No conception: **involution** of CL results in progesterone decline and FSH increase; endometrial sloughing occurs and bleeding begins
      ii. Conception: CL is maintained by **human chorionic gonadotropin (hCG)** until placenta produces progesterone

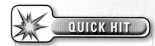

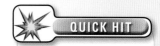

II. Primary Amenorrhea
A. Definition
   1. No menstruation by age 13 years without breast budding
   2. No menstruation by age 15 years with breast budding
B. Etiology
   1. **Gonadal dysgenesis** implies nondeveloped "streak" gonads without germ cells, normal external and internal female genitalia, and deficient estrogen production
     a. **Turner syndrome (45,X)**
       i. Other karyotypes: ring chromosomes; mosaicism, deletions on X chromosome
       ii. Somatic features
         (a) Short stature
         (b) Webbed neck
         (c) Shield-like chest with widely spaced nipples
         (d) Renal and cardiovascular abnormalities
         (e) Autoimmune disorders
     b. **Pure gonadal dysgenesis:** lack of Turner-like features
       i. 46,XX
       ii. 46,XY (Swyer syndrome): intra-abdominal streaks can progress to tumors and should be removed early
     c. **Vanishing testes syndrome (anorchia)**
       i. Regression of testes before 8 weeks: identical to pure gonadal dysgenesis
       ii. Regression 8–13 weeks: ambiguous genitalia, wolffian structures, no Müllerian structures due to early presence of anti-Müllerian hormone (AMH)
   2. Receptor abnormalities
     a. Complete **androgen insensitivity syndrome (AIS)** previously known as *testicular feminization*
       i. **Phenotypic females** (but genetically X,Y) without a uterus and vagina or incomplete vagina; **normal breasts** because estrogen present
       ii. Androgen receptors absent or defective: **no sexual hair**
   3. Enzyme deficiencies
     a. 5α-Reductase deficiency in 46,XY individual
       i. Ambiguous genitalia at birth without Müllerian structures
       ii. Inability to convert testosterone to dihydrotestosterone (DHT) leading to a lack of masculinization at puberty
     b. Congenital adrenal hyperplasias (CAHs) such as 17α-hydroxylase (CYP17) deficiency = no production of adrenal or gonadal sex steroids (see also Chapter 41)
       i. 46,XX female internal and external genitalia (phenotypically normal)
       ii. 46,XY incompletely developed external genitalia

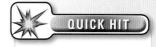

QUICK HIT

Orderly sloughing of the endometrium in a normal ovulatory cycle is triggered by falling progesterone levels on an estrogen-primed endometrium.

QUICK HIT

The normal luteal phase is more constant (14 days) than the follicular phase, which can vary in length.

QUICK HIT

Secondary sexual development is characterized by breasts and pubic/axillary hair.

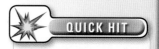

QUICK HIT

The most common cause of primary amenorrhea is gonadal dysgenesis.

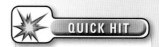

QUICK HIT

Classic presentation of AIS is a phenotypic woman with normal breasts, no pubic hair, and blind vagina.

Amenorrhea and Abnormal Uterine Bleeding

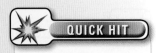

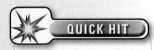

4. Hypothalamic
   a. Constitutional delay of puberty: lack of pulsatile GnRH
   b. Congenital GnRH deficiency; therefore, no FSH or LH
   c. Inability of GnRH to reach pituitary by tumors, infection, radiation, trauma, etc.
   d. Functional hypothalamic hypogonadism (see "Secondary Amenorrhea" section)
5. Congenital anomalies
   a. Imperforate hymen
   b. **Müllerian agenesis (46,XX):** congenital absence of uterus and upper 2/3 of vagina
   c. **Vaginal agenesis:** complete lack of vagina
   d. Transverse vaginal septum
6. Pituitary
   a. Congenital absence is lethal
   b. **Pituitary micro- or macroadenomas** (hyperprolactinemia)
   c. Hypothyroidism
7. Ovarian failure
   a. Gonadal dysgenesis (see previous)
   b. Savage syndrome: gonadotropin-resistant ovaries
   c. Blizzard syndrome: autoimmune ovarian failure
   d. Fragile X premutation carriers

C. Clinical evaluation: important consultations in diagnosis and management may include reproductive endocrinology, pediatric endocrinology, and genetic counselor
   1. History
      a. Past medical history
      b. Family history
      c. Progression of pubertal stages
   2. Physical examination
      a. Secondary sexual characteristics and external genitalia
         i. **Breast development** implies presence of **estrogen**
         ii. **Pubertal hair** implies presence of **androgens**
      b. Presence of vagina, cervix, and uterus typically with ultrasound (U/S) or magnetic resonance imaging (MRI)

D. Diagnostics
   1. **Uterus absent**
      a. XY karyotype
         i. **AIS:** normal male testosterone levels but female phenotype
         ii. **5α-Reductase deficiency:** normal male testosterone levels but male phenotype
         iii. **CAH**
      b. XX karyotype
         i. **Pure gonadal dysgenesis**
         ii. **Müllerian** agenesis: normal female testosterone levels
   2. Uterus present without patent vagina
      a. **Imperforate hymen**
      b. Transverse septum
      c. Vaginal agenesis
   3. Uterus present with patent vagina
      a. **hCG** to rule out pregnancy
      b. **FSH**
         i. High: primary ovarian failure; proceed to karyotyping for Turner syndrome
         ii. Low or normal (hypogonadotropic hypogonadism)
            (a) MRI of head
            (b) Thyroid-stimulating hormone (TSH)
            (c) Prolactin

E. Management
   1. Correct underlying cause if applicable
   2. Patients with **Y chromosomes** require surgical removal of internal gonads

BOX 40.1

Common Causes of Hypogonadotropic Hypogonadism

Psychogenic: anxiety, anorexia nervosa, pseudocyesis (false pregnancy)
Functional: obesity, extreme weight loss, dieting, or exercise
Medication or drug induced: psychoactive drugs (antidepressants), marijuana
Neoplasms: prolactinomas, craniopharyngioma
Other: head injury or chronic medical illness

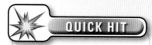

QUICK HIT

Aortic dissection or rupture is a complication in pregnant Turner patients (via oocyte donation); close cardiovascular monitoring is indicated.

3. Infertility treatment is based on specific etiology
4. Turner syndrome patients may achieve pregnancy with donor oocytes and hormonal support
5. Hypoestrogenic patients require estrogen replacement for osteoporosis prevention

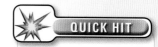

QUICK HIT

The most common cause (95%) of secondary amenorrhea or oligomenorrhea is pregnancy. Always do a serum hCG first!

III. Secondary Amenorrhea

A. *Previously menstruating* woman who has not menstruated for 3–6 months
B. Etiology
  1. Any abnormality involving hypothalamic–pituitary–ovarian (HPO) axis or genital outflow tract
    a. **Pregnancy:** most common cause
    b. **Hypothalamic–pituitary dysfunction** (Box 40.1)
      i. State of **estrogen deficiency** (hypogonadotropic hypogonadism)
        (a) Alteration of pulsatile GnRH, inhibiting FSH and LH
        (b) No folliculogenesis = no ovulation
        (c) No sex hormone production = no endometrial growth or menstruation
      ii. State of **chronic estrogen: anovulation** or oligoovulation
        (a) Idiopathic
        (b) Polycystic ovarian syndrome (PCOS) is subset of anovulation (Box 40.2)
        (c) Adrenal hyperplasia
        (d) Thyroid dysfunction (hypo- or hyperthyroidism)
        (e) Obesity
    c. **Ovarian dysfunction** or failure
      i. Turner syndrome (45,X)
      ii. Premature ovarian failure (PMOF)
        (a) Idiopathic
        (b) Iatrogenic (chemotherapy, radiation, surgery)
        (c) Autoimmune processes (Blizzard syndrome)
        (d) Fragile X premutation
    d. **Abnormal genital outflow** tract
      i. Primary (see "Primary Amenorrhea" section)
      ii. Secondary
        (a) **Asherman syndrome** (scarring of uterine cavity from infection or dilation and curettage) is *most common anatomic cause of secondary amenorrhea*
        (b) Cervical stenosis

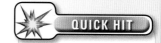

QUICK HIT

Female athletes with low percentile body fat and strict dietary requirements frequently present with amenorrhea or AUB.

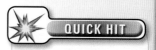

QUICK HIT

Female athlete triad: amenorrhea, disordered eating, and osteopenia.

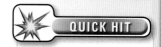

QUICK HIT

If a patient experienced massive postpartum hemorrhage, consider **Sheehan syndrome** (postpartum necrosis of the anterior pituitary).

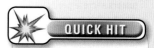

QUICK HIT

PMOF is ovarian failure at age ≤40 years.

BOX 40.2

Polycystic Ovarian Syndrome

Anovulation + androgen excess
- Androgen excess can be either clinical hirsutism or elevated serum testosterone
- Pelvic U/S often reveals ovaries with multiple follicles in varying stages of development in the outer cortex of the ovary (ring-of-pearls sign)
- Etiology unknown but results in chronic, tonic elevated LH levels
- Associated with insulin resistance, HTN, hypercholesterolemia, metabolic syndrome

HTN, hypertension; LH, luteinizing hormone; U/S, ultrasound

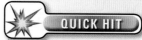

QUICK HIT

Asherman syndrome is most frequently associated with uterine curettage.

FIGURE 40.3 Clinical algorithm for secondary amenorrhea.

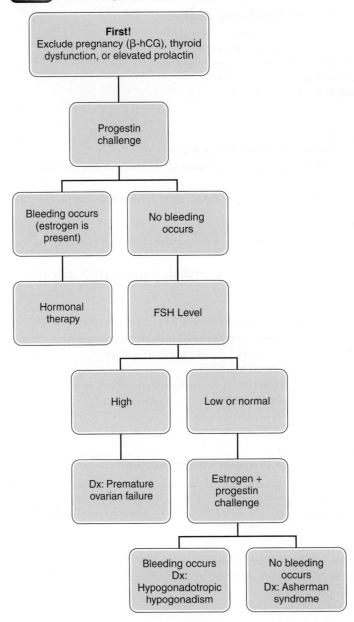

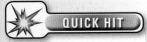

QUICK HIT

PMOF has elevated **FSH levels** with ovarian failure = hypergonadotropic hypogonadism.

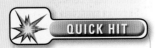

QUICK HIT

About 80% of all **pituitary tumors** secrete prolactin, which causes a milky discharge from the bilateral breast **(galactorrhea)**. Treat with bromocriptine or cabergoline.

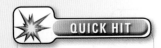

QUICK HIT

PCT essentially mimics ovulation with the administration of exogenous progestin.

C. Diagnosis and management of secondary amenorrhea (Figure 40.3)
1. Laboratory
   a. **hCG**
   b. **TSH**
   c. **Prolactin level**
2. **Progesterone challenge test (PCT):** administer medroxyprogesterone acetate 10 mg by mouth (PO) × 10 days
   a. *If withdrawal bleeding occurs, there was adequate estrogen to proliferate endometrium*
      i. Result is physiologic withdrawal bleeding after exogenous progestin is discontinued
      ii. Anovulatory or oligoovulatory (see Dysfunctional uterine bleeding)
   b. No withdrawal bleeding: obtain FSH
      i. High FSH (>40 mIU/mL) = PMOF
      ii. Low or normal FSH: administer estrogen followed by progestin withdrawal (can use standard combination oral contraceptive)
         (a) Withdrawal bleeding = hypogonadotropic hypogonadism
         (b) No withdrawal bleeding = Asherman syndrome

Amenorrhea and Abnormal Uterine Bleeding

BOX 40.3

Variations of Abnormal Uterine Bleeding

- Pregnancy-related causes
  - Early pregnancy: ectopic, spontaneous abortion (threatened, inevitable, incomplete, complete, or missed)
  - Later pregnancy: placenta previa or abruption, vasa previa, vaginal or vulvar tears or lacerations, cervical ectropions, cervicitis, carcinoma, varicosities
- Oligomenorrhea: reduction in menses frequency (>35 days)
- Polymenorrhea: frequent menses (<21 days)
- Hypomenorrhea: light bleeding during menses
- Menorrhagia (hypermenorrhea): excessive bleeding during menses (>80 mL) or prolonged menstrual bleeding (>7 days)
- Metrorrhagia: breakthrough bleeding (bleeding between cycles)
- Menometrorrhagia: metrorrhagia + menorrhagia

IV. Abnormal Uterine Bleeding (AUB)

A. Irregularity or unpredictability of menstrual cycle (any variation in frequency, duration, or amount of menstrual bleeding) (Box 40.3)

B. Classification

1. **Dysfunctional uterine bleeding (DUB)**: anovulatory or oligoovulatory bleeding not attributable to anatomic or organic causes
   a. **Anovulation with normal estrogen** production
      i. State of **chronic estrous: constant, noncyclic estrogen levels** without interruption by progesterone
      ii. Stimulates endometrial proliferation or overproliferation, which results in **unpredictable bleeding** (duration, interval, and amount)
   b. **Anovulation without estrogen** production
      i. State of estrogen deficiency
      ii. Results in **endometrial atrophy and amenorrhea**
   c. Luteal phase defects
      i. Abnormal CL function: <14 days of progesterone production or inadequate amount of progesterone
      ii. Results in shortened menstrual cycle
2. **Anatomic** causes of AUB
   a. **Malignancy:** endometrial, myometrial, cervical, endocervical, vaginal
   b. **Endometrial cavity** disorders: leiomyomas (fibroids), endometrial polyps, foreign body (e.g., intrauterine device [IUD]), adenomyosis, uterine septum, endometrial hyperplasia
   c. **Infection:** endometrial, cervical, vaginal
   d. **Pregnancy-related:** miscarriage (spontaneous abortion), ectopic pregnancy, gestational trophoblastic disease (GTD)
3. **Organic** causes of AUB
   a. **Coagulopathies** (e.g., von Willebrand disease)
   b. Liver disease can affect coagulation and estrogen metabolism
   c. Hypothyroidism
   d. Sepsis
   e. **Medications:** anticoagulants, exogenous hormones

C. **Diagnosis** (Figure 40.4)

1. **Pelvic exam** to evaluate for anatomic causes of irregular bleeding
   a. Speculum exam to evaluate vagina and cervix
   b. Uterine size, irregularity, tenderness, and adnexa
2. Laboratory
   a. Urine or serum β-hCG to exclude pregnancy
   b. **TSH**: free T_4 if abnormal
   c. **Prolactin** level to exclude pituitary problem or prolactinoma
   d. **CBC** to exclude anemia from severe bleeding

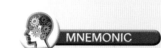

Cycles are commonly irregular (anovulatory) during the first 3 years after menarche (first menses) and during the 3 years prior to menopause.

MNEMONIC

Think of the unpredictable arrival of metro rides when remembering metrorrhagia.

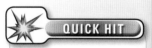

Midcycle spotting (at time of ovulation) is attributed to the sudden decline in estrogen levels.

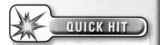

Midcycle pain (at time of ovulation) is called **mittelschmerz.**

QUICK HIT

Anovulation or oligoovulation can cause either DUB or secondary amenorrhea.

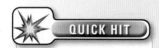

Women with **unopposed estrogen** (chronic estrous) may develop **endometrial hyperplasia**, increasing their risk for endometrial cancer.

QUICK HIT

Patients with anatomic causes of AUB typically have regular (ovulatory) cycles with menorrhagia or intermenstrual bleeding. Dysmenorrhea is also frequently present.

Amenorrhea and Abnormal Uterine Bleeding

FIGURE 40.4 Clinical algorithm for abnormal uterine bleeding.

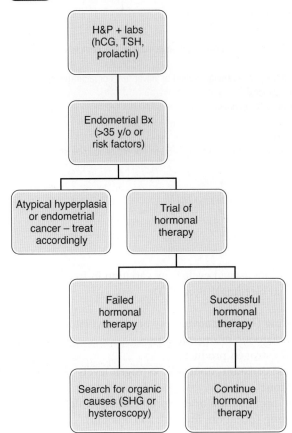

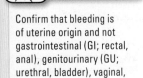

QUICK HIT

Confirm that bleeding is of uterine origin and not gastrointestinal (GI; rectal, anal), genitourinary (GU; urethral, bladder), vaginal, or vulvar.

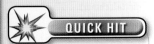

QUICK HIT

Remember that a patient presenting with any post-menopausal bleeding needs an endometrial biopsy to exclude endometrial cancer (unless it is a withdrawal bleed from exogenous hormones).

MNEMONIC

OLD AUNT: obesity, late menopause, diabetes, age, unopposed estrogen, nulliparity, tamoxifen.

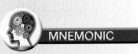

QUICK HIT

Do not confuse SHG with HSG. A hysterosalpingogram (HSG) is the use of radiopaque dye into the endometrial cavity, used mainly to assess tubal patency.

3. **Endometrial biopsy:** if patient is age >35 years or has risk factors for endometrial cancer (Box 40.4)
4. Imaging
    a. **Pelvic ultrasound** (abdominal and transvaginal)
       i. Uterine dimensions, masses
      ii. Endometrial thickness (**endometrial stripe** [EMS])
     iii. Adnexal masses
    b. Sonohysterography (SHG): transcervical saline instillation into uterine cavity
    c. Hysteroscopy: fiber-optic scope visualizes uterine cavity; can remove polyps or submucosal fibroids
D. Management of AUB
   1. Hormonal therapy
    a. **Combination oral contraceptives**
    b. **Cyclical progestin** therapy for 10–12 days each month

---

BOX 40.4

Endometrial Cancer Risk Factors

Postmenopausal
Unopposed estrogen
Chronic anovulation
Nulliparity
Obesity
Diabetes mellitus
Tamoxifen use (selective estrogen receptor modulator)

    c. **Continuous progestin** therapy

       i. Progestin-only pills

      ii. Depot medroxyprogesterone acetate (Depo-Provera)

     iii. Subcutaneous progestin implant (Implanon)

     iv. Progestin (levonorgestrel)-releasing IUD

    d. Ovulation induction (if conception desired)

2. **Surgical**

    a. Hysteroscopic resection of polyps, pedunculated fibroids

    b. Endometrial ablation for menorrhagia

    c. Myomectomy for fibroids

    d. Hysterectomy: bleeding refractory to other management

E. Management of **acute excessive blood loss**

1. Hormonal

    a. **High-dose intravenous estrogen**: typically controls or ceases bleeding within 24 hours

    b. **Accelerated** regimen of **combination oral contraceptives**: twice a day (bid) for 10 days followed by daily dosing for another 3 weeks

2. Surgical

    a. Dilation and curettage with or without hysteroscopy

    b. Uterine artery embolization

    c. Hysterectomy

3. If cycles are irregular

    a. Progesterone challenge: administer medroxyprogesterone acetate 10 mg PO × 10 days or progesterone 200 mg PO

    b. If *withdrawal bleeding occurs, there are adequate estrogen levels to proliferate endometrium*

       i. Discontinuation of exogenous progestin simulates physiologic end of luteal phase and triggers withdrawl bleeding

      ii. Diagnose patient with DUB (anovulatory or oligoovulatory); needs hormonal therapy to control cycles

    c. No withdrawal bleeding

       i. Inadequate estrogen levels are present to proliferate endometrium and there is no endometrium to shed (hypoestrogenic)

      ii. Proceed to amenorrhea management

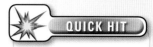

QUICK HIT

The primary goal of treatment of anovulatory bleeding is to ensure a regular slough of the estrogen-primed endometrium and achieve predictable withdrawal bleeding.

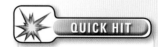

QUICK HIT

Nonsteroidal anti-inflammatory drugs (NSAIDs) inhibit prostaglandins, which are known to affect endometrial vasculature and may reduce bleeding by up to 50%.

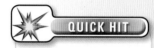

QUICK HIT

A **total** hysterectomy is removal of the **entire uterus** (does not include removal of ovaries/fallopian tubes, which would add the term salpingo-oophorectomy).

Amenorrhea and Abnormal Uterine Bleeding

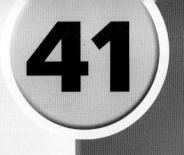

Hirsutism and Virilization

I. Hyperandrogenism

A. Clinical manifestation of excess levels of male hormones in women

B. Hirsutism

    1. Male pattern distribution of excess hair, with conversion of terminal hair to vellus hair

    2. Degree of hirsutism is measured with Ferriman-Gallwey scoring system (Figure 41.1)

        a. Terminal hair: dark, coarse, kinky

        b. Vellus hair: soft, downy, fine

FIGURE 41.1 Modified Ferriman-Gallwey scale for extent of hirsutism.

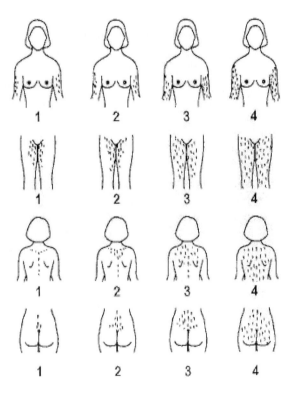

(Modified from Hatch, et al. Hirsutism: implications, etiology, and management. *Am J Obstet Gynecol.* 1981;140:815–830.)

C. Virilization
1. Hirsutism
2. Masculinization of women with marked increase in testosterone levels
   a. Clitoral enlargement
   b. Temporal balding
   c. Voice deepening
   d. Limb-shoulder girdle remodeling

II. Normal Androgen Metabolism

A. Androgen production results from cholesterol metabolism (Figure 41.2)
B. Produced in adrenal glands and ovaries (Table 41.1)
C. Converted to estrogens in fat cells
D. Most are bound to albumin and sex hormone–binding globulin (SHBG) and are clinically inactive
   1. 1%–3% of circulating testosterone is unbound and biologically active
   2. Total testosterone measurement may not reflect amount of biologically active SHBG
   3. Production in liver is stimulated by estrogens
E. Androgen metabolism
   1. Testosterone: converted within hair follicles and within genital skin
   2. Conversion leads to more potent dihydrotestosterone (DHT) via *5α-reductase*
      a. Responsible for constitutional hirsutism
      b. May also be aromatized to estrogens
      c. Primary androgen that causes increased hair growth, acne, and physical changes associated with virilization

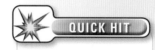

QUICK HIT

Higher estrogen stimulates SHBG, which decreases free active testosterone.

FIGURE 41.2 Adrenal androgen production.

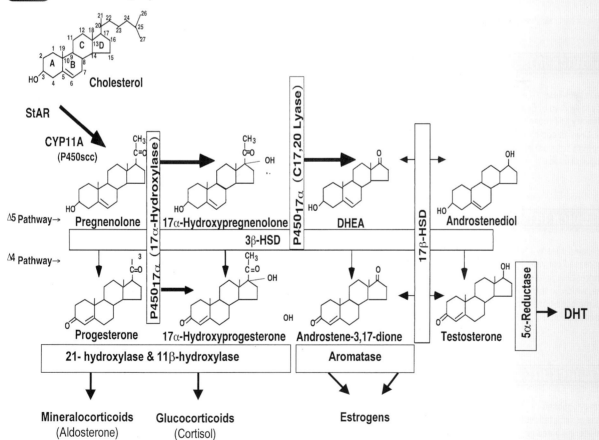

The ovary, the testis, and the adrenal gland produce six common core steroids. The core D5 steroids are pregnenolone, 17-hydroxypregnenolone, and dehydroepiandrosterone. The core D4 steroids are progesterone, 17-hydroxyprogesterone, and androstenedione (androstene-3,17-dione). The core steroids are important precursors for the production of sex steroids, glucocorticoids, and mineralocorticoids. (From Scott JR, Gibbs RS, Karlan BY, Haney AF. *Danforth's Obstetrics and Gynecology.* Baltimore: Lippincott Williams & Wilkins; 2005.)

Hirsutism and Virilization

TABLE **41.1**	Androgen Characteristics		
Androgen	**Activity**	**Secreted By**	**Notes**
Dehydroepiandrosterone (DHEA)	Weak androgen	Adrenal glands (90%)	DHEA-S: sulfated form, has a longer half-life
Androstenedione	Weak androgen	Ovaries (50%) Adrenal glands (50%)	
Testosterone	Potent androgen	Ovaries (25%) Adrenal glands (25%) Extraglandular (50%)	Aromatized to estrone in adipose tissue

DHEA-S, dehydroepiandrosterone sulfate.

F. Adrenal androgen production is controlled by adrenocorticotropic hormone (ACTH)
   1. ACTH stimulates adrenal cortical production of androgens with dehydroepiandrosterone (DHEA) as 1 of precursor molecules (see Figure 41.2)
   2. With enzyme deficiencies within this pathway, precursor molecules like DHEA accumulate
   3. These products can be measured to determine source of enzyme deficiency
   4. DHEA is further metabolized to androstenedione and testosterone
G. Ovarian androgen production
   1. Stimulated by luteinizing hormone (LH) secretion from pituitary gland
   2. LH stimulates theca-lutein cells to secrete androstenedione and testosterone
H. Extraglandular testosterone production occurs in adipocytes
   1. Depends on magnitude of adrenal and ovarian androstenedione production
   2. Obesity increases conversion of androstenedione to testosterone

III. Hyperandrogenic Disorders

A. Polycystic ovary syndrome (PCOS) is most common pathologic cause of hirsutism
   1. Affects 6%–10% of reproductive age women
   2. Etiology: unknown
   3. Symptoms: oligomenorrhea/amenorrhea, acne, hirsutism, infertility
   4. Rotterdam (2003) and Androgen Excess and PCOS Society (2010) criteria
      a. Oligoovulation or anovulation usually marked by irregular menstrual cycles
      b. Biochemical or clinical evidence of hyperandrogenism
      c. Polycystic-appearing ovaries on ultrasound (Figure 41.3)
   5. Need to rule out other endocrine disorders such as congenital adrenal hyperplasia (CAH), Cushing syndrome, hyperprolactinemia
   6. Pathophysiology unclear: appears to be increased LH pulse frequency in patients with PCOS
      a. LH stimulates theca-lutein cells to increase androstenedione production
      b. Androstenedione is aromatized to estrone within adipocytes
      c. With increased androstenedione, coincident increased testosterone production
      d. PCOS is disease of excess androgen and excess estrogen
      e. Elevated androgen levels interfere with normal development of dominant ovarian follicles
      f. Higher estrogen levels (including estrone) disrupt normal pattern of midcycle LH surge resulting in anovulation
      g. Obesity is seen in 50%–60% of patients with PCOS and acquisition of body fat coincides with onset of PCOS; PCOS patients are at high risk for metabolic syndrome
      h. 40% of PCOS patients have impaired glucose tolerance; in PCOS patients, decreased insulin sensitivity in peripheral tissues results in increased insulin secretion (hyperinsulinemia)

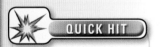

QUICK HIT

Hirsutism is seen less frequently in women of East Asian ethnicity and those who have been on combined contraceptives for most of their postpubertal lives.

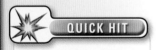

QUICK HIT

With increasing obesity comes increased conversion of androstenedione to estrone, which, in turn, enhances the conditions causing anovulation.

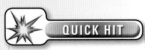

QUICK HIT

Long-term unopposed estrogen is associated with abnormal uterine bleeding, endometrial hyperplasia, and development of endometrial cancer.

Hirsutism and Virilization

FIGURE 41.3 **Polycystic appearance of the ovary on transvaginal ultrasound.**

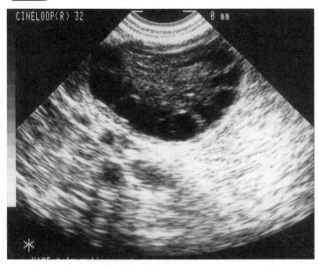

Note the string of subcapsular follicles measuring 2 to 8 mm in diameter, with increased central stromal mass. (From Scott JR, Gibbs RS, Karlan BY, Haney AF. *Danforth's Obstetrics and Gynecology.* Baltimore: Lippincott Williams & Wilkins; 2005.)

    i. 8% have type 2 diabetes mellitus

    j. Lipid abnormalities: elevated triglyceride levels, low high-density lipoprotein (HDL) levels and elevated low-density lipoprotein (LDL) levels, and hypertension (HTN)

B. Acanthosis nigricans (Figure 41.4)

    1. Velvety, hyperpigmented appearance of skin creases

    2. Results from basal layer hyperplasia of epidermal skin from mitogenic effects of insulin

C. Hyperandrogenism, severe insulin resistance, acanthosis nigricans (HAIR-AN) syndrome

    1. Ovaries can appear hyperthecotic

    2. Hyperandrogenism may be severe and can even present with virilization

    3. May be refractory to treatment and to successfully induce ovulation

FIGURE 41.4 **Acanthosis nigricans.**

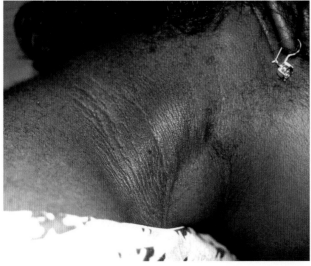

(Courtesy of George A. Datto, III, MD.)

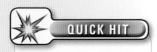

Insulin sensitizers reduce insulin resistance and facilitate ovulation.

D. Therapy
   1. Lifestyle changes: diet and exercise
   2. Oral contraceptives (if pregnancy is not intended)
      a. Suppress pituitary LH production, decreasing androstenedione and testosterone leading to decreased acne, prevention of new hair growth, and decreased androgenic stimulation of existing hair follicles
      b. Decrease circulating estrogen, leading to decreased risk of endometrial hyperplasia and irregular bleeding
   3. If pregnancy is intended
      a. Weight reduction in obese patients can restore regular, ovulatory cycles and lead to spontaneous conception
      b. Ovulation induction with clomiphene citrate
      c. Insulin sensitizers (glucophage) alone or with clomiphene citrate

IV. **Ovarian Neoplasms** (*see also Chapter 50*)
   A. Uncommon, occurring in 1 in 500 hirsute women
   B. Sertoli-Leydig cell tumors (androblastoma, arrhenoblastoma)
      1. Ovarian neoplasms that secrete testosterone
      2. Rapid onset (<6 months) of acne, severe hirsutism (75% of patients), amenorrhea (30% of patients), and virilizing signs
      3. Laboratory markers
         a. Suppressed follicle-stimulating hormone (FSH) and LH
         b. Low plasma androstenedione
         c. Markedly elevated testosterone
      4. Should be no delay in surgical removal of involved ovary to maximize regression of symptoms
   C. Gynandroblastoma: rare, has elements of both granulosa cell and arrhenoblastoma
      1. Virilization is predominant clinical feature
      2. Estrogen production may simultaneously produce endometrial hyperplasia and irregular uterine bleeding
   D. Lipid (lipoid) cell tumors contain sheets of round, clear, pale-staining cells; virilization (or defeminization)
   E. Hilar cell tumors are typically found in postmenopausal women (virilization)

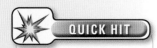

During surgery, the contralateral ovary should be inspected and, if enlarged, should be bisected for gross inspection and possible biopsy.

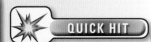

If the clitoris has become enlarged, it does not revert back to its original size. Terminal hair in a sexual distribution will not revert to vellus hair and may need mechanical removal of excess hair.

V. **Adrenal Disorders**
   A. CAH is inborn glandular enzymatic deficiency resulting in precursor (substrate) excess leading to overproduction of steroids
      1. 21-Hydroxylase deficiency: most common enzyme deficiency, affecting 2% of population
         a. Catalyzes conversion of progesterone and 17α-hydroxyprogesterone to desoxycorticosterone and compound S
         b. Deficiency leads to accumulation of progesterone and 17α-hydroxyprogesterone
         c. Alteration in chromosome 6, which contains genes for 21-hydroxylase, leads to disorder
         d. Nonclassic forms are more common
            i. Can appear at puberty or in adulthood (late-onset CAH)
            ii. Clinical manifestations: terminal body hair, acne, subtle alterations in menstrual cycles and infertility
            iii. If presenting in puberty, adrenarche may precede thelarche
         e. Measurement of plasma 17-OH progesterone (preferably fasting level), levels usually are >2,000 ng/dL with this disorder
            i. Those with less severe forms will have mildly elevated basal levels at 200 ng/dL with increase to >1,000 ng/dL with ACTH stimulation
            ii. Dehydroepiandrosterone sulfate (DHEA-S) and androstenedione will also be elevated and contribute to hirsutism and virilization
      2. 11β-Hydroxylase deficiency (catalyzes conversion of desoxycorticosterone to cortisol) also leads to increased androgen production
         a. Clinical presentation: mild hypertension, mild hirsutism
         b. Diagnosis: increased plasma desoxycorticosterone

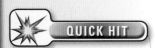

The classic form of CAH manifests with a virilized newborn female infant with ambiguous genitalia as well as life-threatening salt wasting.

Hirsutism and Virilization

3. Treatment goal: restore normal cortisol levels
    a. Decreased cortisol increases ACTH secretion; this in turn leads to oversecretion of precursor molecules proximal to enzymatic block resulting in increased androgen production
    b. In high-grade enzymatic blocks, inadequate amounts of glucocorticoids and mineralocorticoids are made, resulting in salt loss, which can be life-threatening.
    c. Nonclassic CAH can be managed by supplementing glucocorticoids (e.g., prednisone 2.5 mg daily)
    d. With therapy, facial acne improves and ovulation is restored; no new terminal hair growth occurs
B. **Cushing syndrome**
    1. Adrenal disease producing adrenal excess (either from an adrenal neoplasm or an ACTH-producing tumor)
    2. Signs: truncal obesity, moonlike facies, glucose intolerance, skin thinning with striae, osteoporosis, proximal muscle weakness, hyperandrogenism, menstrual irregularities, hypertension, supraclavicular and cervical spinal fat pads
C. Adrenal neoplasms
    1. Characterized by a rapid increase in hair growth associated with severe acne, amenorrhea, and sometimes virilization
    2. Adenomas: produce androgens only
    3. Adrenal carcinomas: may produce large amounts of glucocorticoids and androgens
    4. DHEA-S is usually elevated >6 mg/mL
    5. Diagnosis: adrenal gland computed tomography (CT) scan or magnetic resonance imaging (MRI)
    6. Treatment: surgical removal

VI. Idiopathic Hirsutism (Constitutional or Familial Hirsutism)
A. Most common nonpathologic etiology; responsible for 50% of cases
B. No cause of hirsutism after diagnostic evaluation
C. Present with mild to moderate hirsutism, usually with normal circulating levels of androgens, usually with regular cycles

VII. Iatrogenic Hirsutism: some medications are implicated with hirsutism and virilization (e.g., danazol)

VIII. Other Hirsutism Issues to Consider
A. History and physical examination
    1. Ask about shaving habits (how often, where), as she may shave/use creams to hide
    2. Ferriman-Gallwey score
    3. Assess for thyroid enlargement
B. Laboratory evaluation
    1. Measurement of prolactin and thyroid-stimulating hormone (TSH) can rule out hyperprolactinemia with or without thyroid dysfunction
    2. Measurement of total and free testosterone, DHEA-S
    3. Basal 17-hydroxyprogesterone can rule out 21-hydroxylase–deficient CAH
    4. 24-hour free urinary cortisol or overnight dexamethasone test can diagnose Cushing syndrome if suspected
C. PCOS
    1. If with chronic anovulation and combination contraceptives are contraindicated, patient should have scheduled progestin-induced withdrawal bleeding to reduce risk of endometrial hyperplasia and cancer
    2. Counseling on weight loss, diet and exercise, lifestyle changes to decrease risk of diabetes and cardiovascular disease

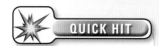

QUICK HIT

Medical therapy for adrenal and ovarian disorders cannot resolve hirsutism; it only suppresses new hair growth. Hair that is already present can be controlled by shaving, bleaching, depilatory creams, electrolysis, and/or laser hair ablation.

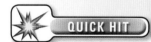

QUICK HIT

Total testosterone >200 or DHEA-S >7,000 ng/mL should prompt a search for adrenal or ovarian androgen-producing tumors.

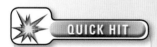

QUICK HIT

An ACTH stimulation test may be done for definitive diagnosis if the results of 17-OH progesterone are over 200 ng/mL.

Hirsutism and Virilization

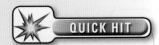

D. Treatment of hirsutism is best achieved by androgen synthesis inhibitors and mechanical removal of excess hair that is already present
   1. Suppress future hair growth but do not immediately cause existing hair to disappear; full effect not evident until 6–48 months
   2. Androgen synthesis inhibitors
      a. Spironolactone 100 mg/day
         i. Competes for testosterone at binding sites
         ii. Inhibits testosterone production by ovary
         iii. Decreases 5α-reductase activity
         iv. Will need to monitor potassium levels
      b. Flutamide
      c. Cyproterone acetate
      d. Finasteride 5 mg daily blocks conversion of testosterone to dihydrotestosterone
   3. Eflornithine hydrochloride 13.9%
      a. Irreversible inhibitor of L-ornithine decarboxylase slows and shrinks hair
      b. Can be used on face

Hirsutism and Virilization

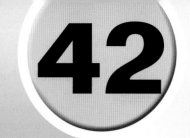

Menopause

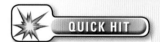

I. Definitions

A. Menopause
1. Defined as last menstrual period, which can only be confirmed after 1 year of amenorrhea
2. Average age in United States is 51 years

B. Perimenopause
1. Defined by North American Menopause Society as a span typically lasting 6 years or more that begins with onset of menstrual cycle changes and other menopause-related symptoms
2. Extends through menopause to 1 year after menopause

C. Premature menopause
1. Menopause before age 40 years

II. Hormone Changes

A. Perimenopause
1. Cycles often shorten
2. Ovulation occurs less frequently
3. Follicle-stimulating hormone (FSH) increases to stimulate follicles (often 20–40 IU/L)
4. Variable to high levels of estradiol

B. Postmenopause (Table 42.1)
1. Increased FSH (typically >40 IU/L)
2. Low estradiol: lower estrogen levels result in lower sex hormone–binding globulin (SHBG), so free testosterone is increased
3. Low estrone, but more estrone than estradiol due to peripheral conversion of androgens in adipose tissue
4. Increased luteinizing hormone
   a. Stimulates ovaries to continue to produce testosterone and androstenedione
   b. Surgical menopause results in lower androgen levels

> **QUICK HIT**
>
> Female life expectancy has increased over the last 100 years, but there has been no change in the age of menopause.

TABLE 42.1 Steroid Hormone Serum Concentrations in Premenopausal Women, Postmenopausal Women, and Women After Oophorectomy

Hormone	Premenopausal (Normal Ranges)	Postmenopausal	Postoophorectomy
Testosterone (ng/dL)	325 (200–600)	230	110
Androstenedione (ng/dL)	1,500 (500–3,000)	800–900	800–900
Estrone (pg/mL)	30–200	25–30	30
Estradiol (pg/mL)	35–500	10–15	15–20

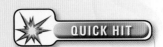

QUICK HIT

Premature menopause occurs before age 40 years.

III. Causes of Premature Menopause

A. Abnormal karyotypes involving X chromosome (Turner syndrome, fragile X syndrome)

B. Autoimmune: polyendocrine syndromes (hypothyroid, adrenal insufficiency, hypoparathyroidism, type 1 diabetes mellitus), myasthenia gravis, rheumatoid arthritis, systemic lupus erythematosus

C. Environmental: pelvic radiation, chemotherapy (especially alkylating agents), hysterectomy even without oophorectomy, uterine artery embolization

IV. Symptoms

A. Hot flashes
1. Incidence
   a. 68%–93% of postmenopausal women
   b. 10%–15% of women consider them severe
2. Definition: momentary sensation of flushing, perspiration, and intense heat, with reddening of face and neck
3. Usually last ~90 seconds
4. Typically begin several years before menopause, peak at menopause, and improve in years after menopause
   a. Last up to 5 years for most women
   b. Can last >10 years
5. Frequency and intensity vary by ethnic groups
6. Other causes of hot flashes include thyroid disease, autoimmune diseases, pheochromocytoma, carcinoid syndrome, panic disorder, epilepsy, infection, insulinoma, and medications (antiestrogens and estrogen agonists/antagonists)
7. Treatment
   a. Lifestyle changes including increased exercise, dressing in layers, calcium supplements, less alcohol, less tobacco, and a low-fat diet
   b. Sleep medications
   c. Hormone therapy (HT): ~90% effective
   d. Selective serotonin reuptake inhibitors/serotonin norepinephrine reuptake inhibitors: ~50%–60% effective
   e. Gabapentin: ~45% effective
   f. Clonidine: "mildly" effective
   g. Soy supplementation: possibly 40%–50% effective
   h. Black cohosh: possibly 40%–50% effective

B. Sleep changes
1. At least partially due to hot flashes at night
2. Result in mood swings and anxiety

C. Weight gain
1. Due to aging and lifestyle changes, not menopause
2. Worsened by sleep deprivation

D. Mood changes
1. Worsened by sleep changes of menopause
2. Depression is common in this age group

E. Skin, nail, and hair changes
1. Lower estrogen levels cause lower SHBG levels, thus more free testosterone, which causes facial hair, scalp hair loss, and acne
2. Skin less elastic; more susceptible to abrasion and trauma
3. Nails more brittle

F. Vaginal dryness
1. Genital tract atrophy due to lack of estrogen
   a. Symptoms of itching, burning, which patient often mistakes for "yeast infection"
   b. Can cause postmenopausal spotting/bleeding
   c. Often causes dyspareunia and relationship difficulties
   d. Treated with over-the-counter lubricants or vaginal estrogen
2. Worsening genital prolapse: damage from childbirth worsened by atrophy of muscles and ligaments, resulting in cystocele, rectocele, and urinary incontinence

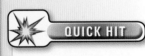

QUICK HIT

Although menopause does not cause obesity, estrogen deprivation is associated with increased adipose tissue in the abdominal region.

V. Disease Risk

A. Cardiovascular disease
1. Lipid profiles worsen
a. Total cholesterol increases
b. High-density lipoprotein cholesterol decreases
c. Low-density lipoprotein cholesterol increases
2. Risk not lessened with HT, and HT should not be used to prevent cardiovascular disease
3. Prevention should focus on lifestyle changes, control of hyperlipidemia, and hypertension

B. Cancer
1. **Breast cancer**: mammograms
2. **Colorectal cancer**
a. Colonoscopy every 10 years for age older than 50 years is preferred
b. Alternatives
i. Flexible sigmoidoscopy every 5 years with fecal occult blood testing annually
ii. Double-contrast barium enema every 5 years

C. Dementia: effect of aging, not menopause

D. Osteoporosis
1. Occurs when reduced bone strength predisposes a patient to fracture
2. National Osteoporosis Foundation (NOF) estimates that 50% of Caucasian women will experience an osteoporotic fracture during their lives
3. Peak bone mass occurs in 3rd decade of life
4. At time of menopause, rapid loss of bone
a. 2% of cortical bone and 5% of trabecular bone lost in 1st 5–8 years after menopause
5. Risk factors include
a. Advanced age
b. Female gender
c. Prior fragility fracture after age 50 years
d. Low bone mineral density (BMD)
e. Corticosteroid use
f. Rheumatoid arthritis
g. Family history of hip fracture
h. Smoking
i. Excessive use of alcohol
j. Use of anticonvulsants
6. Testing guidelines (NOF and American College of Obstetricians and Gynecologists [the College])
a. BMD by central dual-energy X-ray absorptiometry of hip and spine
i. Normal = T score >-1.0
ii. Low BMD (**osteopenia**) = T score -1.0 to -2.5
iii. **Osteoporosis** = T score <-2.5
b. Test all women older than age 65 years
c. Test younger women with risk factors
d. Test all postmenopausal women with fractures
7. FRAX tool
a. Computer calculation that integrates femoral neck BMD with clinical risk factors to estimate fracture risk and determine therapy
b. Gives 10-year probability of hip and major osteoporotic fracture
8. NOF treatment guidelines
a. Treat patients with prior hip or vertebral fracture
b. Treat patients with T score <-2.5
c. Treat patients with T score of -1.0 to -2.5 at high risk of fracture (e.g., steroid use or immobility)
d. Treat patients with a T score of -1.0 to -2.5 and FRAX 10-year risk of hip fracture of $>3\%$
e. Treat patient with T score of -1.0 to -2.5 and FRAX 10-year risk of major osteoporotic fracture of $>20\%$

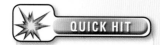

QUICK HIT

Risk of cardiovascular disease increases in postmenopausal women, probably due to loss of the protective effect of natural estrogen.

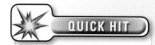

QUICK HIT

Initiating HT within 10 years of menopause for treatment of hot flashes does not increase or decrease risk of coronary heart disease events.

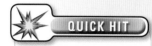

QUICK HIT

Organizations differ on recommendations between ages 35 and 50 years (annually or every 2 years), but all recommend annual mammograms after age 50 years.

Menopause

9. Treatment
   a. All patients advised of calcium supplementation (1,000–1,500 mg/day), adequate vitamin D (800–1,000 IU/day), weight-bearing exercise, and tobacco and alcohol avoidance
   b. Medications
      i. Estrogen agonists/antagonists (raloxifene, bazedoxifene, lasofoxifene)
      ii. Bisphosphonates (alendronate, risedronate, ibandronate, zoledronic acid)
      iii. Receptor activator of nuclear factor-$\kappa\beta$ ligand (RANKL) inhibitor (denosumab)
      iv. Calcitonin
      v. Synthetic parathyroid hormone (teriparatide)
      vi. HT (for prevention only)
   c. Possible complications of medications
      i. Osteonecrosis of jaw
      ii. Atypical fractures

VI. Hormone Therapy

A. Estrogen therapy (ET) if patient does not have uterus
B. Estrogen–progestin therapy (EPT) if patient does have uterus
   1. Progestin converts proliferative to secretory endometrium, thereby preventing hyperplasia and cancer
   2. Progestin can be given cyclically (12–14 days/month) or continuously
C. Estrogen can be given orally, transdermally, vaginally, or intravenously
D. Women's Health Initiative (WHI): assessed long-term risks and benefits of ET and EPT in disease prevention
   1. Risks/benefits of EPT (older patients and prolonged use)
      a. Increased risk of coronary heart disease, stroke, breast cancer, venous thromboembolic disease, and pulmonary emboli
      b. Decreased risk of colorectal cancer and hip fracture
      c. No change in risk of endometrial cancer and total deaths
   2. Risks/benefits of ET (older patients and prolonged use)
      a. Increased risk of stroke
      b. Decreased risk of hip fracture
      c. No change in risk of coronary heart disease, breast cancer, venous thromboembolic disease, pulmonary emboli, colorectal cancer, and total deaths
E. Indications
   1. Treatment of menopausal symptoms and prevention of osteoporosis in patient being treated for menopausal symptoms
   2. Use lowest effective dose for shortest amount of time needed to relieve symptoms
F. Contraindications (Box 42.1)
G. Treatment of vaginal atrophy only: vaginal estrogen (cream, ring, tablets)

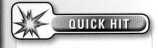

QUICK HIT

The WHI was conducted by the National Institutes of Health to assess the risks and benefits of HT in postmenopausal women.

QUICK HIT

HT should be used to treat symptoms with the lowest effective dose for the shortest amount of time.

BOX 42.1

Contraindications to Hormone Therapy

- Undiagnosed abnormal genital bleeding
- Known or suspected estrogen-dependent neoplasia except in appropriately selected patients
- Active deep vein thrombosis, pulmonary embolism, or a history of these conditions
- Active or recent arterial thromboembolic disease (stroke, myocardial infarction)
- Liver dysfunction or liver disease
- Known or suspected pregnancy
- Hypersensitivity to hormone therapy preparations

Menopause

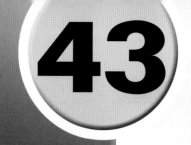

Infertility

I. Definition

A. Failure of couple to conceive after 12 months of unprotected intercourse
B. 15% of reproductive-age couples in United States
C. 85% of infertile couples who undergo treatment can expect to have child

II. Etiology

A. Female factors (65%)
B. Male factors (20%)
C. Unexplained or other conditions (15%)
D. More than 1 factor may be present in partner
E. Common (30%) to find 1 or more conditions in both partners

III. Evaluation

A. Timing
   1. Female partner <35 years of age, after 12 months of attempt
   2. Female partner >35 years of age, initiate evaluation when patient expresses concern, even if it is <12 months of attempt
B. Pertinent points in history taking
   1. Medical disorders
   2. Medications
   3. Prior surgeries
   4. Prior pelvic infections or pelvic pain
   5. History of sexually transmitted diseases
   6. Sexual dysfunction
   7. Environmental and lifestyle factors (e.g., diet, exercise, tobacco, drugs)
C. Investigation of female partner
   1. Ovulation
      a. Presumptive evidence: regular periods with cyclic changes associated with ovulation and progesterone production
         i. Ovulation pain (mittelschmerz)
         ii. Decreased vaginal secretion
         iii. Abdominal bloating
         iv. Increased body weight
         v. Breast fullness/tenderness
         vi. Occasional depression
      b. Indirect evidence
         i. Biphasic basal body temperature chart (postovulation is 0.6°F higher than before ovulation)
         ii. Positive urine ovulation prediction kit (positive urine luteinizing hormone [LH] test 24 hours before ovulation)
      c. Direct evidence
         i. Serum progesterone >3 ng/mL
         ii. Endometrial biopsy shows secretory endometrium

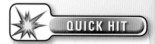

QUICK HIT

The psychological stress associated with infertility must be recognized and addressed accordingly.

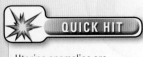

Infertility

QUICK HIT

Uterine anomalies are usually associated with *pregnancy loss* rather than infertility.

2. Anatomic factors
   a. Uterus
      i. Potential abnormalities include leiomyomas, polyps, intrauterine adhesions, and congenital anomalies
      ii. Investigative tools
         (a) Transvaginal ultrasound
         (b) Hysterosalpingography (HSG)
         (c) Hysteroscopy
   b. Fallopian tubes
      i. HSG
      ii. Chromotubation during laparoscopy
      iii. Saline infusion sonography
   c. Peritoneum
      i. Requires laparoscopy
      ii. Pelvic adhesion and endometriosis are most common conditions
D. Investigation of male partner
   1. Semen analysis
      a. 3–5 days of abstinence
      b. Masturbate to collect sample in wide-mouth container
      c. Collect complete sample: most sperm reside in 1st few drops of ejaculate
   2. Normal semen parameters
      a. 1.5–5.0 mL
      b. pH >7.2
      c. >20 million/mL
      d. >50% motile, >25% with rapid progressive movement
      e. >30% normal morphology
   3. Hormonal evaluation of infertile male
      a. Follicle-stimulating hormone (FSH)
      b. LH
      c. Testosterone
      d. Prolactin
   4. Genetic testing for men with azoospermia (no sperm) or severe oligospermia
      a. Cystic fibrosis transmembrane conductance regulator (CFTR)
      b. Karyotype (such as Klinefelter 47,XXY)
      c. Y chromosome microdeletions
   5. Further tests on men with azoospermia
      a. Obstructive azoospermia
         i. Percutaneous epididymal sperm aspiration (PESA)
         ii. Microsurgical epididymal sperm aspiration (MESA)
      b. Nonobstructive azoospermia: testicular biopsy

IV. Unexplained Infertility
A. 15% of infertile couples
B. Likely due to 1 or more mild abnormalities in 1 of above elements
C. Low rate (1%–3% per month) of spontaneous pregnancy

V. Treatment
A. Ovulation induction
   1. Clomiphene citrate
      a. Selective estrogen receptor modulator
      b. Competitively inhibits binding of estrogen to its receptors at hypothalamus and pituitary
      c. Induces release of gonadotropin from pituitary
      d. Start on menstrual cycle days 3, 4, or 5, daily for 5 days
      e. Ovulation occurs 5–12 days after last pill
      f. Ovulation may be triggered using human chorionic gonadotropin injection
      g. May be combined with intrauterine insemination (IUI)
      h. 10% pregnancy is multiple gestation

2. Controlled ovarian hyperstimulation
   a. Use exogenous gonadotropin to stimulate ovaries
   b. Purified FSH and LH (extracted from postmenopausal women's urine) or recombinant human FSH used
   c. Risks include ovarian hyperstimulation syndrome (OHSS) and 25% incidence of multiple gestations
   d. May be combined with IUI

B. IUI
   1. Ejaculated semen specimen washed to recover motile sperm
   2. Sperm resuspended in small amount of medium (usually 0.5 mL)
   3. Sample injected via catheter, which is advanced through cervix into uterus
   4. Benefits couples with unexplained infertility or mild male factor infertility
   5. Does not benefit couples with severe male factor infertility
   6. Total motile sperm <1 million rarely produces pregnancy

C. Assisted reproductive technology (ART) and in vitro fertilization (IVF)
   1. 99% of all ART in United States is IVF
   2. IVF bypasses normal mechanism of gamete transport
   3. IVF may be combined with intracytoplasmic sperm injection (ICSI), by which a single sperm is injected directly into the oocyte
   4. Chance of conception depends on number and quality of embryos transferred
   5. Multiple gestation risk 30%
   6. Spontaneous abortion rate 15%

D. IVF
   1. Essential steps
      a. Ovulation induction to produce multiple follicles
      b. Retrieve oocytes from ovaries
      c. Oocyte fertilization in vitro in laboratory
      d. Embryo incubation for 3–5 days in laboratory
      e. Transfer of embryo to woman's uterus through cervix
      f. Progesterone supplement (until 10 weeks' gestation)
   2. Indications
      a. Absent or blocked fallopian tubes
      b. Severe pelvic adhesion
      c. Severe endometriosis
      d. Severe male factor infertility (combine IVF with ICSI)
      e. Unexplained infertility
      f. Failed treatment with less aggressive therapy

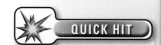

QUICK HIT

IVF success can be as high as 40%–50%; depends on etiology of infertility and age of female partner.

Infertility

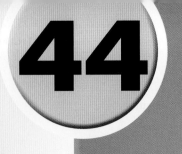

Premenstrual Syndrome and Premenstrual Dysphoric Disorder

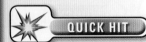

QUICK HIT

Symptoms tend to resolve with initiation of menses and always by the end of menses.

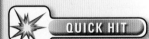

QUICK HIT

PMS and PMDD can present any time during reproductive years (menarche to late 40s). A woman's recognition and acceptance of the symptoms, when present, is the key factor in diagnosis.

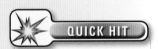

QUICK HIT

Up to 65% of patients with PMDD have a history of major depression.

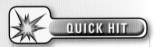

QUICK HIT

There is a relationship between the hormone levels of estrogen and progesterone and symptoms, insofar as menopause and anovulation provide relief.

I. Definition

A. **Premenstrual syndrome (PMS):** mood and behavioral changes affecting aspect of patient's life

B. **Premenstrual dysphoric disorder (PMDD):** severe form of PMS with specific set of diagnostic criteria, which includes depressed mood, anxiety, irritability, or decreased interest in daily activities

C. Both occur regularly and cyclically only during luteal phase of menstrual cycle

II. Incidence

A. Premenstrual symptoms occur in 75%–85% of women

B. PMS occurs in 5%−10% of women

C. PMDD occurs in 3%−5% of women

D. Higher rates present in Mediterranean and Middle Eastern cultures and lower in Asian cultures

E. Genetic component reflected in twin studies

III. Symptoms

A. >200 symptoms have been described

B. Somatic symptoms include bloating, fatigue, mastodynia, headache, acne, nausea, vomiting, diarrhea, and sensitivity to stimuli

C. Behavioral symptoms include emotional liability, change in libido and appetite, hostility, and sleep disturbance

D. Psychological symptoms include irritability, depressed mood, anxiety, easy crying, and loss of interest

E. Sometimes difficult to differentiate from true psychiatric disorders

IV. Etiology

A. No single theory has been found (some include hormonal, endorphins, neurotransmitters, or vitamin or mineral deficiency)

B. Serotonin may be only promising single transmitter directly linked

  1. Progesterone effect on serotonin may be linked by decreasing serotonin availability

  2. γ-Aminobutyric acid (GABA) decreases allopregnenolone (progesterone precursor)

  3. Patients with PMDD and PMS may have dysfunctional neuron response to GABA–progesterone–serotonin interactions

V. Diagnosis

A. Differential diagnosis is extensive (medical and psychiatric)

B. Not all symptoms are PMS or PMDD related just because patient has menses

C. Strict criteria should be met before either diagnosis is made

D. Relationship to luteal phase must be present; all others are unlikely PMS or PMDD

E. For PMS, only 1 symptom is required, but there must be symptom-free phase (Box 44.1)

BOX 44.1

Diagnostic Criteria for Premenstrual Syndrome

1. Premenstrual syndrome can be diagnosed if the patient reports at least one of the following affective and somatic symptoms during the 5 days before menses in each of three menstrual cycles:

Affective Symptoms	**Somatic Symptoms**
Depression	Breast tenderness
Angry outbursts	Abdominal bloating
Irritability	Headache
Anxiety	Swelling of extremities
Confusion	
Social withdrawal	

2. These symptoms are relieved within 4 days of the onset of menses, without recurrence until at least cycle day 13. The symptoms are present in the absence of any pharmacologic therapy, hormone ingestion, or drug or alcohol use. The symptoms occur reproducibly during two cycles of prospective recording. The patient suffers from identifiable dysfunction in social or economic performance.

F. For PMDD, 5 or more symptoms must be present including core symptom, but there must be symptom-free phase (Box 44.2)

G. **Daily symptom record** (Figure 44.1)
 1. Most efficient way to gather information for diagnosis and differentiate from **depression** (symptoms always present)
 2. At least 3 months of diary should be collected before conclusion can be made and cyclic, repetitive luteal phase correlation established

VI. Treatment
 A. Nonpharmacologic
  1. Continue symptoms chart during treatment to monitor progress
  2. Education about normal cycle, lifestyle modifications, and acknowledging that disease are major components

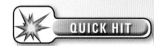

QUICK HIT

Many disorders worsen during the luteal phase and/or menses and are not necessarily PMS or PMDD. Rule out medical or psychiatric conditions before a final diagnosis is made.

PMS and PMDD

BOX 44.2

Diagnostic Criteria for Premenstrual Dysphoric Disorder

A. In most menstrual cycles during the past year, ≥5 of the following were present most of the time during the last week of the luteal phase, began to remit within a few days of menses onset, and were absent in the week postmenses, with at least one of the symptoms being items 1, 2, 3, or 4 ("core symptoms") listed as follows:

 1. Markedly depressed mood, feelings of hopelessness, self-deprecation
 2. Marked anxiety, tension, feelings of being "keyed up" or "on edge"
 3. Suddenly feeling sad or tearful, with increased sensitivity to personal rejection
 4. Persistent and marked irritability, anger, or increased interpersonal conflicts
 5. Decreased interest in usual activities
 6. Subjective sense of having difficulty in concentrating
 7. Lethargy, fatigue, or marked lack of energy
 8. Marked change in appetite and cravings for certain foods
 9. Hypersomnia or insomnia
 10. Feeling overwhelmed or out of control
 11. Other physical symptoms, such as breast tenderness or swelling, headaches, joint or muscle pain, a sensation of "bloating," or weight gain, pain, etc.

B. The disturbance markedly interferes with work or school, or with usual social activities and relationships with others

C. The disturbance is not merely an exacerbation of the symptoms of another disorder, although it may be superimposed on one

D. Criteria A, B, and C must be confirmed by prospective daily ratings during at least 2 consecutive symptomatic cycles (the diagnosis may be made provisionally prior to this confirmation)

(Reprinted with permission from American Psychiatric Association. *The Diagnostic and Statistical Manual of Mental Disorders*, 4th ed. Text Revision. Arlington, VA: American Psychiatric Association; 2000.)

PMS and PMDD

© pending, Jean Endicott, Ph.D. and Wilma Harrison, M.D.

FIGURE 44.1 A sample tool for collection of symptoms.

DAILY RECORD OF SEVERITY OF PROBLEMS

Please print and use as many sheets as you need for at least two FULL months of ratings.

Name or Initials _____

Month/Year _____

Each evening note the degree to which you experienced each of the problems listed below. Put an "x" in the box which corresponds to the severity: 1 - not at all, 2 - minimal, 3 - mild, 4 - moderate, 5 - severe, 6 - extreme.

Enter day (Monday="M", Thursday="R", etc) >

Note spotting by entering "S" >

Note menses by entering "M" >

Begin rating on correct calendar day >   1 2 3 4 5 6 7 8 9 10 11 12 13 14 15 16 17 18 19 20 21 22 23 24 25 26 27 28 29 30 31

1. Felt depressed, sad, "down,", or "blue" or felt hopeless; or felt worthless or guilty

2. Felt anxious, tense, "keyed up" or "on edge"

3. Had mood swings (i.e., suddenly feeling sad or tearful) or was sensitive to rejection or feelings were easily hurt

4. Felt angry, or irritable

5. Had less interest in usual activities (work, school, friends, hobbies)

6. Had difficulty concentrating

7. Felt lethargic, tired, or fatigued; or had lack of energy

8. Had increased appetite or overate; or had cravings for specific foods

9. Slept more, took naps, found it hard to get up when intended; or had trouble getting to sleep or staying asleep

10. Felt overwhelmed or unable to cope; or felt out of control

11. Had breast tenderness, breast swelling, bloated sensation, weight gain, headache, joint or muscle pain, or other physical symptoms

At work, school, home, or in daily routine, at least one of the problems noted above caused reduction of productivity or inefficiency

At least one of the problems noted above caused avoidance of or less participation in hobbies or social activities

At least one of the problems noted above interfered with relationships with others

(From Beckmann CRB, Ling FW, et al. *Obstetrics and Gynecology*, 7th ed. Philadelphia: Lippincott Williams & Wilkins; 2014.)

3. Many treatments including dietary changes (high-carbohydrate diet, raw vegetables, and fruits), vitamins and minerals (B6, D, E, calcium, primrose oil, magnesium), and exercise are suggested

4. Only exercise and calcium 1,200 mg/day with vitamin D has been shown to be effective

5. Relaxation, yoga, massage, and cognitive and light therapy have been tried with inconclusive results

B. Pharmacologic

1. Nonsteroidal anti-inflammatory drugs (NSAIDs) are not useful

2. Spironolactone decreases bloating but not other symptoms

3. Drosperidone (similar molecule to spironolactone precursors) containing oral contraceptives in a 24/4 cycle is U.S. Food and Drug Administration (FDA) approved for PMDD but not PMS

4. Other oral contraceptive combinations are not FDA approved for PMDD

5. Selective serotonin reuptake inhibitors (SSRIs) approved for PMDD (but not PMS)

   a. Include fluoxetine, sertraline, and paroxetine

   b. May be used for luteal phase of cycle monthly or continuously

   c. Significant side effects include stomach upset, insomnia, sexual dysfunction, anxiety, weight gain, etc., and may limit use

6. Danazol and gonadotropin-releasing hormone (GnRH) agonists are useful but long-term benefit unknown, and more side effects may limit use

7. Oophorectomy reserved for most severe cases and is uncommon

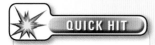

QUICK HIT

Many nonpharmacologic interventions, such as high vegetable and fruit diets and exercise, are part of a healthy lifestyle and should be encouraged even if no true randomized studies exist.

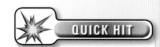

QUICK HIT

Start with nonpharmacologic interventions and move on to more complex treatments in the absence of positive results.

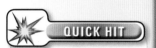

QUICK HIT

If surgical intervention is intended, a trial of "medical menopause" with GnRH agonists may be useful to see the expected effect after removal of the ovaries.

PMS and PMDD

Gynecologic Oncology

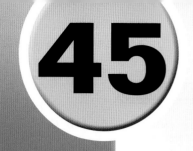

Cell Biology and Principles of Cancer Therapy

I. Cell Cycle

A. 4 cell cycle phases (Figure 45.1)

1. **G1: postmitotic phase**
   a. Key events: RNA and protein synthesis, cell growth, and DNA repair
   b. Agents that work in this phase: asparaginase and actinomycin D
2. **S: synthesis phase**
   a. Key events: DNA replication
   b. Agents that work in this phase: antimetabolites, antifolates, antipyrimidines, antipurines
3. **G2: additional synthesis phase**
   a. Key events: RNA, protein, and specialized DNA synthesis
   b. Agents that work in this phase: bleomycin
4. **M: mitosis phase**
   a. Key events: cell division
   b. Agents that work in this phase: vinca alkaloids (vincristine, vinblastine, and paclitaxel)

FIGURE 45.1 Actions of antineoplastic agents within the cell cycle.

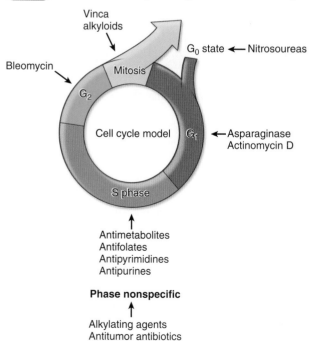

(From Beckmann CRB, Ling FW, et al. *Obstetrics and Gynecology*, 7th ed. Philadelphia: Lippincott Williams & Wilkins; 2014.)

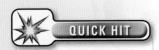

QUICK HIT

Debulking surgery leads to decreased tumor size, causing increased growth fraction and therefore increased vulnerability to chemotherapy and radiation.

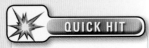

QUICK HIT

In the cell cycle, S and M phases are constant, whereas G1 and G2 vary.

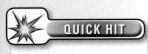

QUICK HIT

G1 time affects a cell's susceptibility to treatment.

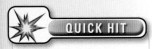

QUICK HIT

First-order kinetics means several doses of chemotherapy are better than one large dose.

5. **G0: resting phase**
    a. Key events: cells exit cell cycle
    b. Cells in this phase are not vulnerable to therapies targeting cell cycle
B. Growth fraction
    1. Definition: portion of cells actively dividing (cells in cell cycle/cells in cell cycle + cells in G0)
    2. As tumor size increases, growth fraction decreases
C. Generation time
    1. Definition: length of cell cycle, M phase to next M phase
    2. Duration
        a. S phase (DNA synthesis) = 7 hours
        b. M phase = 1 hour
    3. G1 time related to G0 phase (4–24 hours)
    4. 1st-order kinetics: dose kills constant fraction

II. **Chemotherapy**
A. Agents (Table 45.1 and Table 45.2)
    1. Cell cycle specific
        a. Best in actively dividing tumors (large growth fraction)
        b. Antimetabolites
            i. Mechanism: structural analogs that compete for binding sites and interfere with normal synthesis enzymes
            ii. S phase
            iii. Side effects: myelosuppression, gastrointestinal (GI) mucositis
            iv. Examples: methotrexate and 5-fluorouracil
        c. Plant (vinca) alkaloids
            i. Mechanism: prevent assembly of microtubules
            ii. M phase
            iii. Side effects: myelosuppression and anaphylactoid reaction
            iv. Examples: vincristine, vinblastine, and paclitaxel
    2. Cell cycle nonspecific
        a. More effective in tumors with low growth fraction
        b. Alkylating and alkylating-like agents
            i. Mechanism: cross-link DNA, interfere with DNA replication
            ii. Phase: nonspecific

TABLE 45.1 **Classes of Chemotherapeutic Drugs**

Class	Mechanism of Action	Primary Toxicity	Representative Drugs	Cell Cycle Phase of Action
Alkylating gents	Cross-link DNA either interstrand, intrastrand, or to proteins; preventing replication and transcription	Hemorrhagic cystitis, alopecia, nephrotoxicity	Cyclophosphamide, isophosphamide, melphalan	Nonspecific
Alkylating-like agents	Cross-link DNA strands (interstrand)	Nephrotoxicity, neurotoxicity, myelosuppression	Cisplatin, carboplatin	Nonspecific
Antitumor antibiotics	Interfere with DNA replication through free radical formation and intercalation between bases	Variable	Bleomycin, actinomycin D	Nonspecific
Antimetabolites	Block enzymes required for DNA synthesis	Gastrointestinal, myelosuppression, dermatologic, and hepatotoxicity	Methotrexate, 5-fluorouracil	S phase
Plant (vinca) alkaloids	Inhibit microtubule assembly	Myelosuppression	Vincristine, vinblastine, paclitaxel	M phase
Topoisomerase inhibitors	Inhibit topoisomerase, resulting in DNA strand breaks	Myelosuppression, alopecia, gastrointestinal	Etoposide, topotecan	Nonspecific

TABLE 45.2 **Major Application and Side Effects of Chemotherapeutic Agents**

Drug	Application	Dose Limiting Toxicity	Other Toxicities
Paclitaxel (mitotic inhibitor)	Ovarian cancer, endometrial cancer (advanced), granulosa cell tumors	Myelosuppression (neutropenia), peripheral neuropathy	Alopecia, myalgias/arthralgias, GI toxicity, hypersensitivity reaction
Carboplatin (alkylating-like agent)	Ovarian cancer, endometrial cancer (advanced), granulosa cell tumors	Myelosuppression (thrombocytopenia)	Nephrotoxicity, ototoxicity, GI toxicity, alopecia, hypersensitivity reaction
Cisplatin (alkylating-like agent)	Cervical cancer, germ cell tumors	Nephrotoxicity	Neurotoxicity, GI toxicity, hypersensitivity reaction
Bleomycin (antibiotic)	Germ cell tumors	Pulmonary fibrosis	Dermatologic (mucositis, hyperpigmentation)
Topotecan (topoisomerase inhibitor)	Ovarian cancer	Myelosuppression (neutropenia)	Alopecia, GI toxicity
Liposomal doxorubicin	Ovarian cancer	Myelosuppression	Palmar-plantar erythrodysesthesia, GI toxicity (stomatitis, N&V), cardiac (minimal)
Gemcitabine hydrochloride (antimetabolite)	Ovarian cancer	Neutropenia	Hepatotoxicity, nephrotoxicity, hemolytic uremic syndrome
Etoposide (topoisomerase inhibitor)	Germ cell tumors, gestational trophoblastic neoplasia	Myelosuppression (neutropenia)	Alopecia, GI toxicity, acute MI, acute leukemia
Ifosfamide (alkylating agent)	Uterine sarcoma	Hemorrhagic cystitis	Nephrotoxicity, GI toxicity, alopecia, mild leukopenia
Methotrexate (antimetabolite)	Gestational trophoblastic neoplasia, molar pregnancies	Myelosuppression (all cell lines)	Hepatotoxicity, nephrotoxicity, dermatologic (photosensitivity, rashes, vasculitis)
Dactinomycin/actinomycin D (antibiotic)	Endometrial cancer, gestational trophoblastic neoplasia	Myelosuppression (all cell lines)	GI toxicity (N&V, mucositis), alopecia, extravasation necrosis
Cyclophosphamide (alkylating agent)	Gestational trophoblastic neoplasia	Myelosuppression	Hemorrhagic cystitis, alopecia, SIADH
Vincristine (plant alkaloid)	Gestational trophoblastic neoplasia	Myelosuppression	Alopecia, GI toxicity, myalgias, peripheral neuropathy

GI, gastrointestinal; MI, myocardial infarction; N&V, nausea and vomiting; SIADH, syndrome of inappropriate secretion of antidiuretic hormone.

    iii. Late G1 and S phase interference
    iv. Side effect: myelosuppression
    v. Examples: cyclophosphamide, ifosfamide, cisplatin, and carboplatin
  c. Antitumor antibiotics
    i. Mechanism: inhibit DNA-directed RNA synthesis and free radical formation
    ii. Phase: nonspecific
    iii. Side effect: myelosuppression
    iv. Examples: bleomycin and actinomycin D
  d. Topoisomerase inhibitors
    i. Mechanism: inhibit topoisomerase I, thus preventing repair of single-strand DNA
    ii. Phase: nonspecific
    iii. Side effects: myelosuppression, alopecia, and GI upset
    iv. Examples: topotecan and etoposide
 3. Endocrine agents
  a. Selective estrogen receptor modulators (SERMs) act like estrogen agonists at some sites and estrogen antagonists at other sites
    i. Mechanism: block estrogen receptors (ERs) in ER+ cancers, competitive inhibitor
    ii. Examples: tamoxifen and raloxifene
    iii. Side effects: uterine cancer and blood clots

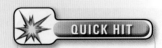

QUICK HIT

The bone marrow is rapidly dividing, so neutropenia, anemia, and thrombocytopenia are common side effects of chemotherapy.

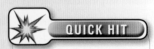

QUICK HIT

Patients presenting with fever, lethargy, or spontaneous bleeding need an Hgb to check for anemia, platelet count to check for thrombocytopenia, and a complete blood count (CBC) with differential to calculate ANC.

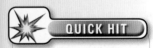

QUICK HIT

Adjuvant chemo aims to kill microscopic disease following optimal surgical debulking. The intent is complete cure.

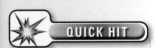

QUICK HIT

Remember: Just like in chemotherapy, first-order kinetics means multiple doses are needed because a standard fraction of tumor cells is killed with each dose.

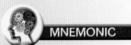

MNEMONIC

4 Rs of radiobiology
1. **R**epair of subepithelial injury: divided dose allows more normal cells to survive
2. **R**epopulation: reactivation of stem cells occurs when radiation stops, allowing healthy tissue to regenerate
3. **R**eoxygenation: cells are most sensitive to radiation with oxygen present; as some of the tumor dies off, surviving cells get closer to capillaries (and thus oxygen)
4. **R**edistribution of the cell cycle: not every tumor cell is actively dividing at any time, so multiple doses over time make it more likely that a cell will be actively dividing

b. Aromatase inhibitors (AIs)
  i. Mechanism: suppress estrogen levels by blocking aromatase and decreasing conversion of androgens to estrogens
  ii. Examples: anastrozole, exemestane, and letrozole
  iii. Side effects: bone loss, joint pain, and menopausal symptoms
c. Progestational agents
  i. Mechanism: inhibits pituitary release of gonadotropins
  ii. Utility in endometrial cancer, early or recurrent; best if low grade and ER/progesterone receptor (PR)+
  iii. Examples: medroxyprogesterone and megestrol

B. Side effects of chemotherapy: rapidly dividing cells (erythroid, myeloid, megakaryocytic) highly sensitive to chemotherapy
  1. **Neutropenia**
    a. Sometimes defined as **absolute neutrophil count (ANC)** <500
    b. Prophylactic antibiotics indicated
    c. Symptoms: fever, diarrhea
  2. **Thrombocytopenia**
    a. Prophylactic transfusion for platelets <5,000–10,000 to prevent spontaneous bleeding
    b. *If bleeding (e.g., gums) or easily bruising, transfuse if ANC <50,000*
  3. **Anemia**
    a. Symptoms: lethargy, shortness of breath, chest pain
    b. Transfuse if Hgb <8 or <8.5 with coronary artery disease
C. Regimens
  1. **Combination chemotherapy:** multiple agents in combination to prevent drug resistance and overcome limitation of toxicity in high-dose single agent treatment; can have additive or even *synergistic* effects (ideally would not antagonize each other)
  2. **Adjuvant chemotherapy:** given *following surgery* in patient with *no evidence of cancer*
  3. **Neoadjuvant chemotherapy:** used to reduce tumor burden prior to surgery or to reduce amount of tumor left behind at initial surgery
  4. **Induction chemotherapy:** using combination chemotherapy in high doses to cause remission
  5. **Maintenance chemotherapy** (also called *consolidation chemotherapy*): long-term, low-dose chemotherapy in *patient already in remission*, meant to maintain remission by suppressing cancer growth

III. Radiation

A. Mechanism of action: ionizing radiation causes production of free radicals, which causes formation of hydrogen peroxide, which disrupts DNA structure
B. 1st-order kinetics and fractionated dosages: 4 Rs of radiobiology
C. Side effects
  1. Acute reactions
    a. Actively dividing cells are most sensitive
    b. Skin, GI tract, bone marrow, bladder mucosa, and reproductive cells
  2. Chronic complications
    a. Present months to years after radiation
    b. Obliteration of blood vessels; fibrosis causes chronic prostatitis, hemorrhagic cystitis, ureterovaginal and vesicovaginal fistula, rectal or sigmoid stenosis, bowel obstruction, and GI fistula formation
D. Delivery
  1. Teletherapy: **external irradiation** (also called *external beam radiation*)
    a. Uses high-energy beams, total dose of therapy 60–80 Gy
    b. Usually given in daily dose of ~2 Gy over course of many weeks
  2. Brachytherapy: local irradiation; preferred because spares bowel and bladder
    a. **Inverse square law:** closer the source of radiation, higher the dose delivered to tissue

b. To get source as close as possible, encapsulated sources of ionizing radiation are placed
   i. Interstitial implants: placed directly into tissue, utilizes iridium-192 or iodine-125 formulated into wires
   ii. Intracavitary implants: placed into natural body cavities (i.e., uterus, cervix, or vagina), which can be low-dose (2 Gy/hr) using cesium-137, or high-dose (>12 Gy/hr) using iridium-192 or cobalt-60
3. Intraoperative radiation: used in patients with previous irradiation and recurrence who would otherwise not be candidates for external radiation

IV. Novel Agents
A. Monoclonal antibodies
   1. Specific molecular targets (e.g., trastuzumab and bevacizumab)
   2. Ongoing investigation will determine final roles of these agents in gynecologic cancer
B. Cancer vaccines: ongoing studies for ovarian cancer vaccine to prevent recurrence; cervical cancer prevention with human papillomavirus (HPV) vaccines
C. Gene therapy: future therapies with p53 under investigation

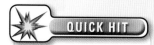

Common side effects of radiation include skin desquamation, enteritis, proctosigmoiditis, bone marrow suppression, and acute cystitis.

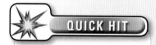

One Gray equals 1 joule per kilogram, which equals 100 rads.

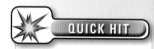

Trastuzumab binds to human epidermal growth factor receptor 2 (HER2), and bevacizumab binds to vascular endothelial growth factor (VEGF), prohibiting angiogenesis.

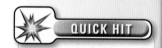

Bevacizumab lost U.S. Food and Drug Administration (FDA) indication for breast cancer use due to lack of efficacy data and serious side effect profile in December 2010.

Cell Biology and Principles of Cancer Therapy

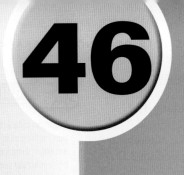

46 Gestational Trophoblastic Neoplasia

I. Introduction: clinical spectrum that includes all neoplasms that derive from abnormal placental (trophoblastic) proliferation
A. Benign disease: hydatidiform molar pregnancy (most common)
B. Malignant disease
   1. Invasive trophoblastic disease, choriocarcinoma, placental site trophoblastic tumors
   2. 20% of patients with benign molar disease develop malignant disease
C. Key clinical features
   1. Clinical presentation as pregnancy
   2. Reliable means of diagnosis by pathognomonic ultrasound findings
   3. Specific tumor marker (quantitative serum human chorionic gonadotropin [hCG])

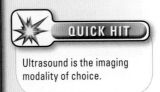

QUICK HIT

Ultrasound is the imaging modality of choice.

II. Epidemiology
A. Incidence ranges from 1/200 in Asia to 1/1,500 in the United States
B. Recurrence rate 1%–2%
C. Associations: older age, low dietary carotene, and vitamin A

III. Hydatidiform Mole
A. Definition: abnormal proliferation of the syncytiotrophoblast and replacement of normal placental trophoblastic tissue by hydropic placental villi
B. Complete mole (Table 46.1)
   1. No identifiable embryonic or fetal structure
   2. Paternal chromosomes: fertilization of **blighted ovum** by 1 haploid sperm that duplicates or fertilization of blighted ovum with 2 sperms
C. Partial mole
   1. Identifiable fetal or embryonic structures
   2. **Dispermic fertilization** of normal ovum
D. Clinical presentation
   1. Vaginal bleeding
   2. Uterine size larger than expected
   3. Lack of fetal heart tones
   4. Excessive nausea/emesis
   5. Marked gestational hypertension, proteinuria
   6. Hyperthyroidism
   7. Theca lutein cyst (enlarged adnexal masses)
   8. Acute hypertensive crisis
E. Diagnosis
   1. Quantitative hCG levels are excessively elevated for gestational age
   2. Ultrasound findings
      a. Complete mole: "snowstorm" appearance and absence of fetal parts (Figure 46.1)
      b. Partial mole: abnormally formed fetus

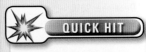

QUICK HIT

Complete mole is more likely to become malignant than a partial mole.

TABLE 46.1 Features of Partial and Complete Hydatidiform Moles

Feature	Partial Mole	Complete Mole
Karyotype	Triploid	46,XX, rarely 46,XY
Pathology		
Fetus	Often present	Absent
Amnion, fetal RBCs	Usually present	Absent
Villous edema	Variable, focal	Diffuse
Trophoblastic proliferation	Focal, slight to moderate	Diffuse
Clinical presentation		
Diagnosis	Missed abortion	Molar gestation
Uterine size	Small or appropriate for gestational age	50% large for gestational age
Theca lutein cysts	Rare	>25% depending on diagnostic modality
Medical complications	Rare	Becoming rare with early diagnosis
Postmolar invasion and malignancy	<5%	15% and 4% respectively

RBCs, red blood cells.
(Table modified from *ACOG Practice Bulletin #53* June 2004. Updated information from Berkowitz RS, Goldstein DP. Gestational trophoblastic disease. In: Hoskins WJ, Perez CA, Young RC, eds. *Principles and Practice of Gynecologic Oncology*, 4th ed. Philadelphia: Lippincott Williams & Wilkins; 2005:1057–1061.)

3. Preoperative evaluation: baseline quantitative hCG level, baseline chest X-ray, complete blood count (CBC), blood type and screen, coagulation studies, thyroid function test

F. Treatment
1. Evacuation of uterine contents by dilation and suction curettage followed by gentle sharp curettage
2. Uterotonic administration after uterine evacuation and blood transfusion if needed

FIGURE 46.1 "Snowstorm" appearance of complete mole on ultrasound examination.

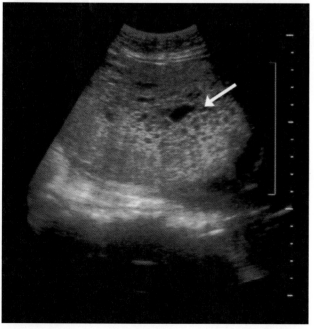

The *white arrow* points to intrauterine tissue. (From Beckmann CRB, Ling FW, et al. *Obstetrics and Gynecology*, 7th ed. Philadelphia: Lippincott Williams & Wilkins; 2014.)

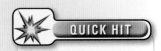

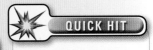

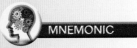

3. Hysterectomy for women who have no interest in further childbearing
4. Theca lutein cysts **do not** require removal and will likely regress

G. Postevacuation management
   1. Quantitative hCG within 48 hours following evacuation and every 1–2 weeks while elevated and at 1–2 months thereafter for a total of 6–12 months
   2. Give Rh immune globulin if Rh negative
   3. Use reliable contraception to prevent pregnancy in the first 6–12 months monitoring hCG
   4. Risk of recurrence after 1 year <1%

IV. **Malignant Gestational Trophoblastic Neoplasia** (*Table 46.2*)
   A. Invasive mole
      1. Invades myometrium, histologically similar to molar pregnancy
      2. Diagnosed months after evacuation of complete mole when hCG levels do not fall appropriately as persistent metastatic or nonmetastatic gestational trophoblastic neoplasia
   B. Choriocarcinoma
      1. Malignant transformation of trophoblastic tissue
      2. Can follow molar pregnancy, normal-term pregnancy, abortion, or ectopic pregnancy
      3. Rapid systemic metastasis results from hematogenous embolization
      4. Sites of metastasis: lungs, vagina, central nervous system (CNS), kidney, liver
      5. Sensitive to chemotherapy
         a. Single-agent chemotherapy (for treating nonmetastatic disease)
            i. Methotrexate or actinomycin D
            ii. Cure rate up to 100%
         b. Combined chemotherapy for treatment of metastatic disease International Federation of Gynecology and Obstetrics (FIGO) score ≥ 7 (Table 46.3)
            i. EMACO
            ii. Cure rate up to 80%–90%
         c. Adjunctive radiotherapy is used for patients with brain metastasis

TABLE 46.2	Clinical Classification of Malignant Gestational Trophoblastic Disease	
Category	**Criteria**	
Nonmetastatic gestational trophoblastic disease	No evidence of metastases; not assigned to prognostic category	
Metastatic gestational trophoblastic disease	Any extrauterine metastasis	
Good prognosis	No risk factors: 1. Short interval from antecedent pregnancy <4 months 2. Pretherapy hCG level <40,000 mIU/mL 3. No brain or liver metastases 4. No antecedent term pregnancy 5. No prior chemotherapy	
Poor prognosis	Any risk factor: 1. >4 months since last pregnancy 2. Pretherapy hCG level >40,000 mIU/mL 3. Brain or liver metastases 4. Antecedent term pregnancy 5. Prior chemotherapy	

(From American College of Obstetricians and Gynecologists. Diagnosis and treatment of gestational trophoblastic disease. *ACOG Practice Bulletin No. 53. Obstet Gynecol.* 2004;103:1365–1377.)

TABLE 46.3 Revised FIGO Scoring System

Finding	FIGO Score			
	0	**1**	**2**	**4**
Age (years)	<40	>40	–	–
Antecedent pregnancy	Hydatidiform mole	Abortion	Term pregnancy	–
Interval from last pregnancy	<4 months	4–6 months	7–12 months	>12 months
Pretreatment hCG level	<1,000	1,000–<10,000	10,000–100,000	>100,000
Largest tumor size including uterus	<3	3–5	>5–	–
Site of metastases	Lung, vagina	Spleen, kidney	Gastrointestinal tract	Brain, liver
Number of metastases	0	1–4	5–8	>8
Previous failed chemotherapy	–	–	Single drug	Two or more drugs

The total score for a patient is obtained by adding the individual scores for each prognostic factor. Total score: 0–6 = low risk and ≥7 = high risk.
FIGO, International Federation of Gynecology and Obstetrics.

C. Placental site tumors
1. Intermediate cytotrophoblastic cells that invade locally at site of placental implantation
2. Secretes small amounts of hCG
3. Rarely metastatic
4. Resistant to standard chemotherapy
5. Hysterectomy is often curative

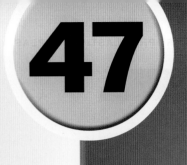

47 Benign Vulvar Disease

I. **Lichen Simplex Chronicus** (*Table 47.1; also see Figure 30.2A*)
   A. General characteristics
      1. Develops secondary to a chronic irritant or contact dermatitis that results in lichenification
      2. Initial causes of pruritus can include detergents, soaps, perfumes, dyes
   B. Clinical features
      1. Chronic scratching and irritation causes excoriations and epidermal thickening, hyperplasia, and inflammation
      2. On exam, labia and perineum may have erythematous areas with occasional hyperpigmented plaques that appear dark and leathery
   C. Diagnosis
      1. Based on history and physical exam, biopsy is usually unnecessary
   D. Treatment
      1. Remove offending irritant
      2. Oral antihistamines (diphenhydramine hydrocloride or hydroxyzine) for pruitis
      3. Topical steroids (hydrocortisone, triamcinolone)
      4. Biopsy of any lesion that persists >3 months is warranted

TABLE **47.1** **Clinical Characteristics of the Common Vulvar Dermatoses**

Disorder	Lesion	Hallmarks
Lichen simplex chronicus	Lichenified, hyperplastic plaques of red to reddish brown	Symmetric with variable pigmentation
Lichen sclerosus	Atrophic, thin, whitish epithelium with frequent perianal halo or "keyhole" distribution	"Cigarette paper," parchment-like skin, halo, or loss of elasticity
Lichen planus	White lacy network (Wickham striae) with flat-topped lilac papules and plaques	Erosive vaginitis with demarcated edges
Psoriasis	Annular pink plaques with silvery scale that bleed if removed (Auspitz sign)	Elbows, knees, scalp also often affected
Dermatitis irritant, allergic, or atopic	Eczematous lesions with underlying erythema	Symmetric with extension into areas of irritant or allergen contact
Seborrheic	Pale red to yellowish pink plaques; often oily appearing, scaly crust	Other hair-bearing areas often affected (scalp and chest, also back and face)

(From Beckmann CRB, Ling FW, et al. *Obstetrics and Gynecology*, 7th ed. Philadelphia: Lippincott Williams & Wilkins; 2014.)

II. Lichen Sclerosus (see Table 47.1 and Figure 30.2B)

A. General characteristics
  1. Etiology unknown; underlying connective tissue disorder
  2. Familial association has been noted
  3. Any age, especially young and old
  4. Risk of concurrent carcinoma approximately 4%; **not** considered a premalignant lesion but associated with squamous cell carcinoma (SCC)

B. Clinical features
  1. Well-demarcated, white "**onion skin**" or "**parchment**" **epithelium**
  2. Can involve both sides of vulva, with most common sites being labia majora, labia minora, clitoral and periclitoral skin, and perineum
  3. Presents with intense vulva **pruritus, dyspareunia**, and/or bleeding with minimal trauma

C. Diagnosis
  1. Clinical, based upon history and physical exam
  2. Punch biopsy can confirm histology and rule out carcinoma
  3. Histologically appears as chronic inflammatory cells, thinning of epithelium, loss of rete pegs, chronic lymphocytic infiltrate, spongiosis, and hyperkeratosis of the surface epithelium

D. Treatment
  1. Topical steroids (commonly clobetasol) for symptomatic relief
  2. Other treatments include topical tretinoin, pimecrolimus, testosterone propionate, and progesterone
  3. Lesions often persist despite therapy, and treatment of symptoms can be indefinite

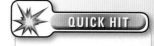

QUICK HIT

Lichen sclerosus requires lifelong treatment because the condition rarely regresses.

III. Lichen Planus (see Table 47.1 and Figure 30.2C)

A. General characteristics
  1. Rare vulvovaginal dermatosis
  2. Often associated with other autoimmune diseases
  3. Usually in women >50 years of age
  4. Can be associated with medications that are known to cause lichenoid reactions (β-blockers, angiotensin-converting enzyme [ACE] inhibitors, nonsteroidal anti-inflammatory drugs [NSAIDs])

B. Clinical features
  1. Intense pruritus, burning, pain, dyspareunia, profuse vaginal discharge
  2. Shiny, violaceous papules and desquamative ulcers on the vulva that can involve the labia and vulvar vestibule
  3. Progressive scarring and shrinkage of involved areas

C. Diagnosis
  1. Usually based on characteristic lesions and patient complaints
  2. 50% of women with vulvovaginal lichen planus will have lichen planus elsewhere on their body (especially gingivae)
  3. Histology of biopsy specimen may show hyperkeratosis with basal layer destruction/liquefaction

D. Treatment
  1. Topical steroids and vaginal steroid suppositories
  2. Discontinuation of lichenoid-causing medications

QUICK HIT

Do *not* treat with vulvectomy, laser, cryo, or loop electrode excision procedure (LEEP).

IV. Psoriasis (see Table 47.1)

A. Autoimmune disorder affecting up to 2.5% of general population
B. Vulvar lesions resemble systemic manifestations: round plaques with an erythematous base and silver scale
C. Minimal pruritus or pain
D. Treatment usually not limited to vulvar lesions; can involve topical coal tar, ultraviolet (UV) light, corticosteroids, and methotrexate

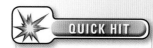

QUICK HIT

The use of vaginal dilators is important to lessen chance of vaginal stenosis.

V. Vestibulitis

A. Unknown etiology
B. Presents as new-onset insertional dyspareunia

Benign Vulvar Disease

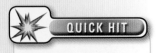

C. Can cause decreased libido or avoidance of sexual activity
D. Thought to be related to inflammation of the vestibular glands (located just proximal to introitus near the hymenal ring)
E. Diagnosis is made by physical exam and history
   1. Pinpoint location of pain with use of a moistened cotton swab
   2. Rule out infection, muscle spasm, or other pelvic floor dysfunction
F. Treatment options include physical therapy, biofeedback, topical anesthetics, topical steroids, tricyclic antidepressants, selective serotonin reuptake inhibitors (SSRIs), and surgical removal of vestibular glands

VI. Squamous Cell Hyperplasia

A. General characteristics
   1. Pruritus
   2. Most common age 30–60 years
   3. Thick, white, keratin surface
   4. Look for allergens
B. Histology
   1. Thickened epithelium
   2. Acanthosis
   3. Deep and broad rete pegs
C. Treatment
   1. Avoid allergens
   2. Avoid panty hose
   3. Wear cotton underwear
   4. Wear nightgowns instead of pajama pants to bed
   5. Topical steroids

VII. Vulvar Neoplasia

A. Vulvar interepithelial neoplasia (VIN)
   1. General characteristics
      a. VIN 1–3 or all "usual type" lesions are likely related to human papillomavirus (HPV) infection
      b. Smoking or secondhand smoke exposure is a risk factor for VIN
   2. VIN 1 (mild dysplasia, low-grade VIN, condyloma acuminata)
      a. Reactive atypia or related to HPV infection
      b. Unlikely to progress to cancer
      c. Includes condylomatous lesions (vulvar warts)
   3. VIN, usual type (VIN 2–3, high-grade VIN, carcinoma in situ)
      a. Represents dysplasia caused by high-oncogenic-risk HPVs (30% of cases)
      b. All have same histologic evidence of dysplasia: atypical mitotic figures, nuclear pleomorphism, lack of cellular maturation
      c. In World Health Organization (WHO) grading system, differences in VIN 2 and 3 are related to the degree of dysplasia present
      d. International Society for the Study of Vulvovaginal Disease (ISSVD) subdivided usual type VIN into warty, basaloid, or mixed subtypes based on histologic features
   4. VIN, differentiated type (VIN 3, simplex type)
      a. Represents keratinizing SCCs, not related to infections with HPV (70% of cases)
      b. Etiology unknown
      c. Usually develops in women with chronic lichen sclerosus or squamous cell hyperplasia
      d. Histologically differentiated from HPV-related VIN by normal-appearing surface epithelium but marked atypia of the basal layer of the epithelium
   5. Clinical presentation
      a. Lesions can be various in location and appearance
      b. Classically presents as chronic vulvar itching with a raised plaque
      c. Appearance can range from dry, raised, demarcated plaques to erythematous, ulcerated patches

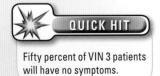

Benign Vulvar Disease

d. Location is classically in hairless areas of the vulva and near the perineal body but entire perineum and perinanal at risk

6. Diagnosis
   a. Lesions made more distinct (white epithelium or increased vascularity) with the application of acetic acid are suspicious for VIN
   b. Definitive diagnosis is made by biopsy

7. Treatment
   a. If invasive cancer is ruled out, treatment involves excision of all VIN lesions
      i. Laser ablation
      ii. Surgical excision
   b. Topical application of 5-fluorouracil or imiquimod may be considered in some cases

B. Vulvar cancer
   1. General characteristics
      a. Majority are SCCs
      b. Melanoma accounts for 2% of vulvar cancers; other types include basal cell carcinoma and adenocarcinoma
      c. Most often presents in postmenopausal women
      d. Risk factors include history of VIN and smoking
   2. Clinical presentation
      a. Most common presenting complaint is vulvar itching
      b. Patients may also describe a white or red lesion or ulcer
      c. Metastasis is usually lymphatic (inguinal and femoral nodes)
   3. Diagnosis
      a. Biopsy
      b. Staging (Table 47.2)
   4. Treatment
      a. Mainstay: surgical excision
      b. Degree of excision depends on stage; options range from radical vulvectomy with pelvic lymphadenectomy to removal of focal lesions
      c. Radiation with and without adjuvant chemotherapy

C. Other vulvar cancers
   1. Melanoma
      a. 7%–10% of all vulvar malignancies
      b. Classically presents as pigmented, pruritic lesion

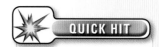

QUICK HIT

Twenty-five percent to 30% of the time, VIN (usual type) is found next to invasive SCC.

Benign Vulvar Disease

TABLE **47.2**	2009 FIGO Staging of Vulvar Cancer
Stage	**Definition**
1A	Tumor confined to the vulva or perineum, ≤2 cm in size with stromal invasion ≤1 mm, negative nodes
1B	Tumor confined to the vulvar or perineum, >2 cm in size with stromal invasion >1 mm, negative nodes
II	Tumor of any size with adjacent spread (1/3 lower urethra, 1/3 lower vagina, anus), negative nodes
IIIA	Tumor of any size with positive inguino-femoral lymph nodes (i) 1 lymph node metastasis greater ≥ 5 mm (ii) 1–2 lymph node metastasis(es) of less than 5 mm
IIIB	(i) 2 or more lymph nodes metastases ≥5 mm (ii) 3 or more lymph nodes metastases less than 5 mm
IIIC	Positive node(s) with extracapsular spread
IVA	(i) Tumor invades other regional structures (2/3 upper urethra, 2/3 upper vagina), bladder mucosa, rectal mucosa, or fixed pelvic bone (ii) Fixed or ulcerated inguino-femoral lymph nodes
IVB	Any distant metastasis including pelvic lymph nodes

FIGO, International Federation of Gynecology and Obstetrics.

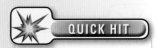

c. Diagnosed and treated with wide local excision
d. Node dissection is of questionable benefit
2. Vulvar (extramammary) Paget disease
   a. Histology of vulvar Paget disease is similar to that of the breast disease and includes apocrine glands
   b. May be associated with underlying adenocarcinoma or another primary carcinoma (especially colon)
   c. Presents as bright red lesion with areas of white hyperkeratosis
3. Bartholin gland carcinoma
   a. Rare cancer that arises from the Bartholin gland
   b. Histologically, can present as SCC, adenocarcinomas, adenosquamous carcinoma, adenoid cystic carcinoma, or transitional cell carcinoma
   c. Presents as a painless vulvar mass
   d. Treatment is radical vulvectomy and lymphadenectomy

VIII. Vaginal Neoplasia

A. Vaginal intraepithelial neoplasia (VAIN)
   1. 3 primary types
      a. VAIN 1: first 1/3 of epithelium
      b. VAIN 2: up to 2/3 of the vaginal epithelium
      c. VAIN 3: more than 2/3 of the vaginal epithelium
      d. Carcinoma in situ (CIS) encompasses the full thickness of the epithelium and is included with VAIN 3

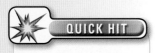

   2. Highly associated with HPV infections, especially HPV subtypes 16 and 18
   3. Commonly located in proximal 1/3 of vagina
   4. Lesions are usually asymptomatic
   5. Like cervical intraepithelial neoplasia (CIN), colposcopy with the application of acetic acid to lesions causes acetowhite changes to VAIN, and suspicious lesions should be biopsied
   6. Diagnosis is histologic
   7. VAIN I (and sometimes VAIN II) managed with surveillance
   8. VAIN III (and some VAIN II) treated with surgical therapy, CO_2 laser ablation, or topical treatment (5-flourouracil or imiquimod cream)
B. Vaginal cancer
   1. Approximately 3% of gynecologic cancers
   2. Greater than 80% of vaginal cancers are SCC, with the remainder comprising adenocarcinoma, sarcoma, or melanoma
   3. Risk factors for SCC of the vagina are the same for cervical cancer: multiple sexual partners, smoking, HPV infection (again, especially subtypes 16 and 18)
   4. Staging is nonsurgical (Table 47.3)

TABLE 47.3	FIGO Staging of Carcinoma of the Vagina
Stage	**Definition**
I	Carcinoma limited to the vaginal wall
II	Carcinoma involving subvaginal tissue but not extending to the pelvic wall
III	Carcinoma extends to the pelvic wall
IVA	Carcinoma invades beyond the true pelvis or has involved the mucosa of the bladder or rectum (bullous edema is not sufficient evidence to classify tumor as stage IV)
IVB	Spread to distant organs

FIGO, International Federation of Gynecology and Obstetrics.

5. Treatment almost always includes radiation therapy, with radical hysterectomy and upper vaginectomy and pelvic lymph node dissection or pelvic exenteration and radical vulvectomy reserved for more advanced stages or vulvar involvement

C. Sarcoma botryoides

1. Classically presents as "grape-like" polyps protruding from the vagina and bloody discharge in an infant female
2. A type of embryonic rhabdomyosarcoma that arises from within the vaginal wall or wall of the bladder
3. Metastasis is local but it may also exhibit hematogenous spread
4. Chemotherapy has replaced aggressive surgical excision

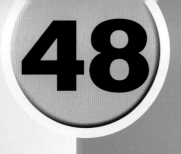

48 Cervical Dysplasia and Carcinoma

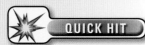

QUICK HIT

Ninety percent of lower genital tract neoplasias arise at the SCJ.

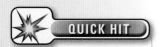

QUICK HIT

Metaplastic cells in the TZ are least mature and most vulnerable to oncogenic change.

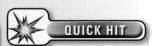

QUICK HIT

HPV is responsible for cervical cancer and CIN.

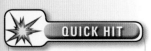

QUICK HIT

Majority of CIN is caused by high-risk HPV types 16, 18, 31, and 35.

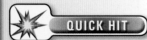

QUICK HIT

Low-risk HPV types 6 and 11 are associated with genital warts.

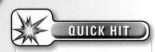

QUICK HIT

Average time from HPV infection until development of invasive cervical cancer is 20 years.

I. Anatomy *(Figure 48.1A–C)*

A. Internal os: portion of cervix abutting endometrial cavity

B. External os: portion of cervix opening into vagina

C. Exocervix: exterior portion of cervical canal

D. Endocervical canal: interior portion of cervical canal

E. Cervical epithelium is columnar (glandular) and squamous

  1. Squamocolumnar junction (SCJ): where these epithelia meet

  2. Prior to puberty, the SCJ is within the external os

  3. During puberty, metaplasia causes the SCJ to "roll-out" to the cervical surface

  4. Transformation zone (TZ): area between original SCJ and active SCJ

II. Epidemiology

A. Cervical cancer

  1. United States: 3rd most common gynecologic cancer

  2. Worldwide

    a. 2nd most common cancer in women

    b. 3rd most common cause of cancer-related death

    c. Most common cause of mortality from a gynecologic cancer

  3. One of few cancers for which vaccine exists

  4. 80% of cases are squamous cell carcinomas (SCCs)

  5. 15% are adenocarcinoma or adenosquamous carcinoma

  6. Average age for development = 50 years

B. Cervical intraepithelial neoplasia (CIN)

  1. Precursor to cancer

  2. Often regresses with no treatment (only 15% progress)

C. Risk factors for cervical neoplasia (Box 48.1)

III. Cervical Cytology *(Tables 48.1 and 48.2)*

A. Classified using Bethesda system

  1. Squamous lesions

  2. Glandular lesions

B. Evaluation of abnormal Pap test

  1. Visual inspection for gross lesion

  2. Colposcopy (looking at cervix through microscope)

    a. Biopsy at abnormal locations

    b. Endocervical curettage (sampling cells from endocervical canal) if entire SCJ not seen

C. Human papillomavirus (HPV) testing

  1. Determines need for colposcopy in atypical squamous cells of undetermined significance (ASCUS) and low-grade squamous intraepithelial lesion (LSIL) in older women

  2. Determines whether Pap smears for women age >30 years can be spaced out

FIGURE
48.1 Anatomy of the cervix.

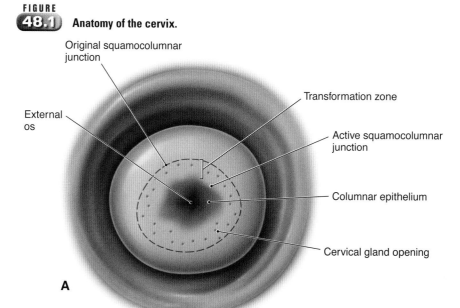

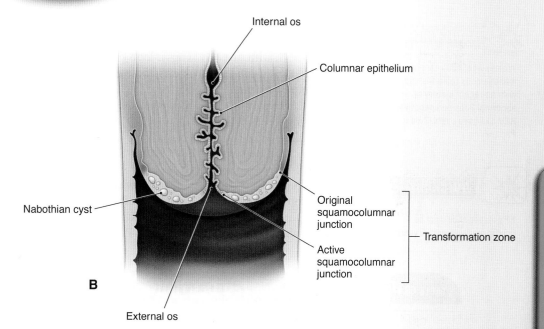

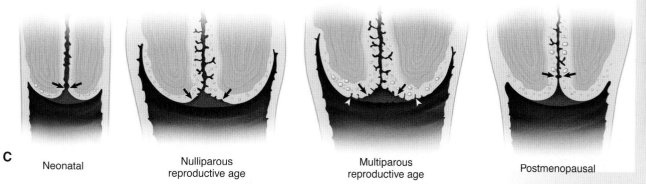

(A) The cervix and the transformation zone. **(B)** Anterior view of the cervix and exocervix. **(C)** Different locations of the transformation zone and the squamocolumnar junction during a woman's lifetime. The *arrows* mark the active transformation zone. (From Beckmann CRB, Ling FW, et al. *Obstetrics and Gynecology*, 7th ed. Philadelphia: Lippincott Williams & Wilkins; 2014.)

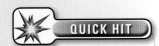

QUICK HIT

Begin Pap screening at age 21 years.

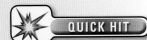

QUICK HIT

A colposcopic examination is termed satisfactory if entire SCJ is seen.

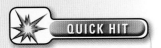

QUICK HIT

Any immunocompromised person is at greater risk to develop cervical cancer.

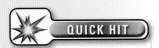

QUICK HIT

Women age >30 years in monogamous relationships with no recent history of abnormal Paps and negative HPV can have every-3-year Pap testing.

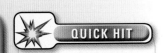

QUICK HIT

HPV testing should not be used in women age <30 years.

BOX 48.1

Risk Factors for Cervical Cancer

- More than one sexual partner or have a male sexual partner who has had sex with >1 person
- First intercourse at an early age (<18 years)
- Male sexual partner who has had a sexual partner with cervical cancer
- Smoking
- Human immunodeficiency virus (HIV) infection
- Organ (especially kidney) transplant
- Sexually transmitted disease (STD) infection
- Diethylstilbestrol (DES) exposure
- History of cervical cancer or high-grade squamous intraepithelial lesion (HSIL)
- Infrequent or absent Pap screening tests

(From Beckman CRB, Ling FW, et al. *Obstetrics and Gynecology*, 7th ed. Baltimore: Lippincott Williams & Wilkins; 2014.)

IV. Abnormal Cytology Management

    A. ASCUS

        1. Positive HPV: needs colposcopy and biopsy of abnormal findings

        2. Negative HPV: repeat Pap in 1 year

    B. LSIL, HSIL (high-grade squamous intraepithelial lesion)

        1. Colposcopy and biopsy of abnormal findings

        2. If HSIL with negative biopsy, loop electrode excision procedure (LEEP)/ cold knife cone for diagnosis and treatment (may have missed the lesion on colposcopy and biopsy)

    C. CIN 1 managed by close observation and repeat cytology for most. **Rarely** ablative measures used in older age.

        1. Ablation/destruction of tissue such as cryotherapy

        2. Excision: removal of tissue such as LEEP

    D. CIN 2

        1. Women age <30 years managed with observation

        2. Women age >30 years managed ideally with excisional method

    E. CIN 3 managed with excisional method

    F. After ablative or excisional method, Pap tests every 6 months for 2 years

---

TABLE 48.1 Comparison of Pap Test Descriptive Conventions

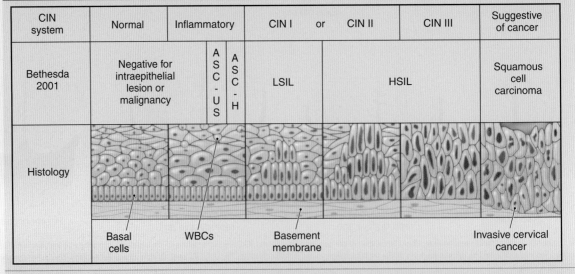

CIN system	Normal	Inflammatory		CIN I or CIN II		CIN III	Suggestive of cancer
Bethesda 2001	Negative for intraepithelial lesion or malignancy	ASC-US	ASC-H	LSIL		HSIL	Squamous cell carcinoma
Histology	Basal cells	WBCs		Basement membrane			Invasive cervical cancer

(From Beckman CRB, Ling FW, et al. *Obstetrics and Gynecology*, 7th ed. Baltimore: Lippincott Williams & Wilkins; 2014.)
ASC-US, atypical squamous cells of undetermined significance; CIN, cervical intraepithelial neoplasia; HSIL, high-grade squamous intraepithelial lesion; LSIL, low-grade squamous intraepithelial lesion; WBCs, white blood cells.

TABLE 48.2 Cervical Cancer Screening Guidelines for Average-Risk Women[1]

	American Cancer Society (ACS), American Society for Colposcopy and Cervical Pathology (ASCCP), and American Society for Clinical Pathology (ASCP)[2] 2012	U.S. Preventive Services Task Force (USPSTF)[3] 2012	American College of Obstetricians and Gynecologists (ACOG)[4] 2009
When to start screening[5]	Age 21. Women aged <21 years should not be screened regardless of the age of sexual initiation or other risk factors. (Strong recommendation)	Age 21. (A recommendation) Recommend against screening women aged <21 years. (D recommendation)	Age 21 regardless of the age of onset of sexual activity. Should be avoided <21 years. (Level A evidence)
Statement about annual screening	Women of any age should not be screened annually by any screening method. (Strong recommendation)	Individuals and clinicians can use the annual Pap test screening visit as an opportunity to discuss other health problems and preventive measures. Individuals, clinicians, and health systems should seek effective ways to facilitate the receipt of recommended preventive services at intervals that are beneficial to the patient. Efforts also should be made to ensure that individuals are able to seek care for additional health concerns as they present.	Physicians should inform their patients that annual gynecologic examinations may be appropriate. (Level C evidence)[6]
Screening method and intervals[7]			
Cytology (conventional or liquid based) 21–29 years of age	Every 3 years.[8] (Strong recommendation)	Every 3 years. (A recommendation)	Every 2 years. (Level A evidence)
30–65 years of age	Every 3 years.[8] (Strong recommendation)	Every 3 years. (A recommendation)	May screen every 3 years with a history of 3 negative cytology tests. (Level A evidence)
HPV co-test (cytology + HPV test administered together) 21–29 years of age	HPV co-testing should not be used for women aged <30 years.	Recommend against HPV co-testing women aged <30 years. (D recommendation)	Not recommended for women aged <30 years.
30–65 years of age	Every 5 years (Strong recommendation); this is the preferred method (Weak recommendation).	For women who want to extend their screening interval, HPV co-testing every 5 years is an option. (A recommendation)	Every 3 years if cytology normal, HPV test negative. (Level A evidence)
Primary HPV testing[9]	For women aged 30–65 years, screening by HPV testing alone is not recommended in most clinical settings. (Weak recommendation)[10]	Recommends against screening for cervical cancer with HPV testing (alone or in combination with cytology) in women aged <30 years. (D recommendation)	Not addressed.
When to stop screening	Women aged >65 years with adequate screening history should not be screened.[10] Women aged >65 years with a history of CIN2, CIN3, or AIS should continue screening for at least 20 years after spontaneous regression or appropriate management. (Weak recommendation)	Women aged >65 years with adequate recent screening with normal Pap tests, who are not otherwise at high risk for cervical cancer. (D recommendation)[11]	Between 65–70 years of age with 3 consecutive normal cytology tests and no abnormal tests in the past 10 years (Level B evidence). An older woman who is sexually active and has multiple partners should continue to have routine screening.

(continued)

Cervical Dysplasia and Carcinoma

Cervical Dysplasia and Carcinoma

TABLE 48.2 Cervical Cancer Screening Guidelines for Average-Risk Women[1] (continued)

	American Cancer Society (ACS), American Society for Colposcopy and Cervical Pathology (ASCCP), and American Society for Clinical Pathology (ASCP)[2] 2012	U.S. Preventive Services Task Force (USPSTF)[3] 2012	American College of Obstetricians and Gynecologists (ACOG)[4] 2009
Screening post-total hysterectomy	Women who have had a total hysterectomy (removal of the uterus and cervix) should stop screening, unless the hysterectomy was done as a treatment for cervical pre-cancer or cancer. Women who have had a hysterectomy without removal of the cervix (supra-cervical hysterectomy) should continue screening according to guidelines. *(Strong recommendation)*	Recommend against screening in women who have had a hysterectomy with removal of the cervix and who do not have a history of a high-grade precancerous lesion (CIN2 or CIN3) or cervical cancer. *(D recommendation)*	If removal for benign disease and no history of high-grade CIN or worse, may discontinue screening. *(Level A evidence)* Women for whom a negative history cannot be documented should continue to be screened. *(Level B evidence)*
The need for a bimanual pelvic exam	Not addressed in 2012 guidelines but was addressed in 2002 ACS guidelines.[12]	Addressed in USPSTF ovarian cancer screening recommendations (draft).[13]	Physicians should inform their patients that annual gynecologic examinations may be appropriate. *(Level C evidence)*[6]
Screening among those immunized against HPV 16/18	Women at any age with a history of HPV vaccination should be screened according to the age-specific recommendations for the general population.	The possibility that vaccination might reduce the need for screening with cytology alone or in combination with HPV testing is not established. Given these uncertainties, women who have been vaccinated should continue to be screened.	Recommendations remain the same regardless of vaccination status. *(Level C evidence)*

HPV, human papillomavirus; CIN, cervical intraepithelial neoplasia

[1] These recommendations do not apply to women who have received a diagnosis of a high-grade precancerous cervical lesion (CIN 2 or 3) or cervical cancer, women with in utero exposure to diethylstilbestrol, or women who are immunocompromised, or are HIV positive.

[2] Saslow D, Solomon D, Lawson HW, et al. American Cancer Society, American Society for Colposcopy and Cervical Pathology, and American Society for Clinical Pathology screening guidelines for the prevention and early detection of cervical cancer. *CA Cancer J Clin.* 2012 Mar 14. Available at http://www.cancer.org/Cancer/CervicalCancer/DetailedGuide/cervical-cancer-prevention

[3] USPSTF. Screening for Cervical Cancer. 2012. Available at http://www.uspreventiveservicestaskforce.org/uspstf11/cervcancer/cervcancers.htm. These recommendations apply to women who have a cervix, regardless of sexual history.

[4] ACOG Practice Bulletin No. 109: Cervical cytology screening. ACOG Committee on Practice Bulletins-Gynecology. *Obstet Gynecol.* 2009 Dec;114(6):1409-20.

[5] Since cervical cancer is believed to be caused by sexually transmissible human papillomavirus infections, women who have not had sexual exposures (e.g., virgins) are likely at low risk. Women aged >21 years who have not engaged in sexual intercourse may not need a Pap test depending on circumstances. The decision should be made at the discretion of the women and her physician. Women who have had sex with women are still at risk of cervical cancer. 10%–15% of women aged 21–24 years in the United States report no vaginal intercourse (Saraiya M, Martinez G, Glaser K, et al *Obstet Gynecol* 2009. 114 (6)). Providers should also be aware of instances of non-consensual sex among their patients.

[6] More specific guidance from 2003 states an annual pelvic examination is a routine part of preventive care for all women aged ≥21 years even if they do not need cervical cytology screening. *(Level C evidence)*

[7] Conventional cytology and liquid-based cytology are equivalent regarding screening guidelines, and no distinction should be made by test when recommending next screening.

[8] There is insufficient evidence to support longer intervals in women aged 30-65 years, even with a screening history of consecutive negative cytology tests.

[9] Primary HPV testing (HPV testing alone) is defined as conducting the HPV test as the first screening test. It may be followed by other tests (like a Pap) for triage.

[10] No further explanation of which clinical settings HPV testing should be used to screen women aged 30–65 years as a standalone test.

[11] Current guidelines define adequate screening as three consecutive negative cytology results or two consecutive negative co-tests within 10 years before cessation of screening, with the most recent test performed within 5 years, and are the same for ACS and USPSTF.

[12] 2002 guidelines statement: The ACS and others should educate women, particularly teens and young women, that a pelvic exam does not equate to a cytology test and that women who may not need a cytology test still need regular health care visits including gynecologic care. Women should discuss the need for pelvic exams with their providers. Saslow D, Runowicz CD, Solomon D, et al. American Cancer Society Guideline for the Early Detection of Cervical Neoplasia and Cancer. *CA Cancer J Clin* 2002;52:342–362.

[13] The bimanual pelvic examination is often conducted (usually annually) in part to screen for ovarian cancer, although its effectiveness and harms are not well known and were not a focus of this review. No randomized trial has assessed the role of the bimanual pelvic examination for cancer screening. In the PLCO Trial, bimanual examination was discontinued as a screening strategy in the intervention arm because no cases of ovarian cancer were detected solely by this method and a high proportion of women underwent bimanual examination with ovarian palpation in the usual care arm.

V. Cervical Cancer Staging

A. Clinical staging
   1. Exam
   2. X-ray of chest and skeleton
   3. Intravenous pyelography
   4. Cystoscopy

B. Surgery and additional imaging do not change the initial stage
   1. Stage I = carcinoma confined to the cervix
      a. IA = microscopic invasion
         i. IA1 = Measured stromal invasion ≤ 3 mm in depth and ≤ 7 mm in horizontal spread
         ii. IA2 = Measured stromal invasion 3–5 mm in depth with a horizontal spread ≤ 7.0 mm
      b. IB = clinically visible lesion confined to the cervix or microscopic lesion > IA2
   2. Stage 2 = carcinoma extends beyond cervix but has not extended to pelvic wall; lower 1/3 of vagina not involved
      a. IIA = no parametrial invasion or involvement of the lower 1/3 of vagina
         i. IIA1 = clinically visible lesion ≤ 4cm with involvement of > upper 2/3 of vagina
         ii. IIA2 = clinically visible lesion > 4.0 cm with involvement of < upper 2/3 of vagina
      b. IIB = obvious parametrial involvement
   3. Stage III = extension onto pelvic sidewall and/or involves lower 1/3 of vagina; and/or causes hydronephrosis or nonfunctioning kidney
      a. IIIA = no sidewall extension but involves lower 1/3 of vagina
      b. IIIB = extension onto pelvic sidewall and/or causes hydronephrosis or nonfunctioning kidney
   4. Stage IVA = invades mucosa of bladder or rectum and/or extends beyond the true pelvis

C. Spread via local extension and lymphatics

VI. Cervical Cancer Treatment

A. Stage IA can be treated by conization in some cases, but most should have simple hysterectomy

B. Stages IB and IIA can be treated with radical surgery in some cases

C. Survival rates vary greatly with stage at diagnosis (Table 48.3)

VII. Prevention

A. Condoms

B. Regular Pap smears and gynecologic examination

C. HPV vaccination
   1. 3 doses over 6 months
   2. Boys and girls ages 9–26 years
   3. HPV testing before vaccination is not indicated
   4. Continue regular Pap smears starting at age 21 years

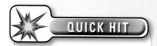

QUICK HIT

Cervical excisional procedures increase the risk of preterm labor, low-birth-weight infants, and Cesarean deliveries.

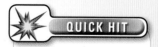

QUICK HIT

Cervical cancer is clinically staged.

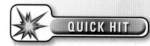

QUICK HIT

The International Federation of Gynecology and Obstetrics (FIGO) does not recognize positron emission tomography (PET), magnetic resonance imaging (MRI), or computed tomography (CT) in staging.

TABLE 48.3 Five-Year Survival Rates for Cervical Cancer

Stage	5-Year Survival Rate
IA	>95%
IB1	Approximately 90%
IB2	80%–85%
IIA/B	75%–78%
IIIA/B	47%–50%
IV	20%–30%

(From Beckman CRB, Ling FW, et al. *Obstetrics and Gynecology,* 7th ed. Baltimore: Lippincott Williams & Wilkins; 2014.)

Cervical Dysplasia and Carcinoma

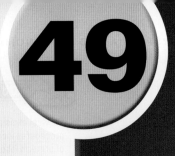

49 Cancer of the Uterine Corpus

MNEMONIC

"Old aunt" = endometrial cancer:
Obesity
Late-onset menopause
Diabetes
Age (older) and/or **a**novulation
Unopposed estrogen (early-onset menses)
Nulliparity
Tamoxifen therapy

QUICK HIT

Abnormal uterine bleeding occurs in 90% of cases.

QUICK HIT

Tamoxifen is a weak estrogen and can cause endometrial hyperplasia, the precursor to endometrial cancer.

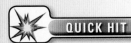
QUICK HIT

Patients with endometrial cancer tend to be obese, postmenopausal women of low parity.

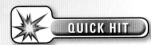
QUICK HIT

Endometrial cancer can be caused by prolonged exposure to endogenous or exogenous estrogen in the absence of opposing progesterone.

I. Epidemiology

A. Most common gynecologic cancer in United States; 4th most common cancer (after breast, bowel, and lung carcinoma)
   1. 47,000 cases each year
   2. Nearly 8,000 deaths each year
   3. Occurs in 2%–3% of all women
B. Occurs in premenopausal (25%) and postmenopausal (75%) women
C. Median age: 61 years
D. Decreasing mortality due to symptoms at a low grade and stage
E. Risk factors (relative risk in parentheses)
   1. Nulliparity (3)
   2. Menopause after age 55 years (2–3)
   3. Older age (2–3)
   4. Obesity (2–5)
   5. Unopposed estrogen therapy (10–20)
   6. Anovulatory cycles (e.g., as seen with polycystic ovarian syndrome) (3)
   7. Tamoxifen use (3–7)
   8. Diabetes mellitus (2)
   9. Estrogen-secreting tumors (e.g., as seen with granulosa-theca cell tumors where concurrent endometrial cancer occurs in 25% of cases)
   10. Hereditary nonpolyposis colon cancer (Lynch syndrome) (27%–71% lifetime risk)
F. Protective factors (relative risk in parentheses)
   1. Combined oral contraceptive pills for >12 months (0.6)
   2. Smoking after menopause ([0.7] because smoking is antiestrogenic)
   3. Multiparity

II. Pathogenesis

A. Estrogen stimulation of endometrium, without opposing progesterone, leads to hyperplasia (supposed precursor) and then to carcinoma (because anovulation is ovarian source for estrogen)
   1. Endogenous sources = ovarian, peripheral conversion by aromatase
   2. Exogenous sources = pills, patches, vaginal creams/rings
B. Two types of endometrial cancer
   1. Type I most common and estrogen dependent
      a. Progresses from endometrial hyperplasia
      b. Favorable prognosis
   2. Type II estrogen independent
      a. Not progressive from endometrial hyperplasia
      b. Poor prognosis
      c. High grade

C. Endometrial hyperplasia
  1. Thought to represent a precursor to endometrioid adenocarcinoma
  2. World Health Organization (WHO) subtypes
    a. Simple hyperplasia without atypia
    b. *Excessive* proliferation of glandular and stromal elements = 1% risk of progression to carcinoma
    c. Complex hyperplasia without atypia
      i. *Abnormal* proliferation of glandular elements
      ii. Risk of progression to carcinoma = 3%
    d. Simple hyperplasia with atypia
      i. Excessive proliferation of glandular and stromal elements *and* disordered maturation of cells
      ii. Risk of progression to carcinoma = 8%
    e. Complex hyperplasia with atypia
      i. Abnormal proliferation of glandular elements *and* disordered maturation of cells
      ii. Risk of progression to carcinoma = 29%
  3. Histology of uterine corpus cancer
    a. Grade ranges from well-differentiated, to moderately differentiated, to poorly differentiated
    b. Depth of invasion is the 2nd most important prognostic factor
    c. Histologic subtypes
      i. Most common is endometrioid adenocarcinoma (80%)
      ii. Mucinous carcinoma (5%)
      iii. Clear cell carcinoma (5%)
      iv. Papillary serous carcinoma (4%)
      v. Squamous carcinoma, sarcoma, mixed mesodermal tumors (rare)
    d. Estrogen receptor (ER) and progesterone receptor (PR)–positive tumors are associated with better outcomes
D. Metastasis
  1. Lymphatic spread can occur to pelvic and periaortic nodes
  2. Hematogenous spread can occur to liver, lungs (most common), and bone

III. Clinical Presentation
  A. Irregular bleeding
  B. Obesity, hypertension, diabetes, and metabolic syndrome are common findings
  C. Pelvic examination is typically *normal* in early stages
  D. Differential diagnosis
    1. Postmenopausal bleeding: polyps, leiomyoma, endometrial hyperplasia, exogenous estrogen use, atrophic vaginitis

IV. Diagnosis
  A. Screening is *not* indicated (exception: patients with hereditary nonpolyposis colorectal cancer [HNPCC, Lynch syndrome])
  B. Endometrial sampling
    1. Dilation and curettage (D&C)
    2. In office endometrial biopsy (accuracy is 90%–98% compared to D&C or hysterectomy)
  C. Cervical screening with Pap smear: only 30%–40% of women with endometrial cancer will have abnormal Pap smears
  D. Pelvic ultrasound
    1. Endometrial thickness of >5 mm in postmenopausal women or polypoid mass suggests need for endometrial sampling
    2. Thickness <5 mm does not exclude possibility of carcinoma and sampling should be considered in a woman with persistent bleeding
    3. Not as valuable in premenopausal woman

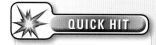

QUICK HIT

Grade is the most important prognostic factor.

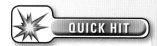

QUICK HIT

The uncommon subtypes (adenocarcinoma) of endometrial cancer are associated with poorer prognosis.

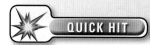

QUICK HIT

Metastasis most commonly occurs by direct extension.

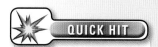

QUICK HIT

Postmenopausal bleeding is defined as bleeding after 6 months of amenorrhea in a patient who has been diagnosed as menopausal.

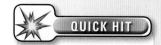

QUICK HIT

Irregular bleeding is the most common symptom (occurs in 90% of cases).

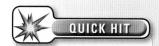

QUICK HIT

Postmenopausal bleeding, perimenopausal intermenstrual bleeding, or premenopausal bleeding in the setting of anovulation should raise the suspicion of endometrial cancer.

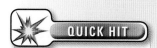

QUICK HIT

In-office endometrial biopsies can have up to a 10% false-negative rate. A negative endometrial biopsy in a high-risk, symptomatic patient should be followed by a D&C in the operating room.

Cancer of the Uterine Corpus

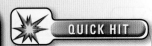

QUICK HIT

All postmenopausal women with abnormal uterine bleeding or premenopausal women with abnormal bleeding and risk factors (family history of breast, colon, or gynecologic cancer; obesity; prior hyperplasia; unopposed estrogen therapy/anovulation) should have endometrial sampling.

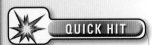

QUICK HIT

Any Pap smear that shows atypical glandular cells of undetermined significance (AGCUS) requires endometrial sampling.

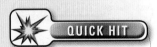

QUICK HIT

Complete surgical staging is not only important in treatment planning but also associated with improved patient survival.

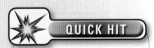

QUICK HIT

Depth of myometrial invasion and tumor grade are important risk factors for metastatic disease and risk of recurrence.

V. Treatment

A. Endometrial hyperplasia
  1. Low-grade lesions treated with **progestins**
     a. Decreases estrogen receptors, causes endometrial thinning and stromal decidualization, stimulates estrogen breakdown
     b. Options
        i. Cyclic medroxyprogesterone acetate
        ii. Depot-medroxyprogesterone acetate
        iii. Mirena intrauterine device (may be the best treatment)
  2. Hysterectomy in persistent hyperplasia or cases of atypia
B. Endometrial cancer
  1. Staging (as recommended by the International Federation of Gynecologists and Obstetricians [FIGO])
     a. Surgically staged with total abdominal hysterectomy and bilateral salpingo-oophorectomy (TAH/BSO) with pelvic and periaortic lymph node dissection
     b. Preoperative Ca-125 level can be a useful marker for patients with advanced disease
     c. Designation (5-year survival): Table 49.1
  2. Postoperative radiation therapy/chemotherapy in high risk for recurrence
  3. High-dose progestins for advanced or recurrent disease
     a. Megace (megestrol)
     b. Provera (medroxyprogesterone)
  4. Chemotherapy for high-risk/advanced disease

TABLE **49.1** **FIGO Surgical Staging System for Endometrial Cancer**

FIGO Stages	Primary Tumor (T) (Surgical/Pathologic Findings)
I	Tumor confined to corpus uteri
IA	Tumor limited to endometrium or invades less than 1/2 of the myometrium
IB	Tumor invades 1/2 or more of the myometrium
II	Tumor invades stromal connective tissue of the cervix but does not extend beyond uterus
IIIA	Tumor involves serosa and/or adnexa (direct extension or metastasis)
IIIB	Vaginal involvement (direct extension or metastasis) or parametrial involvement
IVA	Tumor invades bladder mucosa and/or bowel mucosa (bullous edema is not sufficient to classify a tumor as T4)
	Regional Lymph Nodes
IIIC1	Regional lymph node metastasis to pelvic lymph nodes
IIIC2	Regional lymph node metastasis to para-aortic lymph nodes, with or without positive pelvic lymph nodes
	Distant Metastasis
IVB	Distant metastasis (includes metastasis to inguinal lymph nodes, intraperitoneal disease, or lung, liver, or bone; excludes metastasis to para-aortic lymph nodes, vagina, pelvic serosa, or adnexa)

FIGO, International Federation of Gynecology and Obstetrics.

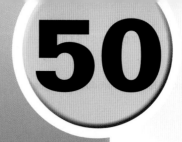

Ovarian and Adnexal Disease

I. Anatomy (Figure 50.1)

A. Adnexa: space between the pelvic sidewall and uterine cornua containing the ovaries, fallopian tubes, broad ligament, and mesosalpinx

B. Adjacent systems that can cause pathology
1. Urologic system (cystitis/pyelonephritis/nephrolithiasis)
2. Gastrointestinal (GI) disorders (appendicitis/irritable bowel syndrome [IBS]/inflammatory bowel disease [IBD]/diverticular disease/carcinoma)

II. Age Considerations in Physical Exam

A. "Normal" is age dependent

B. Reproductive-age women: palpable ovaries in 50% of patients
1. Less commonly when taking combined oral contraceptive pills (OCPs)
2. Most adnexal masses are functional cysts
3. Postmenopausal women: more concerning to have a palpable ovary
   a. 25% of ovarian tumors are malignant in postmenopausal women
   b. Serum tumor markers include CA-125, He4, and Ova1 when mass is discovered
4. Assess mass for size, mobility, discomfort, consistency
5. Ultrasound (U/S) preferred imaging modality
6. Any mass that is simple, unilocular, and <10 cm wide is likely benign and can be followed clinically

III. Functional Ovarian Cysts (Figure 50.2)

A. Cysts arise from normal ovarian function

B. Discovered either incidentally or as a result of symptoms (pain)

C. Follicular cysts
1. Arise from a failure of rupture during follicular maturation
2. Cyst fluid is rich in estrogen from **granulosa cells**
   a. Can alter cycle length: excess estrogen
   b. Produces pain from size
   c. Cysts may "rupture," producing pain from fluid in peritoneum
   d. On exam, unilateral tenderness with mobile, adnexal mass
3. On U/S, will be unilocular *without* thick septations
4. Management: reexamine in 6 weeks to ensure cyst resolution
5. If cyst persists, further workup/evaluation is warranted

D. **Corpus luteum (CL) cyst**: postovulatory cyst
1. Size >3 cm
2. Persistent CL cyst may produce dull lower quadrant pain
3. Associated with delayed menses

E. **Hemorrhagic CL (corpus hemorrhagic)**
1. Seen in late luteal phase
2. Hemoperitoneum on U/S
3. Manage surgically if patient becomes unstable via cyst resection

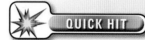

QUICK HIT

Premenstrual and postmenopausal females should never have palpable ovaries.

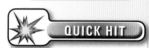

QUICK HIT

CA-125 elevation in a postmenopausal female is cancer until proven otherwise; however, it has many false positives and should *not* be looked upon as a screening test.

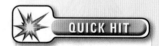

QUICK HIT

U/S cannot tell you if a mass is cancer, but it can tell you if it is not.

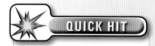

QUICK HIT

Appendicitis is often confused with a ruptured/leaking ovarian cyst.

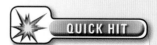

QUICK HIT

Must rule out ectopic pregnancy—check urine pregnancy test and hCG!

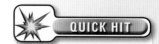

QUICK HIT

Consider coagulopathy workup for recurrent hemorrhagic CL.

FIGURE 50.1 Internal female reproductive organs.

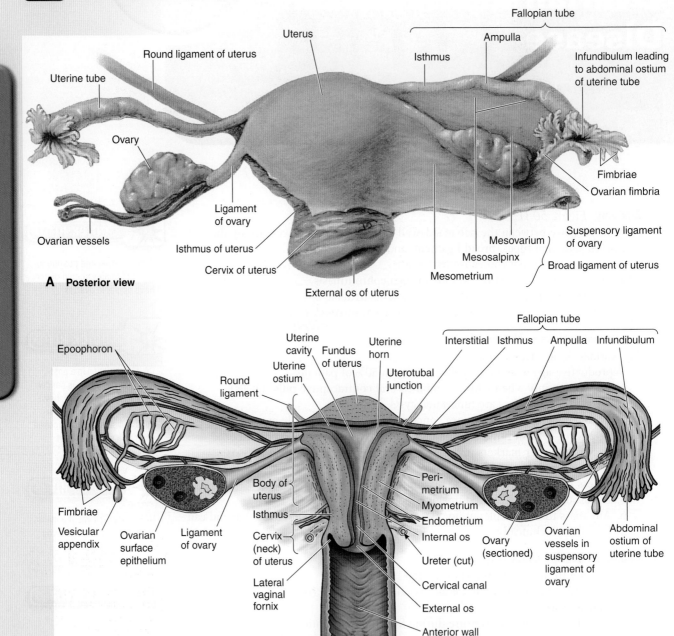

A Posterior view

B Posterior view, cross section

(From Moore KL, Dalley AF. *Clinically Oriented Anatomy*, 5th ed. Baltimore: Lippincott Williams & Wilkins; 2006: Fig. 3.39A&B.)

F. **Theca lutein cyst**
   1. Less common than CL and follicular cysts
   2. Seen in pregnancy; usually **bilateral**
   3. Seen in conditions with elevated human chorionic gonadotropin (hCG)
      a. Multiple gestations
      b. Trophoblastic disease

FIGURE
50.2 Benign ovarian cyst.

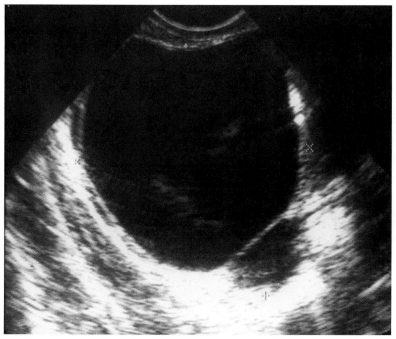

(Courtesy of Wesley C. Fowler, Jr., MD.)

    c. Assisted reproductive technologies (ART)+/ovulation induction with clomiphene citrate
  4. Often large and multicystic
  5. Resolve spontaneously in most cases

IV. Benign Ovarian Neoplasms

  A. Divided into 3 categories based on cell type (Box 50.1)
    1. Epithelial cell tumor
    2. Germ cell tumor
    3. Stromal cell tumors
  B. Key features of all benign ovarian neoplasms
    1. More common than malignant ovarian tumors at all ages
    2. Risk of malignant transformation increases with age
    3. Consider conservative surgery if fertility is desired
  C. Benign epithelial cell tumors: arise from **glandular epithelial cells**
    1. **Serous cystadenoma**: most common epithelial cell neoplasm
      a. 70% benign
      b. 10% low malignant potential (LMP)
      c. 20% malignant
      d. Treat surgically (based on possibility of malignancy)
      e. May attempt unilateral oophorectomy/cystectomy if fertility is desired, or proceed with hysterectomy and bilateral salpingo-oophorectomy (BSO) (especially in postmenopausal women) because of risk of recurrence
    2. **Mucinous cystadenoma**: 2nd most common epithelial cell tumor
      a. Lower malignancy rate (15%) than serous cystadenoma
      b. Can be extremely large, filling pelvic/abdominal cavity
      c. May have multilocular septations on U/S
      d. Treat surgically like serous cystadenomas
    3. **Endometrioid tumor**
      a. Benign form most commonly **endometrioma**

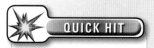

QUICK HIT

Treat with surgical resection; if left untreated, it can lead to torsion or malignant transformation.

BOX 50.1

Histologic Classification of All Ovarian Neoplasms

From coelomic epithelium (epithelial)
    Serous
    Mucinous
    Endometrioid
    Brenner

From gonadal stroma
    Granulosa theca
    Sertoli–Leydig (arrhenoblastoma)
    Lipid cell fibroma

From germ cell
    Dysgerminoma
    Teratoma
    Endodermal sinus (yolk sac)
    Choriocarcinoma

Miscellaneous cell line sources
    Lymphoma
    Sarcoma
    Metastatic
        Colorectal
        Breast
        Endometrial

(From Beckmann CRB, Ling FW, et al. *Obstetrics and Gynecology*, 7th ed. Philadelphia: Lippincott Williams & Wilkins; 2014.)

---

    b. Histologic features similar to endometrial carcinoma
    c. Occurs with endometriosis or with endometrial cancer of the uterus
  4. **Brenner cell tumor:** least common of benign epithelial cell tumors
    a. Large amounts of stroma and fibrotic tissue
    b. More common in postmenopausal women; smaller tumor size
    c. Rarely malignant
  5. **Benign germ cell neoplasms:** arise from primary germ cells
    a. Most commonly: benign **cystic teratoma (dermoid cyst)**
    b. Has differentiated structures
      i. Tissue arising from all 3 embryonic germ layers (ectoderm, mesoderm, and endoderm)
      ii. Hair and bone often seen
    c. 80% occur in reproductive-age women, median age = 30 years
    d. 10%–20% are **bilateral**
    e. High fat content from ectodermal tissue (sebum, sebaceous glands) causing characteristic appearance on computed tomography (CT)
    f. Increased buoyancy predisposes to **torsion**
    g. Management/treatment
      i. Low rate of malignant transformation (1%)
      ii. Surgical removal to prevent torsion and rupture
  6. **Benign stromal cell neoplasms**
    a. Solid tumors from gonadal specialized sex cord stroma
    b. 2 types, both "**functioning tumors**" = hormone production with malignant potential
      i. Estrogenic (**granulosa-theca cell**) tumors: precocious puberty; postmenopausal bleeding
      ii. Androgenic (**Sertoli-Leydig cell**) tumors: virilization/hirsutism
    c. **Ovarian fibroma:** excessive **collagen** from **ovarian spindle cells**
      i. Most common during middle age
      ii. No sex steroid synthesis

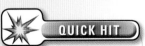

QUICK HIT

Rarely, ovarian tumor can contain thyroid tissue and is called *stroma ovarii*.

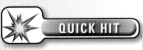

QUICK HIT

Meigs syndrome is a triad of (1) ovarian fibroma, (2) ascites, and (3) right pleural effusion.

**FIGURE
50.3** Ovarian cancer.

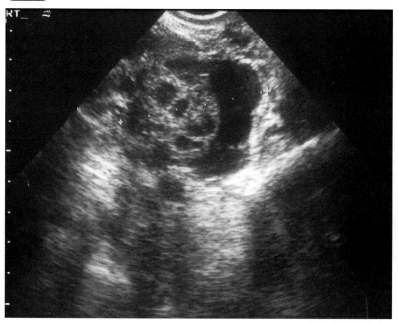

(Courtesy of Wesley C. Fowler, Jr., MD.)

V. Malignant Ovarian Neoplasms *(Figure 50.3)*

A. Ovarian cancer facts
1. 2nd most common gynecologic cancer
2. Highest mortality rate of all gynecologic cancers
3. 22,000 new cases per year, with 5-year survival rate of only 30%–40%
4. 2/3 of new diagnoses have advanced disease
5. Overall lifetime risk for women is 1/70

B. Risk factors
1. Age (more common in postmenopausal age)
2. Genetics (Tables 50.1 and 50.2)
   a. *BRCA1* and *BRCA2*: ~10% of all ovarian cancer
   b. Hereditary nonpolyposis colorectal cancer (HNPCC) = 13-fold greater risk
   c. Western European ancestry

TABLE 50.1 Risk Factors for Ovarian Cancer

Risk Factor	Ovarian Cancer Risk Increase
First-degree relative with ovarian epithelial carcinoma	5% overall lifetime risk of epithelial carcinoma
Two first-degree relatives with ovarian epithelial carcinoma	20%–30% lifetime risk of epithelial carcinoma, often with earlier onset of disease
Breast/ovarian familial cancer syndrome (multiple first- and second-degree relatives with epithelial ovarian and breast cancers)	Two to three times increase from baseline lifetime risk of epithelial ovarian and bilateral breast carcinoma
BRCA1	85% lifetime risk of breast cancer and 50% lifetime risk of ovarian epithelial carcinoma
Ashkenazi Jewish ancestry (have 1% carrier frequency of *BRCA1*)	Ten times increase from baseline lifetime risk of breast and ovarian epithelial carcinoma
HNPCC	13-fold increase in lifetime risk of ovarian epithelial cancer

HNPCC, hereditary nonpolyposis colorectal cancer.

Ovarian and Adnexal Disease

TABLE 50.2 Genetic Risks for Common Diseases

Average Risk	Moderate Risk	High Risk
• No known family history, *or* • Only one second-degree or more distantly related relative	• One first-degree relative (FDR) with onset of disease at an average age, *or* • Two second-degree relatives (SDRs)[a]	• Premature disease or unusual presentation in an FDR • ≥2 affected FDRs[a] • ≥2 SDRs, with at least one having premature onset[a] • ≥3 affected relatives[a] • Moderate risk status on both sides of the family

[a]Relatives must be on the same side of the family.

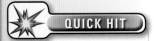

QUICK HIT

Ovulatory infertility confers greater risk for developing ovarian cancer.

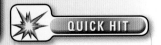

QUICK HIT

Lifetime risk of ovarian cancer is reduced by 50% with 5 years or more of ovulation suppression.

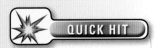

QUICK HIT

Symptoms are typically vague and overlap with other organ systems, which often leads to delayed diagnosis and advanced disease.

    3. Nulliparity
    4. Primary infertility
    5. Endometriosis
  C. Protective factors
    1. *Long-term ovulation suppression* (such as with OCPs)
    2. African American and East Asian ancestry
  D. Presenting symptoms (Box 50.2)
  E. Pathogenesis and diagnosis
    1. Disease extension via cell sloughing from ovaries into adjacent space; this explains frequent peritoneal dissemination at diagnosis
    2. Epithelial cell ovarian cancers have capacity to spread via **lymph** and **blood**, but primarily via direct extension
    3. No effective screening test
      a. CA-125 used to monitor response to therapy
      b. CA-125 elevated in multiple benign conditions (leiomyomata, adenomyosis, pregnancy, pelvic inflammatory disease [PID], endometriosis, menstruation), limiting its usefulness in premenopausal women
      c. He4 and Ova1 are other tumor markers for ovarian cancer
  F. Histology: similar classification system to benign ovarian tumors
    1. Malignant epithelial cell: **most common**
    2. Malignant germ cell tumors
    3. Malignant stromal cell tumors
  G. Staging
    1. Based on surgical staging
    2. The International Federation of Gynecology and Obstetrics (FIGO) staging system (Table 50.3)

BOX 50.2

Early Warning Signs of Ovarian Cancer

Increase in abdominal sizes
Abdominal bloating
Fatigue
Abdominal pain
Indigestion
Inability to eat normally
Urinary frequency
Constipation
Back pain
Urinary incontinence of recent onset
Unexplained weight loss

(From Beckmann CRB, Ling FW, et al. *Obstetrics and Gynecology*, 7th ed. Philadelphia: Lippincott Williams & Wilkins; 2014.)

Stage	Description
TABLE 50.3	**International Federation of Gynecology and Obstetrics (FIGO) Staging for Primary Carcinoma of the Ovary**
I	Growth limited to the ovaries
Ia	Growth limited to one ovary; no ascites containing malignant cells; no tumor on the external surface; capsule intact
Ib	Growth limited to both ovaries; no ascites containing malignant cells; no tumor on the external surface; capsule intact
Ic	Tumor involves one or both ovaries
Ic1	Surgical spill
Ic2	Capsule rupture before surgery or tumor on ovarian surface
Ic3	Malignant cells in the ascites or peritoneal washings
II	Growth involving one or both ovaries with pelvic extension or primary peritoneal cancer
IIa	Extension and/or metastases to the uterus and/or tubes
IIb	Extension to other pelvic tissues
III	Tumor involving one or both ovaries with peritoneal implants outside the pelvis and/or positive retroperitoneal or inguinal nodes; superficial liver metastasis equals stage III; tumor is limited to the true pelvis, but histologically proven malignant extension is to small bowel or omentum
IIIa	Positive retroperitoneal lymph nodes and/or microscopic metastasis beyond the pelvis
IIIa1	Positive retroperitoneal lymph nodes only
IIIa1(i)	Metastasis ≤ 10 mm
IIIa1(ii)	Metastasis > 10 mm
IIIa2	Microscopic, extrapelvic peritoneal involvement ± positive retroperitoneal lymph nodes
IIIb	Macroscopic, extrapelvic, peritoneal metastasis ≤ 2 cm ± positive retroperitoneal lymph nodes; includes extension to capsule of liver/spleen
IIIc	Macroscopic, extrapelvic, peritoneal metastasis > 2 cm ± positive retroperitoneal lymph nodes; includes extension to capsule of liver/spleen
IV	Distant metastasis excluding peritoneal metastasis
IVa	Pleural effusion with positive cytology
IVb	Hepatic and/or splenic parenchymal metastasis, metastasis to extraabdominal organs (including inguinal lymph nodes and lymph nodes outside of the abdominal cavity)

(From Prat J. Staging classification for cancer of the ovary, fallopian tube, and peritoneum. *Int J Gynaecol Obstet.* 2014 Jan;124(1):1–5. doi: 10.1016/j.ijgo.2013.10.001.)

H. Borderline ovarian tumors
   1. Previously called "tumors of low malignant potential"
   2. Usually confined to 1 ovary
   3. Occur in younger women (age 30–50 years)
   4. Treated surgically
I. Epithelial cell ovarian carcinoma (Box 50.3)
   1. 90% of ovarian malignancies
   2. Derived from **mesothelial** cells of coelomic epithelium
   3. Familial risk factors (see Tables 50.1 and 50.2)
J. Malignant epithelial serous tumors (serous cystadenocarcinomas)
   1. Most common
   2. ~50% derived from benign cystadenomas
   3. ~30% are bilateral at time of presentation

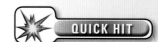

QUICK HIT

Ten percent of benign epithelial cell tumors have histologic evidence of intraepithelial neoplasia.

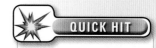

QUICK HIT

May treat tumors of low malignant potential with fertility-sparing surgery (unilateral oophorectomy with staging) as long as patient desires fertility and understands small risk or reoccurrence in contralateral ovary.

Ovarian and Adnexal Disease

BOX 50.3

Histologic Classification of the Common Epithelial Tumors of the Ovary

Serous Tumors
Serous cystadenomas
Serous cystadenomas with proliferating activity of the epithelial cells and nuclear abnormalities but with no
infiltrative destructive growth (low potential malignancy)
Serous cystadenocarcinoma

Mucinous Tumors
Mucinous cystadenomas
Mucinous cystadenomas with proliferating activity of the epithelial cells and nuclear abnormalities but with no
infiltrative destructive growth (low potential malignancy)
Mucinous cystadenocarcinoma

Endometrioid Tumors (similar to adenocarcinomas in the endometrium)
Endometrioid benign cysts
Endometrioid tumors with proliferating activity of the epithelial cells and nuclear abnormalities but with no
infiltrative destructive growth (low potential malignancy)

Adenocarcinoma
Brenner Tumor
Unclassified Carcinoma

(From Beckmann CRB, Ling FW, et al. *Obstetrics and Gynecology*, 7th ed. Philadelphia: Lippincott Williams & Wilkins; 2014.)

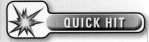

Histology reveals psammoma bodies: calcified, laminated structures.

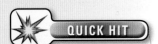

Malignant mucinous tumors of the ovary are rare; GI malignancy must be eliminated as a source.

4. Features
    a. Multiloculated
    b. External excrescences on smooth capsules
K. **Malignant mucinous epithelial tumor** (mucinous cystadenocarcinoma)
    1. ~1/3 of all epithelial ovarian tumors are from this cell type, with **5%** of these mucinous tumors being malignant
    2. Lower rate of bilateral manifestation
    3. Can be large in size (>20 cm)
L. Endometroid tumors
    1. More often malignant than other epithelial tumors
    2. Contain histologic features similar to endometrial carcinoma
    3. Seen with **endometriosis**
    4. Often co-occur with endometrial cancer of uterus
M. Other malignant epithelial cell ovarian carcinomas: less common
    1. **Clear cell** carcinomas: arise from **mesonephric** elements
    2. **Brenner tumors**: arise from benign counterpart and may co-occur with **mucinous cystadenoma**
N. Germ cell tumors
    1. Most common ovarian cancers in women age <20 years
    2. Tumors may be functional with **hCG** or **α-fetoprotein (AFP)** production (follow these levels as tumor markers)
    3. **Dysgerminoma** and **immature teratomas** are most common
    4. Other, less common types
        a. Mixed germ cell
        b. Endodermal sinus
        c. Embryonal tumors
    5. Show a strong response to chemo and radiation therapy
    6. **Dysgerminomas**
        a. Unilateral; most common germ cell tumor
        b. Arise from **gonadoblastoma** (benign), seen in patients with gonadal dysgenesis
        c. Responsive to chemo and radiation therapy with 95% 5-year survival when presentation is unilateral
        d. Surgical treatment is unilateral oophorectomy (unless tumor >10 cm or evidence of extra-ovarian extension)

e. Attempt to preserve fertility as this affects young women

f. Spread via lymphatics: pelvic and periaortic lymph node

7. **Immature teratoma**

a. Malignant form of dermoid

b. Unilateral, rapidly growing

c. Pain from hemorrhage and necrosis

d. Discomfort leads to early diagnosis with good prognosis

e. Treatment: unilateral oophorectomy/chemotherapy

O. Endodermal sinus tumors (produces AFP) and embryonal cell carcinomas (produces AFP and hCG)

1. Previously had poor prognosis, but recent improvements have increased 5-year survival to >60%

2. Seen in childhood/adolescence

3. Treatment: surgical resection followed by chemotherapy

P. Gonadal stromal cell tumors

1. All tumors in this group produce hormones = functioning tumors

2. Typically sex hormones, but may be **adrenal**

3. Granulosa cell tumor: most common

a. Prognosis is better in older patients

b. Surgical treatment (if disease confined to intact capsule, may proceed with fertility-preserving staging)

c. Larger tumors are more likely to recur

d. **Sertoli-Leydig** cell tumors

i. Rarer, testosterone secreting

ii. Consider in older patients, especially with virilization

4. Fibroma/thecomas with malignant versions of fibrosarcoma and malignant thecoma

Q. Ovarian lymphoma: rarely, ovaries can be the primary site of lymphoma

R. Malignant mesodermal sarcomas (carcinosarcoma):

1. Rare, aggressive, often diagnosed with progressive disease

2. Survival rates are poor

S. Cancer metastatic to the ovary

1. Infiltrative, mucinous carcinoma: **signet-ring cell type**

2. Bilateral; widespread metastatic disease

3. Can have uterine bleeding or virilization

VI. Surgical Management of Ovarian (and Fallopian Tube) Cancers

A. **Cytoreductive** or **tumor debulking surgery** is indicated in most ovarian malignancies

B. Chemotherapy more effective when all tumor masses are <1 cm

C. **Chemotherapy**

1. Taxanes and platin are 1st-line adjunctive treatment

2. 2nd line: ifosfamide, doxorubicin, topotecan, gemcitabine, etoposide, vinorelbine, hexamethylmelamine, and tamoxifen

3. Radiation has limited role

4. Follow up with examination, imaging, and tumor markers (CA-125)

VII. Fallopian Tube Cancer

A. Benign disease: usually small and symptomatic

1. Paraovarian cysts: develop in mesosalpinx from vestigial Wolffian duct structures, tubal epithelium, and peritoneum inclusions

2. Paratubal cysts: found near fimbria and are very common; also called **hydatid cysts of Morgagni**

B. Carcinoma of fallopian tube

1. Primary fallopian tube carcinoma is most commonly **adenocarcinoma** (less commonly adenosquamous carcinoma or sarcoma)

a. ~1% of all gynecologic cancers

b. Occurs mostly in postmenopausal women

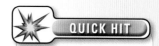

QUICK HIT

Immature teratoma is most often seen in women age <25 years.

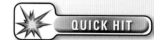

QUICK HIT

Presence of increased estrogen from the tumor may produce endometrial hyperplasia/carcinoma; therefore, the endometrium must be sampled.

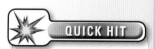

QUICK HIT

Krukenberg tumors are metastatic from primary GI or breast tumors to the ovary.

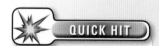

QUICK HIT

About 10% of malignant ovarian cancer is found to be nonovarian.

Ovarian and Adnexal Disease

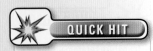

Hydrops tubae profluens: profuse serosangineous discharge associated with fallopian tube carcinoma.

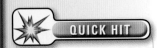

Women with *BRCA1/BRCA2* mutation have a 5% risk of developing primary peritoneal cancer even after prophylactic oophorectomy.

    c. Large, with appearance similar to hydrosalpinx on gross examination; usually unilateral

    d. Histologically, most similar to **ovarian papillary serous cystadenocarcinomas**

    e. Present with postmenopausal bleeding or discharge

    f. Staging identical to ovarian carcinoma with similar progression of disease (intraperitoneal metastases and ascites)

        i. Often see lymphatic spread to pelvic and para-aortic lymph nodes

        ii. 70% of cases are identified at stage I or II

        iii. Overall 5-year survival rate = 40%

        iv. Initial treatment is surgery then chemotherapy

  2. Metastatic spread to fallopian tubes from primary uterine or ovarian is more common than primary fallopian tube carcinoma

VIII. Primary Peritoneal Carcinoma

  A. Cancer of cells lining peritoneum (abdominal cavity)

  B. Usually have widespread intra-abdominal disease with only surface involvement of ovaries

  C. Treated as per ovarian cancer

Index

Page numbers followed by *f, t,* and *b* indicate figures, tables, and boxed material, respectively.